INSTRUCTOR'S RESOURCE MANUAL

for

Beare/Myers

Adult

Health Nursing

THIRD EDITION

INSTRUCTOR'S RESOURCE MANUAL
for

Beare/Myers

Adult Health Nursing

THIRD EDITION

Prepared by

Golden M. Tradewell, MSN, MA, RN

Assistant Professor
College of Nursing
McNeese State University
Lake Charles, Louisiana

Test Bank by

Judith C. Trotti, MSN, RN, CS, CNOR
Clinical Instructor
University of Texas Health Science Center
San Antonio, Texas

Acknowledgements for past contributors:

Linda K. Wendling, MA
Carole A. Broxon, RN, PhD
Carolyn A. Patiño, RN, MSN
Donita T. Qualey, RN, MN

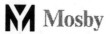 Mosby

St. Louis Baltimore Boston Carlsbad Chicago Minneapolis New York Philadelphia Portland
London Milan Sydney Tokyo Toronto

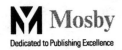

Mosby
Dedicated to Publishing Excellence

A Times Mirror
Company

Publisher   Sally Schrefer
Editor   Michael S. Ledbetter
Associate Developmental Editor   Kristin Geen
Project Manager   Gayle Morris
Manufacturing Manager   Betty Mueller
Design and Layout   DocuComp Services
Cover Design   Amy Buxton

Printed in the United States of America

Mosby–Year Book, Inc.
11830 Westline Industrial Drive
St. Louis, Missouri 63146

International Standard Book Number 0-8151-1008-1
29578

97 98 99 00 01 / 9 8 7 6 5 4 3 2 1

Contents

Instructor's Resources

The Instructor's Resources portion of this manual contains the following features for each chapter: **Learning Objectives**, **Key Terms**, a **Chapter Outline** along with related **Lecture Strategies**, and **Related Skills** and **Related Clinical Skills**. Included throughout the Lecture Strategies are references to the following media teaching tools designed to supplement traditional medical-surgical coursework:

TA: **TRANSPARENCY ACETATES** consist of 102 full-color figures and tables selected from the ADULT HEALTH NURSING text to enhance lectures and class discussion.

VIDEO: **MOSBY'S MEDICAL-SURGICAL NURSING VIDEO SERIES** consists of 12 videos covering the nursing management of common medical-surgical disorders. These videos are designed to enhance critical thinking skills and synthesize the nursing process in actual patient situations.

VIEWSTUDY: **MOSBY'S MEDICAL-SURGICAL NURSING VIEWSTUDY** is a CD-ROM containing over 500 full-color images. Instructors may create custom slide shows, export images to use in word processing programs and to create tests and quizzes, and enlarge images for projection or for making transparencies. Appendix B contains a complete list of images in VIEWSTUDY.

1   Infection

LEARNING OBJECTIVES

1 Characterize the microorganisms that cause infections in the body.
2 Describe the processes involved in host-agent interaction that produce infection
3 Identify the clinical manifestations associated with the five stages of a primary acute infection.
4 Identify the unique characteristics of nosocomial and opportunistic infections.
5 Compare the clinical manifestations of infection in the older adult with those that occur in the younger adult.
6 Apply the nursing process to the management of the patient with an infection.
7 Identify the immunizations recommended for adults and the elderly.
8 Describe the role of standard precautions and isolation techniques in the prevention and management of infection.

KEY TERMS

carriers
incubation
isolation
methicillin-resistant
    *Staphylococcus
    aureus* (MRSA)
nosocomial infections

opportunistic infections
pathogenic
septicemia
shift to the left
standard precautions
superimposed infections

Chapter Outline	Lecture Strategies

Infection
    Definition/etiology
        Viruses
        Bacteria
        Mycoplasmas
        Rickettsiae
        Chlamydia
        Fungi
        Protozoa
    Pathophysiology
    Exposure
    Dose
    Entry
    Multiplication
    Spread
	Identify the term *infection* as referring to those diseases that produce dysfunction because of the presence of a living organism in or on the human body. Ask students to suggest what is meant by *pathogenic* organisms.
	
	Critical Thinking: Give an example of an infection in each of the seven categories of microorganisms that cause infections.
	
	Critical Thinking: How do the agent and host interact to produce an infection?
	
	Identify the body's defenses against pathogen binding on epithelial cells.

Chapter Outline	Lecture Strategies
Tissue damage	Describe the two primary mechanisms through which microorganisms produce tissue damage.

Clinical manifestations
    Primary acute infection
    Unique primary infections
        Nosocomial infections
        Drug-resistant nosocomial infections
        Opportunistic infections
    Other types of infection
	Critical Thinking: Describe the five stages of a primary acute infection in terms of clinical manifestations.
	
	Identify clients at risk for nosocomial infections.
	
	Critical Thinking: Describe the etiology of nosocomial and opportunistic infections. What are common sources of these infections?

Nursing management of the patient with an infection
    Assessment
        Risk factors
        Local signs and symptoms
	Critical Thinking: Of the factors that increase the older adult's susceptibility to infection, which one increases the risk of pneumonia in a patient in a nursing home?
	
	Critical Thinking: What is the importance of a person's nutritional needs during an infection process?

Systemic signs and symptoms	**Critical Thinking:** What is the importance of accurate fever assessment in the patient with an infection?
Laboratory data	Use **TA 1** to discuss laboratory tests. **Critical Thinking:** What is the significance of a shift to the left in the patient's differential WBC count?
Nursing diagnosis Planning/expected outcomes Implementation	**Critical Thinking:** What is the key nursing intervention used to protect the patient from pathogens?

Immunizations
    Nutrition
    Sleep and rest
    Skin integrity
    Handwashing
    Standard precautions
    Isolation precautions
	Critical Thinking: Why are immunizations important for adults and the elderly?
	
	Describe the appropriate use and procedures for standard precautions in a variety of situations.
	
	Critical Thinking: How are standard precautions and isolation techniques used in the care of a patient with an infection?

Pharmacologic management
    Antipyretics
    Antimicrobial therapy
Evaluation/documentation
Continuity of care
	Critical Thinking: Discuss the use of pharmacologic agents in the management of the patient who has an infection.

Related Skills

1 Demonstrate proper gowning, gloving, and disposal of linens, used equipment, and supplies in a simulated isolation setting.
2. Demonstrate proper handwashing technique in a variety of settings.

Related Clinical Skills

1. Assess and document an infectious process in the clinical area.

2 Fluids, Electrolytes, and Acid-Base Balance

LEARNING OBJECTIVES

1 Describe the basic physiologic mechanisms responsible for maintaining fluid, electrolyte, and acid-base balance.
2 Describe the distribution of body fluids and electrolytes in the body.
3 Identify the major causes of electrolyte imbalance and their clinical manifestations.
4 List significant nursing assessments for a patient with risk for or actual fluid-electrolyte imbalance.
5 Describe the nursing management of patients with actual or risk for fluid imbalances.
6 Describe the nursing management of patients with actual or risk for electrolyte imbalances.
7 Compare pathophysiology, treatment, and nursing management of acidosis with that of alkalosis.
8 Discuss the nursing management of the elderly patient with fluid, electrolyte, or acid-base imbalance.

KEY TERMS

acidosis
alkalosis
buffers
diffusion
dissociate
electrolyte
extracellular
filtration
homeostasis
hydrostatic pressure
hypercalcemia
hyperkalemia
hypermagnesemia
hypernatremia
hyperphosphatemia
hypocalcemia
hypokalemia
hypomagnesemia
hyponatremia
hypophosphatemia
intracellular
osmolality
osmosis
permeable
sodium-potassium pump

Chapter Outline	Lecture Strategies
Body fluids	**Critical Thinking:** Name three compartments where fluid is found in the body.
	VIEWSTUDY image #49 demonstrates differential assessment of extracellular fluid volume.
	VIEWSTUDY image #50 shows isotonic gains and losses.
Electrolytes	Ask students to recall the definition for *electrolyte*.

Fluid and electrolyte transportation
  Active transport
  Fluid volume shifts
	Critical Thinking: What are the means by which fluids move in the body?

	Critical Thinking: Describe diffusion, facilitated diffusion, filtration, and osmosis.
	VIEWSTUDY image #45 illustrates diffusion.

Chapter Outline	Lecture Strategies
	Critical Thinking: List the function of the following electrolytes: sodium, potassium, calcium, magnesium, and phosphate.
	VIEWSTUDY image #46 shows the sodium-potassium pump.
Regulation of fluid volume	**Critical Thinking:** Describe how aldosterone influences fluid volume.
	VIEWSTUDY image #47 demonstrates the influences of aldosterone secretion.
	VIEWSTUDY image #142 illustrates the mechanisms of action of aldosterone.
	Critical Thinking: Describe the function of the antidiuretic hormone (ADH) in the regulation and maintenance of fluid and electrolyte imbalance.
	VIEWSTUDY image #48 illustrates the effects of stress on fluid and electrolyte balance
Regulation and maintenance of fluid and electrolyte balance	

Role of organ systems in regulating fluid volume
   Kidney
      Glomerular filtration pressure
      Colloid osmotic pressure and filtration
   Neuroendocrine system, heart, and blood vessels
      Central nervous system ischemic response
      Baroreceptor reflex
      Volume receptor mechanism
      Renin-angiotensin-aldosterone mechanism
	Critical Thinking: When diuretic medications are given, what might be the effect on electrolyte balance?

Nursing management of the patient with fluid and electrolyte problems Assessment	**Critical Thinking:** Of all the factors that might lead to fluid or electrolyte imbalance, describe signs and symptoms that might be seen in an elderly person.

Fluid volume imbalances
   Fluid volume deficit
      Definition
      Pathophysiology
      Abnormal gastrointestinal fluid loss
      Abnormal fluid loss via skin
      Increased water vapor loss via lungs
      Conditions that increase renal excretion of fluids
      Decrease in fluid intake
	Critical Thinking: What are the common causes of fluid volume deficit? overload? clinical signs and symptoms?
	
	If possible, obtain as many types of venous access devices as you have access to; demonstrate their use.
	
	It is important to remember that significant amounts of fluid can be lost from the various body systems.

Chapter Outline	Lecture Strategies
Third-space fluid loss Significant laboratory tests Collaborative management	Use common conditions (burns, plastic surgery) to illustrate third-space fluid loss.

Nursing management of the patient with fluid volume deficit
  Assessment
  Nursing diagnosis
  Implementation
	Critical Thinking: If you are given a report that a 55-year-old patient had 400 ml of urine output for the past 24 hours, what would you want to find out next?
	
	Critical Thinking: List the important assessment areas to evaluate the fluid status of a patient.

Types of venous access devices and equipment necessary for home maintenance
  Peripheral venous access devices
    Peripheral vein intermittent infusion devices
  Central venous catheters
    Central vein intermittent infusion devices
  Implantable devices	

Fluid volume excess
  Definition
  Pathophysiology
  Significant laboratory tests
  Collaborative management
	Critical Thinking: If you are caring for Mr. Jones, who weighed 171 pounds yesterday, and 180 pounds today, what would you find out next? What might this represent?

Nursing management of the patient with fluid volume excess
  Assessment
  Nursing diagnosis
  Implementation	

Electrolyte imbalances: Sodium
  Hypernatremia
    Definition
    Pathophysiology
    Significant laboratory tests
    Collaborative management
	Ask students to recall what occurs when sodium and water are in excess.
	
	Critical Thinking: Describe the likely causes, signs and symptoms, and collaborative management for potassium deficit, sodium excess, magnesium deficit, and calcium excess.

Nursing management of the patient with hypernatremia
  Assessment
  Nursing diagnosis
  Implementation	

Hyponatremia
  Definition
  Pathophysiology
  Significant laboratory data
  Collaborative management
	Discuss how diuretics can cause hyponatremia.

Chapter Outline	Lecture Strategies
Nursing management of the patient with hyponatremia 　　Assessment 　　Nursing diagnosis 　　Implementation Electrolyte imbalances: Potassium 　　Hyperkalemia 　　　　Definition 　　　　Pathophysiology 　　　　Significant laboratory tests 　　　　Collaborative management	**TA 2** shows causes and effects of hyperkalemia. **Critical Thinking:** In discussing potassium imbalances, describe the three mechanisms necessary to maintain normal hydrogen ion concentration in the body. Include the following body systems: buffer, respiratory, and renal.
Nursing management of the patient with hyperkalemia 　　　　Assessment 　　　　Nursing diagnosis 　　　　Implementation 　　Hypokalemia 　　　　Definition 　　　　Pathophysiology 　　　　Significant laboratory tests 　　　　Collaborative management 　　Nursing management of the patient with hypokalemia 　　　　Assessment 　　　　Nursing diagnosis 　　　　Implementation	Ask the students to speculate on which system is dysfunctional if potassium imbalance occurs. **TA 3** shows causes and effects of hypokalemia. Review food sources rich in potassium. Students will be able to define *hypokalemia* by considering the word parts.
Electrolyte imbalances: Calcium 　　Hypercalcemia 　　　　Definition 　　　　Pathophysiology 　　　　Significant laboratory tests 　　　　Collaborative management 　　Nursing management of the patient with hypercalcemia 　　　　Assessment 　　　　Nursing diagnosis 　　　　Implementation 　　Hypocalcemia 　　　　Definition 　　　　Pathophysiology 　　　　Significant laboratory tests 　　　　Collaborative management 　　Nursing management of the patient with hypocalcemia 　　　　Assessment 　　　　Nursing diagnosis 　　　　Implementation	**TA 4** shows causes and effects of hypocalcemia. Because of similarities in the way that they sound, stress that hypokalemia and hypocalcemia are separate states. Review food sources rich in calcium.

Chapter Outline	Lecture Strategies
Electrolyte imbalances: Magnesium	Review food sources high in magnesium.

Hypermagnesemia
    Definition
    Pathophysiology
    Significant laboratory tests
    Collaborative management	

Nursing management of the patient with hypermagnesemia
    Assessment
    Nursing diagnosis
    Implementation	

Hypomagnesemia
    Definition
    Pathophysiology
    Significant laboratory tests
    Collaborative management	

Nursing management of the patient with hypomagnesemia
    Assessment
    Nursing diagnosis
    Implementation
	Ask students to speculate on signs and symptoms of hypomagnesemia.

Electrolyte imbalances: Phosphorus
    Hyperphosphatemia
        Definition
        Pathophysiology
        Significant laboratory tests
        Collaborative management
	Review food sources high in phosphorus.

Nursing management of the patient with hyperphosphatemia
    Assessment
    Nursing diagnosis
    Implementation	

Hypophosphatemia
    Definition
    Pathophysiology
    Significant laboratory tests
    Collaborative management	

Nursing management of the patient with hypophosphatemia
    Assessment
    Nursing diagnosis
    Implementation	

Chapter Outline	Lecture Strategies
Acid-base balance	
Henderson-Hasselbalch equation	
Acid-base regulatory mechanisms	
Chemical buffer systems	
Bicarbonate system	
Phosphate system	
Protein system	
Hemoglobin system	
Lungs	
Kidneys	
Arterial blood gas analysis	**TA 5** is a table showing ABG comparisons of acid-base disorders.
Acid-base imbalance	Present the normal ABG values and then present problems in acid-base balance, using abnormal values.
Metabolic acidosis	
Definition	
Pathophysiology	**Critical Thinking:** Describe the probable causes and effects of metabolic acidosis, metabolic alkalosis, respiratory acidosis, and respiratory alkalosis.
Significant laboratory tests	
Collaborative management	
Nursing management of the patient with metabolic acidosis	
Assessment	
Nursing diagnosis	
Implementation	
Metabolic alkalosis	**Critical Thinking:** Differentiate among simple, compensated, acute, and chronic respiratory or metabolic acidosis and alkalosis.
Definition	
Pathophysiology	
Significant laboratory tests	
Collaborative management	
Nursing management of the patient with metabolic alkalosis	
Assessment	
Nursing diagnosis	
Implementation	
Respiratory acidosis	Stress the need to maintain low-flow oxygen rates in patients with chronic CO_2 retention with respiratory acidosis.
Definition	
Pathophysiology	
Significant laboratory tests	
Collaborative management	
Nursing management of the patient with respiratory acidosis	Compare and contrast the clinical manifestation of respiratory alkalosis/acidosis.
Assessment	
Nursing diagnosis	
Implementation	
Respiratory alkalosis	
Definition	
Pathophysiology	
Significant laboratory tests	
Collaborative management	

Chapter Outline	Lecture Strategies

Nursing management of the patient with respiratory alkalosis
    Assessment
    Nursing diagnosis
    Implementation
Imbalances in the elderly
    Respiratory
    Cardiovascular
    Gastrointestinal
    Cognitive-perceptual
    Musculoskeletal
    Urinary
	Critical Thinking: Describe the causes, signs and symptoms, and collaborative management for patients with acid-base imbalance.
	
	Critical Thinking: Identify nursing implications for the elderly patient in relationship to fluid, electrolyte, and acid-base imbalance.

Related Skills

1. Discuss collection of blood for arterial blood gases.
2. Arrange for a visit to a laboratory to observe the analysis of blood for ABGs and of serum samples for electrolytes.
3. Demonstrate IV solutions that are isotonic, hypertonic, and hypotonic to be used for IV hydration.
4. Demonstrate types of venous access devices and their uses.

Related Clinical Skills

1. Assign students to patients at risk for developing an acid-base imbalance. Discuss the clinical reasons for the imbalance and the collaborative and nursing management.
2. Review a chart of a patient with an acid-base imbalance. Discuss the clinical reasons for the imbalance and the collaborative and nursing management.
3. Demonstrate intravenous techniques. Have students successfully initiate an intravenous site.
4. Assign students to a patient who is receiving an IV solution being administered for IV hydration. Ensure that students understand the rationale for the type of solution being used in relation to the fluid volume deficit.

3 Pain

LEARNING OBJECTIVES

1 Identify three reasons for undertreatment of patients in pain.
2 Describe the nurse's role in pain management.
3 List three factors that influence a patient's pain experience.
4 Differentiate between acute and chronic pain.
5 Explain the transmission of pain.
6 Discuss the two most current theories of pain.
7 Assess a patient in pain using a pain assessment tool.
8 Describe the use of nonopioid analgesics in pain management.
9 Discuss and compare opioid analgesics, using an equianalgesic chart.
10 Discuss four routes of analgesic administration.
11 Describe three major noninvasive pain relief measures and their nursing implications.
12 Describe three invasive pain relief measures and their nursing implications.

KEY TERMS

acute pain
adjuvant medication
algology
chronic pain
continuous subcutaneous opioid infusion (CSI)
cutaneous stimulation
endorphins
intravenous continuous opioid infusion (ICO)
opioid
patient-controlled analgesia (PCA)
placebo
referred pain
tolerance
transcutaneous electrical nerve stimulation (TENS)

Chapter Outline	Lecture Strategies

Scope of the problem
    Reasons for undertreatment
    Inadequate education
 	
    Attitudes and misconceptions
        Who is the authority on pain?
        Addiction, tolerance, and physical dependence
        Placebos
	Critical Thinking: Why are some patients in pain undertreated?
	
	Ask student to describe experiences with and attitudes toward individuals in pain.

The role of the nurse in pain management	**Critical Thinking:** Discuss some ways the nurse can improve the problems of pain. **TA 6** depicts a conceptual model of pain.

Factors affecting an individual's response to pain
    Anxiety
    Past experience with pain
    Culture and religion
	Critical Thinking: In caring for two patients with the exact same diagnosis (e.g., first day postoperative chole-cystectomy), why may their pain experiences vary? What factors contribute to an individual's perception of pain?

Chapter Outline	Lecture Strategies
Acute and chronic pain	Use **TA 7** to discuss the characteristics of acute and chronic pain. **Critical Thinking:** A patient in the emergency room has severe pain in the right side. The physician diagnoses the condition as renal colic. Would this be acute or chronic pain? How do these types of pain differ? What is the difference in pain management?

Pain transmission
    The gate-control theory
    The endorphin/enkephalin theory
	Critical Thinking: How are pain impulses carried to the brain? What part of the brain perceives pain?
	
	VIEWSTUDY image #8 shows how peripheral terminals are sensitive to direct heat, mechanical pressure, and chemicals released in response to tissue damage.
	
	VIEWSTUDY image #9 shows dorsal root nociceptive afferents.
	
	VIEWSTUDY image #10 is a schematic representation of two pathways that lead to the production of chemicals that cause the peripheral afferent nociceptors to be more easily excited.
	
	VIEWSTUDY image #12 demonstrates nociceptive pathways and synaptic connections of selected pain pathways.
	
	VIEWSTUDY image #13 shows descending pain-modulation system at receptors in the dorsal horn of the spinal cord.
	
	Use **TA 8** to demonstrate neurologic transmission of pain stimulus.
	
	Critical Thinking: As the nurse is teaching a patient about relaxation techniques, the patient asks, "How will these techniques help my pain?" How might the nurse clearly explain the gate-control theory to this patient?
	
	VIEWSTUDY image #14 illustrates the descending pathway and endorphin response.
	
	Consider and discuss other situations in which the gate is "closed."

Chapter Outline	Lecture Strategies
Pain assessment	**Critical Thinking:** Why is assessment of pain an integral component of pain management? What points should be covered when finding out about a patient's pain?
Components of pain assessment	
Location	
Intensity	**VIEWSTUDY** image #7 demonstrates the five components of pain.
Comfort	
Quality	
Chronology	**VIEWSTUDY** image #11 shows typical areas of referred pain.
Patient's view of pain	
	Critical Thinking: How does the nurse explain that patients should NOT wait until pain is intolerable to ask for pain medication?
	VIEWSTUDY image #16 demonstrates the mechanism of acute pain.
Management of pain	**Critical Thinking:** What are the similarities between aspirin and acetaminophen? How do they differ? What are NSAIDs? How do they decrease pain?
Pharmacologic approaches to pain management	
Nonopioid analgesics	
Acetaminophen	
Aspirin	Aspirin is useful in conditions such as arthritis, in which both pain and inflammation are present.
Nonsteroidal antiinflammatory drugs (NSAIDs)	Present broad classes and common side effects of NSAIDs, and then more specific information.
Opioids	**Critical Thinking:** Why are the following opioid doses most likely to be ineffective? Explain the rationale using an equianalgesic chart.
	Hydromorphone 1.5 mg PO q4h
	Meperidine 50 mg PO q4h
	Morphine 15 mg PO q4h
Equianalgesic chart	Compare the equianalgesic dosages of drugs that are commonly used in the students' clinical facility.
Side effects of opioids	
Nausea and vomiting	
Constipation	
Sedation	
Tolerance	
Respiratory depression	
Timing of analgesics	Occasionally, patients will request that analgesics not be given regularly. It is important to ensure that they have the necessary knowledge and to respect their decision.
Routes of administration	
Oral	
Intramuscular	
Rectal	
Intravenous bolus	
Intravenous continuous opioid infusion	**Critical Thinking:** What is the nurse's role when administering a continuous opioid infusion? In patient-controlled analgesia?
Patient-controlled analgesia	
Continuous subcutaneous opioid infusion	

Chapter Outline	Lecture Strategies

Spinal administration
Adjuvant analgesics
 	
Noninvasive pain-relief techniques
    Cutaneous stimulation
    Heat and cold application
    Transcutaneous electrical nerve stimulation
	Design bingo cards placing names of adjuvant analgesics in squares. Students will attempt to fill in bingo cards from randomly drawn descriptions of drugs.Noninvasive techniques can be useful alone or as adjuncts in the management of pain.
	
	TA 9 shows a patient with a TENS unit in place.
	
	Critical Thinking: How might TENS, heat and cold, and massage help a patient in pain? What is the nurse's role when using these techniques for pain management?

Massage
    Distraction
    Relaxation
Invasive approaches to pain management
    Nerve blocks
    Neurosurgical procedures
    Acupuncture
Pain clinics
	VIEWSTUDY image #15 shows sites of commonly used pharmacologic and nonpharmacologic analgesic therapies.
	
	Critical Thinking: A patient is scheduled for a nerve block for chronic low-back pain. Discuss the different types of nerve blocks and how they might help decrease pain. What types of patients might be considered good candidates for nerve block treatment?
	
	VIEWSTUDY image #17 shows sites of neurosurgical procedures for pain relief.

Related Skills

1. Review and practice principles of hot and cold applications.
2. Obtain examples of pumps for drug administration so that students may examine them.
3 Demonstrate the technique of massage and have students practice the skill.
4. Assign students to a pain control center if possible and observe different techniques in pain management.
5. Have the students develop a teaching plan of nonpharmacologic techniques for a homebound patient with chronic pain.

Related Clinical Skills

1. Assign students to patients with mild to moderate pain. Have students design, implement, and evaluate a plan for teaching the patients about pain control.
2. Assign students to a patient with either a PCA pump or TENS unit. Have them explain to the patient the use of these devices.

4 Neoplasia

LEARNING OBJECTIVES

1 Compare and contrast cellular characteristics that distinguish cancerous tissue from normal tissue.
2 Relate the process of carcinogenesis to both environmental and host risk factors.
3 Describe the tissue classification system for cancers.
4 List the mechanisms by which cancers metastasize.
5 Discuss current incidence of cancers and trends in mortality.
6 Describe screening procedures for early cancer detection.
7 Explain concepts of staging and grading neoplastic disease.
8 Compare and contrast the four major treatment methods, including their indications, limitations, side effects, and safety issues.
9 Explain nursing management for patients with symptoms common to neoplastic disease, treatment, and emergency conditions.
10 Discuss interventions that promote continuity of care, for time of diagnostic workup to the terminal stage of disease.

KEY TERMS

alopecia
anaplasia
biologic response
  modifier (BRM)
  therapybiopsy
brachytherapy
carcinogenesis
chemotherapy
cytotoxic
dysplasia

grading
hyperplasia
metastasis
neoplasm
oncogene
staging
stomatitis
teletherapy
xerostomia

Chapter Outline	Lecture Strategies

Epidemiology
Cancer biology
  Cellular alterations
  Characteristics of cancer cells
    Metabolism
    Growth and spread
 	
  Structural changes
	Critical Thinking: Discuss trends in cancer incidence.
	
	Critical Thinking: Describe the five differences between benign and malignant tumors.
	
	TA 10 can help students check their own answer to the last critical thinking question.
	
	Critical Thinking: Explain the cellular characteristics of a malignant cell.
	
	VIEWSTUDY image #42 illustrates the process of cancer development.
	
	TA 11 shows common metastatic sites.

Chapter Outline	Lecture Strategies
Carcinogenesis	**Critical Thinking:** What are the three events in carcinogenesis?
Risk factors	**Critical Thinking:** Describe six environmental risk factors for cancer.
Tobacco Alcohol Occupational exposure Radiation	The increase in lung cancer has paralleled increases in the incidence of cigarette smoking in women. Ask students how nurses might help reduce the incidence of smoking.
Diet Viruses Drugs Host factors	**Critical Thinking:** Describe dietary modifications suggested to decrease the risk for cancer. Ask students to indicate how many have decreased their fat intake, increased their fiber intake, and so on, over the past year.

Tumor immunology
   Tumor antigenicity
   Failure of the immune response
Classification
Metastasis
   Mechanisms
	Critical Thinking: Explain how the immune system is believed to be a surveillance network against cancer cells.
	
	Critical Thinking: Describe three potential mechanisms of metastasis.
	
	VIEWSTUDY image #43 demonstrates routes of metastasis.
	
	TA 12 is useful in discussing cancer and the cell cycle.

Prevention and early detection
   Prevention
 	
   Early detection
Diagnosis
   Cytologic examination
   Biopsy
   Imaging
   Tumor markers
Staging and grading of tumors
Treatment methods
   Surgery
   Radiation therapy
     Therapeutic goals
     Clinical application
       External therapy
       Internal therapy
 	
   Radiation safety
	Critical Thinking: What are some measures that can reduce an individual's risk for cancer?
	
	Critical Thinking: What are the seven warning signals of cancer?
	
	Review cancer screening guidelines.
	
	Critical Thinking: What are the three major goals of cancer treatment?
	
	VIEWSTUDY image #44 demonstrates goals of cancer treatment.
	
	Critical Thinking: Discuss nursing considerations in the care of the patient undergoing brachytherapy (internal radiation therapy).
	
	Stress that dislodged implants must not be handled with bare hands.

Chapter Outline	Lecture Strategies
Side effects	Summarize the side effects of radiation.
Chemotherapy	
Cellular effects	Summarize cancer cell response to chemotherapy.
Classification of agents	
Collaborative goals	
Combination chemotherapy	**Critical Thinking:** Why is it important to give repeated doses of chemotherapy?
Side effects and toxic effects	
	VIEWSTUDY image #40 illustrates cell life cycle and metabolic activity.
	VIEWSTUDY image #41 shows normal cellular differentiation.
Drug administration	**Critical Thinking:** Describe the nursing implications of handling chemotherapeutic drugs.
Biologic response modifier therapy	
Classifications	
Side effects and toxic effects	Discuss the most commonly used agents in your facility with regard to toxicities, and nursing activities associated with drug therapy.
Other treatment approaches	
Photodynamic therapy	Ask students to speculate as to the effects of heat on cancer cells.
Gene therapy	
	Ask students to consider if patients should be encouraged to seek treatment even if the quality of life is diminished.
Clinical trials	Ask students to discuss their responses to clinical trials.
Unproven methods of treatment	
Management of symptoms and complications	**Critical Thinking:** What should be included in a patient-teaching plan regarding clinical trials?
Altered protective mechanisms	**Critical Thinking:** Explain potential risk factors for infection in the cancer patient.
Nursing management of the patient with altered protective mechanisms	
Assessment	
Nursing diagnosis	
Planning/expected outcomes	
Implementation	Ask students to describe interventions for preventing infection.
Evaluation/documentation	
Bleeding	
Nursing management of the patient with bleeding	
Assessment	
Nursing diagnosis/planning	
Implementation	
Evaluation/documentation	
Anemia	
Nursing management of the patient with anemia	
Assessment	
Nursing diagnosis/planning	
Implementation	
Evaluation/documentation	

Chapter Outline	Lecture Strategies
Alopecia	
Nursing management of the patient with alopecia	
Assessment	
Nursing diagnosis	
Planning/expected outcomes	
Implementation	
Evaluation/documentation	
Oral complications	
Nursing management of the patient with oral complications	
Assessment	
Nursing diagnosis	
Planning/expected outcomes	
Implementation	
Evaluation/documentation	
Nausea and vomiting	
Nursing management of the patient with nausea and vomiting	
Assessment	
Nursing diagnosis/planning	
Implementation	
Evaluation/documentation	
Diarrhea	**Critical Thinking:** Explain how chemotherapy and radiation therapy can induce diarrhea.
Nursing management of the patient with diarrhea	
Assessment	
Nursing diagnosis/planning	Ask students how they would manage constipation.
Implementation	
Evaluation/documentation	
Constipation	
Nursing management of the patient with constipation	
Assessment	
Nursing diagnosis/planning	
Implementation	
Evaluation/documentation	
Sexual dysfunction	
Nursing management of the patient with sexual dysfunction	
Assessment	
Nursing diagnosis/planning	
Implementation	
Evaluation/documentation	
Alterations in nutrition	
Pain	**Critical Thinking:** Describe three categories of pain syndromes that occur in cancer patients.
Nursing management of the patient with pain	
Oncologic emergencies	Ask students to prioritize nursing interventions for each emergency.
Continuity of care	
Rehabilitation and survivorship	Ask students to predict their reactions to being told that they have cancer.
Secondary malignancy	
	Critical Thinking: What supportive care measures could be used to assist the patient in the diagnostic and treatment phase of disease?

Chapter Outline	Lecture Strategies
	Invite members of support groups to discuss their programs. **Critical Thinking:** What are potential obstacles to successful rehabilitation of the cancer patient?
Outpatient and home care The terminally ill patient	**Critical Thinking:** What must be assessed when determining appropriateness of home treatment and care for the patient?
Nursing management of the terminally ill patient Assessment Nursing diagnosis/planning Implementation Evaluation/documentation	**Critical Thinking:** What nursing interventions could be used to provide comfort for the terminally ill patient?

Related Skills

1. Ask students to discuss what they would do tomorrow and next year if they were diagnosed with cancer. Use the discussion to draw out fears and perceptions related to cancer.
2. Discuss oral hygiene for the cancer patient.
3. Review care of the patient receiving radiation.
4. Review care of the patient undergoing chemotherapy.

Related Clinical Skills

1. Assign students to patients with cancer. Encourage the students to listen very carefully to expressed and unexpressed needs of the cancer patients and families. Ask students to detail comfort measures and pain management for the chronically ill patient in the home or hospice setting.

CHAPTER 5

Shock

LEARNING OBJECTIVES

1 Differentiate the three types of shock according to definition, etiology, and pathophysiologic alterations.
2 Summarize the cellular changes common to all forms of shock.
3 Compare the characteristics and clinical evidence of the four stages of shock.
4 Explain the neural, hormonal, and chemical changes that occur during the compensatory stage of shock.
5 List the clinical findings and laboratory abnormalities present in the compensatory and progressive stages of shock.
6 Differentiate definitive and supportive therapy for the major types of shock.
7 Review specific nursing actions to prevent the major types of shock.
8 Explain the components of the nursing assessment of the shock patient, including clinical findings and invasive hemodynamic parameters.
9 Identify appropriate nursing diagnoses for the shock patient.
10 Formulate a nursing care plan for the shock patient, including expected patient outcomes and specific nursing interventions.

KEY TERMS

anaphylactic shock
cardiogenic shock
central venous pressure (CVP)
coronary cardiogenic shock
distributive shock
hypovolemic shock
intraarterial blood pressure
neurogenic shock
noncoronary cardiogenic shock
pulmonary wedge pressure (PWP)
right atrial pressure
septic shock
shock

Chapter Outline	Lecture Strategies
	Relate shock to the students' experience by asking if they have been involved with individuals with severe heat stroke, vomiting, or hemorrhage.
Definitions of shock	**Critical Thinking:** Define shock in terms of tissue perfusion.
Classifications of shock	**TA 14** depicts shock classified by cause.
Hypovolemic shock Pathophysiology	**TA 13** shows pathophysiologic alterations in hypovolemic shock.

Chapter Outline	Lecture Strategies

Cardiogenic shock
   Pathophysiology
Distributive shock
  Neurogenic shock
    Pathophysiology
  Anaphylactic shock
    Pathophysiology
  Septic shock
    Causative microorganisms
    Pathophysiology
	In discussing cardiogenic shock, ask, "Under what circumstances would the heart fail to pump adequate blood?"
	
	Critical Thinking: List in separate columns those patients at risk to develop hypovolemic, cardiogenic, neurogenic, anaphylactic, and septic shock. Compare collaborative management of each.

Common cellular changes in shock Progression of shock Initial stage	**Critical Thinking:** Explain the cellular changes in the shock patient. **Critical Thinking:** Differentiate the major pathophysiologic changes in hypovolemic, cardiogenic, and septic shock.

Compensatory stage
    Neutral compensation
    Hormonal compensation
    Chemical compensation
    Clinical manifestations
	In reviewing the compensatory stage, ask students to recall basic knowledge of fight-or-flight response.
	
	Critical Thinking: Review the effects of compensatory mechanisms by:
	  a. Listing five effects of sympathetic nervous system stimulation
	  b. Describing the action of three hormones released during compensation
	  c. Explaining the effects of decreased pulmonary blood flow on arterial oxygen and carbon dioxide tensions

Progressive stage
  Effects on other organ systems
    Brain
    Kidneys
    Gastrointestinal tract
    Liver
    Pancreas
    Lungs
    Clinical manifestations
  Refractory stage
    Clinical manifestations
	Critical Thinking: Summarize the effects of shock on the following organs/systems:
	  a. Brain
	  b. Kidneys
	  c. Heart
	  d. Liver
	  e. Pancreas
	  f. Lungs

Collaborative management
  Definitive measures
    Hypovolemic shock
    Cardiogenic shock
    Neurogenic shock
	Critical Thinking: Differentiate each of the following as either definitive or supportive therapy for shock:
	  a. Administering antibiotics
	  b. Opening the airway
	  c. Initiating mechanical ventilation
	  d. Receiving a human heart transplantation
	  e. Surgically correcting a bleeding problem
	  f. Administering parenteral fluids
	  g. Providing adequate nutrition

Chapter Outline	Lecture Strategies
	Critical Thinking: A 65-year-old patient is admitted for an acute myocardial infarction. His blood pressure shortly after admission is 80/50 mm Hg. Is this patient in shock? Explain.
Anaphylactic shock	To introduce a discussion of anaphylactic shock, ask whether anyone in the class experienced a severe allergic reaction.
	Relate the alterations in anaphylactic shock to the students' knowledge of the inflammatory process and antigen-antibody reaction.
Septic shock	**Critical Thinking:** List the laboratory changes that develop in the advanced stage of shock.

Supportive measures
    Ventilation and oxygenation
    Red blood cell volume
    Atrial oxygen saturation
    Intravascular volume
    Cardiac output
    Arterial blood pressure
    Metabolic balance
	Critical Thinking: What causes the massive vasodilation in neurogenic, anaphylactic, and septic—distributive—shock?

	Critical Thinking: A 60-year-old patient with septic shock shows the following changes:
	  a. His blood pressure has decreased from 120/90 mm Hg to 70/50 mm Hg.
	  b. His skin has changed from pink and warm to cold and pale.
	  c. His cardiac output has decreased from 5 L/min to 2.8 L/min.

	Explain the significance of these changes.

Nursing management of the shock patient
  Prevention
    Hypovolemic shock
    Cardiogenic shock
    Neurogenic shock
    Anaphylactic shock
    Septic shock
  Assessment
	Critical Thinking: How can the nurse prevent hypovolemic, cardiogenic, neurogenic, anaphylactic, and septic shock?

	Critical Thinking: The nurse caring for a patient in shock must assess many clinical parameters. What findings should the nurse anticipate in advanced shock when checking the:
	  a. Blood pressure
	  b. Level of consciousness
	  c. Urine output
	  d. Peripheral pulses
	  e. Skin
	  f. Bowel sounds

Invasive hemodynamic parameters Intraarterial blood pressure	**Critical Thinking:** Explain why the shock patient may need an intraarterial catheter to monitor arterial blood pressure. What are potential dangers of this invasive catheter?
	VIEWSTUDY image #355 illustrates the components of a pressure-monitoring system.

Chapter Outline	Lecture Strategies
	TA 15 can help students visualize the position of an intraaortic balloon catheter.
	TA 16 shows pulmonary artery catheter placement.

Pulmonary artery pressures
Central venous (right atrial) pressure
    Cardiac output
    Venous oxygen saturation
	Critical Thinking: A pulmonary artery catheter can be used to monitor the cardiovascular status of a shock patient. Explain the purpose of each of the four lumens of the quadruple-lumen pulmonary artery catheter.

	VIEWSTUDY image #356 is an illustration of a venous infusion port pulmonary artery catheter.
	Critical Thinking: Compare the advantages and disadvantages of a central venous catheter and a pulmonary artery catheter.
	Critical Thinking: List the normal values for the central venous pressure, the pulmonary artery diastolic and systolic pressures, the pulmonary wedge pressure, the cardiac output, and the venous oxygen saturation.
	VIEWSTUDY image #357 demonstrates the position of the pulmonary artery flow–directed catheter.

Hemodynamic data in shock
    Hypovolemic shock
    Cardiogenic shock
    Neurogenic shock
    Anaphylactic shock
    Septic shock	

Nursing diagnoses, planning, and interventions	**Critical Thinking:** Review, by listing, possible nursing diagnoses for the shock patient.

Nursing diagnosis
    Rationale
    Expected patient outcomes
    Nursing interventions
	Critical Thinking: Summarize specific nursing interventions related to three of the nursing diagnoses listed in the last question.

	Review the nursing diagnoses, outcomes, and interventions for patients in shock. For example: What nursing diagnosis would result from inadequate intravascular or maldistribution of blood volumes?

Nursing diagnosis
    Rationale
    Expected patient outcomes
    Nursing interventions
Nursing diagnosis
    Rationale
    Expected patient outcomes
    Nursing interventions
Psychologic needs
Additional nursing diagnoses
Evaluation/documentation	

Related Skills

1. In the laboratory setting, review the procedure and describe how readings are taken and the correct procedure for dressing change, medication, and fluid administration.

Related Clinical Skills

1. Assign students to a patient with a central line, either a CVP or pulmonary arterial catheter. Have the student develop a care plan and demonstrate how readings are taken and relate the significance of the readings to the patient problem.

The Critically Ill Adult with Multiple Organ Dysfunction Syndrome

LEARNING OBJECTIVES

1 Define systemic inflammatory response syndrome (SIRS), including the two major types of pathologic insults and typical clinical conditions associated with its development.
2 Explain the hyperdynamic clinical findings in SIRS.
3 Outline the pathophysiologic links of between SIRS and multiple organ dysfunction syndrome (MODS), including mediator release, maldistribution of circulating volume, imbalance of oxygen supply and demand, and alterations in metabolism.
4 Describe how translocation of bacteria and toxins may contribute to the development and progression of SIRS/MODS.
5 Define, differentiate, and explain the relationship between primary and secondary MODS.
6 State the goals of management for patients with SIRS/MODS based on the pathophysiologic changes.
7 Develop a nursing care plan for the patient with SIRS/MODS, including nursing diagnoses, expected patient outcomes, and nursing interventions.
8 List potential discharge planning needs for the critically ill patient with SIRS/MODS.

KEY TERMS

endogenous inflammatory mediator
endotoxin
hyperdynamic state
multiple organ dysfunction syndrome
multisystem organ failure (MSOF)
sepsis syndrome
systemic inflammatory response syndrome (SIRS)
translocation phenomenon

Chapter Outline	Lecture Strategies
Multiple organ dysfunction syndrome 　Definition 　Etiology/epidemiology 　Pathophysiology 　Systemic inflammatory response syndrome 　　Description 　　Relationship of SIRS to MODS 　　Primary events in SIRS	**Critical Thinking:** List the primary events that contribute to the release of mediators into the circulation. **Critical Thinking:** Define multiple organ dysfunction syndrome (MODS) in relation to the inflammatory response. **VIEWSTUDY** image #362 depicts the causes of systemic inflammatory response syndrome and multiple organ dysfunction syndrome.

Chapter Outline	Lecture Strategies
Pathophysiologic changes leading to MODS	**VIEWSTUDY** image #363 illustrates the pathophysiology of systemic inflammatory response syndrome and multiple organ dysfunction syndrome.
	Explain the etiology and pathophysiology of the following assessment findings of the hyperdynamic state: a. Increased cardiac output b. Decreased SVR c. Tachycardia d.. Hypotension

Clinical manifestations of SIRS/MODS
    Cardiovascular system
    Respiratory system
     Gastrointestinal and hepatic systems
    Central nervous system
    Renal system
    Hematologic system
    Endocrine system
    Laboratory values
Collaborative management
	Critical Thinking: Mr. Smith has generalized peripheral edema, yet his PCWP and urine output are low. Therefore, he is not volume overlooked; what is the source of his edema?

Oxygen supply/demand balance	**TA 17** illustrates the causes and effects of the imbalance between oxygen supply and demand.

Cardiac output
    Hemoglobin
    Arterial saturation
    Decreased oxygen demand	

Nutritional support
    Individual organ support
    Investigational therapies
	VIEWSTUDY image #3 shows neurochemical links among the nervous, endocrine, and immune systems.
	
	VIEWSTUDY image #19 illustrates vascular response in inflammation.
	
	VIEWSTUDY image #20 demonstrates cellular response in inflammation.
	
	VIEWSTUDY image #21 shows the margination, diapedesis, chemotaxis of white blood cells.
	
	VIEWSTUDY image #22 demonstrates sequential activation and biologic effects of the complement system.
	
	VIEWSTUDY image #23 illustrates the pathway of arachidonic acid oxygenation and generation of prostaglandins and leukotrienes.
	
	VIEWSTUDY image #24 shows how when monocytes and macrophages are activated, they secrete interleukin-1.

Nursing management of the critically ill patient
    Assessment
        Central nervous system
        Cardiovascular system
        Respiratory system
        Renal system
        Gastrointestinal system
        Laboratory values
        Psychosocial considerations	

Chapter Outline	Lecture Strategies
Nursing diagnosis Planning/expected outcomes Implementation	**Critical Thinking:** What is the major goal of therapy for the critically ill patient?
Evaluation/documentation	**Critical Thinking:** Why is individual organ support (e.g., hemodialysis and mechanical ventilation) alone not effective in the treatment of MODS?
Continuity of care Discharge planning	**TA 18** is useful in discussing evidence of impending organ dysfunction.

Related Skills

1. Have the students practice reading CVP and Swan-Ganz arterial line measurements.

Related Clinical Skills

1. Assign the students with a nurse to patients in the critical care setting. Develop care plans that focus on the interaction of body systems as they compensate for illness or disease.

7   Preoperative Nursing

LEARNING OBJECTIVES

1 Describe the nursing activities in the preoperative period.
2 Classify surgery according to intent or purpose and degree of urgency.
3 Discuss physiologic disruptions that occur as a result of surgery.
4 Describe common preoperative psychologic concerns and nursing support measures.
5 Identify potential risk factors or abnormalities during a preoperative patient assessment.
6 Formulate an individualized plan of nursing care for the preoperative patient.
7 Prepare an individualized teaching plan for the preoperative patients.
8 Evaluate the preoperative patient's readiness for surgery.

KEY TERMS

ambulatory surgery
anesthesia
outpatient surgery
perioperative period
preoperative period
same-day surgery

Chapter Outline	Lecture Strategies
The preoperative environment	**Critical Thinking:** Define the preoperative period, and list nursing goals for this time.
Surgery	**Critical Thinking:** List two methods of classifying surgery and, using both methods, classify the surgery for a patient scheduled to undergo a laparoscopy to evaluate chronic pelvic pain.
Anesthesia	The practice of anesthesia involves making a patient insensible to pain and then managing a patient who is under the influence of anesthesia.
	Ask students to identify the kind of patient who is classified as a Class VI patient by The American Society of Anesthesiologists.
Ambulatory surgery	Obtain and discuss preadmission procedures, charting forms, and patient education sheets for a common outpatient surgery in the students' clinical facility.

Chapter Outline	Lecture Strategies
	Critical Thinking: What criteria must be met for a patient to have ambulatory surgery?
	Critical Thinking: What are some of the advantages of ambulatory surgery?
	Ask students to delineate between outpatient surgery and short-stay surgery.
Preoperative receiving area	**Critical Thinking:** Identify nursing care that is commonly performed in the preoperative receiving area.
	Critical Thinking: What factors would affect the process of informed consent?
Preoperative period Physiologic response to surgery	**Critical Thinking:** What physiologic changes may occur as a result of surgical stress?
	TA 19 illustrates metabolic response to surgery.
Psychologic response to surgery	**Critical Thinking:** Identify fears commonly associated with surgery, and explain how you might respond to them.
	It is essential not to judge the rightness or wrongness of the fears. Attempt to gain more information from the patient about experiences that have influenced the response to surgery.
Nursing management of the preoperative patient Assessment	**Critical Thinking:** Describe the purpose of the preoperative assessment.
Physical assessment Surgical and anesthetic history Medications Preexisting disease	Document and report abnormal findings during the physical assessment. **Critical Thinking:** What preoperative laboratory tests would most likely be needed for a 55-year-old male patient who smokes but has no other history suggestive of systemic disease?
Mental and psychosocial assessment	**Critical Thinking:** What questions would you ask as part of the psychosocial assessment of the preoperative patient?
Planning and implementation Nutrition Elimination Hygiene	Institutions usually produce guidelines for the intent and location of hair removal for various surgeries.
Valuables and prostheses	**Critical Thinking:** If a patient wanted to wear jewelry into the operating room, what would your response be?

Chapter Outline	Lecture Strategies
Medications Psychologic preparation of the patient	Discuss the common preoperative drugs in terms of their action. Research suggests that patients with a high internal locus of control require a great deal of information. These patients are characterized by higher levels of independence.
Teaching Respiratory care Turning and body movement Pain management Emergencies Evaluation/documentation Informed consent Patient record	**Critical Thinking:** List information that you would include in a general teaching plan for the preoperative patient. **Critical Thinking:** How would you evaluate a patient's readiness for surgery?

Related Skills

1. Take the students through a tour of the preoperative and postanesthesia areas, much in the same way that you would take a patient through the areas.

2. Assign students to uncomplicated surgical patients. Before caring for the patients, students will research the surgeries and demonstrate knowledge of the surgery, preoperative and postoperative care, and medications used.

Intraoperative Nursing

LEARNING OBJECTIVES

1 Describe the roles of the surgical team members and the importance of the team approach.
2 Differentiate among the different forms of anesthesia.
3 Contrast the effects of common surgical positions on the respiratory system, cardiovascular system, peripheral nerves, and skin.
4 Apply the principles of surgical asepsis to intraoperative nursing care.
5 Recognize breaks in surgical aseptic technique.
6 Identify common threats to the safety of the intraoperative patient.
7 List nursing measures to decrease intraoperative heat loss.
8 Demonstrate appropriate emotional support and care of the operative patient.
9 Identify information the should be shared between the operating room and recovery unit when the patient is transferred after surgery.

KEY TERMS

anesthesia
caudal anesthesia
circulating nurse
epidural anesthesia
general anesthesia
local anesthesia

malignant hyperthermia
regional anesthesia
scrub nurse
spinal anesthesia
surgical asepsis

Chapter Outline	Lecture Strategies
The intraoperative environment	
The operating room environment	
The surgical team	**Critical Thinking:** What are the roles of the surgical team members? Discuss the importance of the team approach.
Anesthesia care provider	
Surgeon	
Surgical assistants and allied personnel	
Anesthesia	**Critical Thinking:** What are the advantages and disadvantages of the various types of anesthesia?
General anesthesia	
Anesthetic hazards	
Regional anesthesia	
Spinal anesthesia	
Epidural and caudal anesthesia	
Peripheral nerve blocks	
Local anesthesia	Some students may have experienced local anesthesia during dental procedures.
Local anesthetics	
Monitored anesthesia care	
Malignant hyperthermia	Discuss the signs and symptoms of malignant hyperthermia.

Chapter Outline	Lecture Strategies
Nursing management of the intraoperative patient Assessment Nursing diagnosis Planning/expected outcomes Implementation Emotional support and care	**Critical Thinking:** What kind of emotional support should the nurse provide the operative patient?
Patient safety	**Critical Thinking:** What are the common threats to the safety of the intraoperative patient? Ask students to list safety precautions that would be necessary for the unconscious patient.
Patient positioning Asepsis Skin preparation Electrical hazards	**Critical Thinking:** What are the effects of common surgical positions on the following body systems: respiratory, cardiovascular, peripheral nervous, integumentary?
Laser safety Chemical burns	Discuss nursing interventions for preventing laser damage to the skin, eyes, and respiratory system.
Temperature Evaluation/documentation	**Critical Thinking:** List nursing measures to decrease intraoperative heat loss. Summarize factors responsible for heat loss and measures to decrease heat loss. **Critical Thinking:** If the final sponge count or instrument count differs from the initial count, what is the nurse's responsibility?
Transfer from the operating room	**Critical Thinking:** What information should be shared between the operating room and the recovery unit when a patient is transferred after surgery?

Related Clinical Skills

1. Have students observe a patient undergoing surgery and identify the roles and responsibilities of the circulating and the scrub nurse. Have students identify the instrument and sponge count record and relate why accuracy is so important.

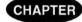
CHAPTER

9

Postoperative Nursing

LEARNING OBJECTIVES

1 Describe nursing assessment of the patient in the postanesthesia care unit, including postanesthesia recovery score.
2 Discuss the elements and implementaion of the postanesthesia "wakeup" regimen.
3 Identify common postanesthesia problems and related nursing care.
4 Describe the process of discharging and transferring a patient out of the postanesthesia care unit.
5 Identify common problems in the later postoperative period.
6 Describe nursing activites to prevent postoperative complications and promote healing.
7 Apply principles of postoperative nursing to develop a plan of nursing care for the postoperative patient.

KEY TERMS

acute parotitis
anabolic phase
atelectasis
catabolic phase
dehiscence
evisceration
paralytic ileus
postanesthesia care unit
    (PACU)
primary intention
secondary intention
tertiary intention

Chapter Outline	Lecture Strategies
Immediate postoperative period	
Recovery from anesthesia	
Family	
Nursing management of the patient during the immediate postoperative period	
Assessment	**Critical Thinking:** Discuss nursing assessment of the patient in the postanesthesia care unit (PACU).
	Critical Thinking: What is the postanesthesia recovery score? How is it used?
Postanesthesia recovery score	
Nursing diagnosis	
Planning/expected outcomes	
Implementation	
"Wake-up" regimen	
Promoting gas exchange	
Positioning and mobilization	
Pain relief	Use **TA 20** to discuss postoperative pain treatment.
Care of patients after anesthesia	
Regional or local anesthesia	
Spinal or epidural anesthesia	
Patient safety	
Common postanesthesia problems	**Critical Thinking:** What are common postanesthesia problems? Describe the related nursing care.

Chapter Outline	Lecture Strategies
Evaluation/documentation	
Continuity of care	**Critical Thinking:** What are the steps in discharging and transferring a patient from the PACU?
Transfer of patient from PACU	
Sending the patient home	
Later postoperative period	Ask the students why written instructions are desirable.
Nursing management of the patient during the later postoperative period	
Assessment	
Nursing diagnosis	
Planning/expected outcomes	
Implementation	**Critical Thinking:** What are common problems in the later postoperative period?
Postoperative pain	
Alterations in gas exchange	**VIEWSTUDY** image #51 depicts potential problems in the postoperative period.
	Critical Thinking: What nursing activities prevent postoperative complications and promote healing?
	VIEWSTUDY image #52 shows etiology and relief of airway obstruction.
Wound healing	**VIEWSTUDY** image #53 shows postoperative atelectasis.
Dehiscence and evisceration	
Factors altering healing	**VIEWSTUDY** image #25 illustrates types of wound healing.
Nutrition	
Circulation and oxygenation	
Drains	**Critical Thinking:** Outline the steps in the wound healing process.
Infection	
Dressings	**TA 21** presents an hour-by-hour view of the wound healing process (primary intention).
	VIEWSTUDY image #54 illustrates techniques for splinting a wound when the patient is coughing.
	VIEWSTUDY image #55 shows postoperative leg exercises.
Maintaining circulation	Review carefully patients who are at risk for development of venous thrombosis.
Thrombosis	
Embolism	
Maintaining metabolic equilibrium	
Nutrition	
Fluids and electrolytes	
Maintaining urinary function	
Urinary retention	
Urinary tract infection	

Chapter Outline	Lecture Strategies

Maintaining gastrointestinal function
  Acute parotitis
  Nausea and vomiting
  Hiccoughs
  Paralytic ileus
  Constipation
 	
Evaluation/documentation
	Ask students to delineate nursing measures that will alleviate constipation.

Related Skills

1. Demonstrate and have students practice sustained maximal inspiration (SMI) maneuver and the cascade cough. With students working in pairs, have them practice instruction of patients in these techniques.
2. Demonstrate and have students practice initial mobilization of postoperative patients.
3. Demonstrate and have students return a satisfactory demonstration of a sterile dressing.

Related Clinical Skills

1. Assign students to patients in the later postoperative period. Encourage them to articulate rationales for their nursing activities.
2. Assign students to preoperative patients for whom they will provide preoperative teaching, and whom they will follow through surgery and the PACU experience and care for in the later postoperative phase. As part of the experience, have the student discharge a patient from PACU to the floor.
3. Assign students to observe a surgical procedure and the PACU (or recovery room).
4. Assign students to an elderly patient receiving an outpatient surgical procedure. Follow the patient to the home setting. Develop a teaching plan to prevent postoperative complications.

10 Nursing Assessment of the Respiratory System

LEARNING OBJECTIVES

1. Understand the structure and function of the respiratory system.
2. Describe the physical principles of respiratory gas transport.
3. Obtain a complete and concise history from the patient with a respiratory disorder.
4. Accurately examine a patient with a respiratory disorder in an organized manner to obtain appropriate objective data.
5. Record history and physical findings of the patient with a respiratory disorder in a concise, accurate, and logical manner.
6. Differentiate normal from abnormal history and physical findings of the patient with a respiratory disorder.
7. Describe procedures and tests used in the detection and diagnosis of disorders of the respiratory system.
8. Describe patient preparation and care related to diagnostic procedures of the respiratory system.

KEY TERMS

alveoli
bronchophony
bronchoscopy
crackles
dissolved oxygen
egophony
expiration
flow-volume loop analysis
fremitus
inspiration
lower respiratory tract
Mantoux test
mediastinoscopy
minute volume
perfusion lung scan
pleural friction rubs
Schick test
spirometry
thoracentesis
upper respiratory tract
ventilation lung scan
vital capacity
wheezes

Chapter Outline	Lecture Strategies
Anatomy and physiology Ventilation	Use anatomic models to aid in description.
Anatomy of respiratory tract	**VIEWSTUDY** image #82 depicts structures of the respiratory tract.
	VIEWSTUDY image #83 illustrates landmarks and structures of the chest wall.
	VIEWSTUDY image #84 shows a portion of the respiratory membrane greatly magnified.
Pulmonary ventilation	Allowing a balloon to deflate is a useful visual illustration of the passive process of expiration.

Chapter Outline	Lecture Strategies
	VIEWSTUDY image # 85 illustrates the frontal section of the chest, showing movement of the lungs and chest wall during inspiration and expiration.
Lung volumes Gas transport Physical principles	Ask students to forcibly inspire or expire to illustrate inspiratory and expiratory reserve volumes. Ask students to actively recall these concepts from anatomy and physiology classes.
Blood transport of carbon dioxide Blood transport of oxygen	**Critical Thinking:** How is oxygen carried in the blood? **VIEWSTUDY** image #112 shows the normal gas exchange unit in the lung. **VIEWSTUDY** image #113 shows a gas exchange unit illustrating V/Q mismatch.
Homeostasis of carbon dioxide and oxygen Intrinsic control mechanisms	**Critical Thinking:** Describe the homeostatic function of the respi ratory system.
Extrinsic control mechanisms Voluntary control of respiration	Question: What effect does temperature have on the respiratory rate?
Assessment Subjective	**VIEWSTUDY** image #89 demonstrates the relationship of lung volumes and capabilities. Severe respiratory distress requires immediate intervention even if a health history is not complete. **Critical Thinking:** Compose at least three questions to ask patients regarding risk factors for respiratory impairment.

Objective
        General assessment
        Integumentary
        Cardiovascular
	Ask students to distinguish between S1, S2, S3 and S4 cardiovascular sounds.

Respiratory	**Critical Thinking:** Design a logical plan for assessing the thorax and lungs of a patient in respiratory distress, setting priorities of assessment to allow for immediate intervention if indicated. **Critical Thinking:** Discuss possible psychosocial concerns of patients with respiratory alterations. **VIEWSTUDY** image #86 demonstrates the sequence for examination of the chest.

Chapter Outline	Lecture Strategies
	VIEWSTUDY image #87 is a diagram of percussion areas and sounds in the anterior side of the chest.
	VIEWSTUDY image #88 is a diagram of percussion areas and sounds in the posterior side of the chest.
	TA 23 shows normal auscultatory sounds.
	Students should be able to define *fremitus, crackles, rhonchi, pleural friction rubs, bronchophony,* and *egophony.*
Laboratory and diagnostic tests	
Radiography	
Chest roentgenogram (chest x-ray film)	Bring x-ray films to class to demonstrate common abnormalities that may be detected by chest films.
Patient preparation	
Tomography (body-section roentgenography, planigraphy, and laminagraphy)	Use **TA 22** to show the difference in diameter between a normal and a barrel chest.
Esophagram (barium swallow and esophagraphy)	
Patient preparation	**Critical Thinking:** Discuss the preparation and care of a patient undergoing bronchography.
Bronchography (bronchogram)	
Patient preparation	
Postprocedure care	
Pulmonary angiography	
Patient preparation	
Postprocedure care	
Computed tomography scan	
Patient preparation	
Magnetic resonance imaging	Ask, "For what kinds of patients is MRI contraindicated? Why?"
Radioisotope procedures	
Lung scintiscanning	
Endoscopy procedures	
Bronchoscopy/bronchial biopsy	
Patient preparation	
Postprocedure care	
Mediastinoscopy	
Patient preparation	
Pleural fluid examination	
Thoracentesis	
Patient preparation	
Postprocedure care	
Lung biopsy (pleural biopsy)	
Pulmonary function tests	
Spirometry	
Flow-volume loop analysis	
Determination of diffusing capacity	
Maximal inspiratory pressure	
Pulse oximetry	Students should be able to describe the function of a pulse oximetry test.
Patient preparation	

Chapter Outline	Lecture Strategies
Sputum examination Throat culture Patient preparation	Newer methods for detecting GABHS—latex agglutinations, enzyme-linked immunoabsorbent assay (ELISA), and coagglutination—are faster but not as sensitive as culture methods, which should still be used as a follow-up to negative test results.

Skin tests
    Tuberculin skin testing (Mantoux)
        Patient preparation
        Interpretation of results
    Schick test
Blood serum tests
	Ask students to explain how misleading or false-negative Mantoux test results can occur.

Related Skills

1. Have the students practice respiratory assessment in pairs. Before clinical assignments, have the students return a satisfactory demonstration of respiratory assessment skills.
2. Arrange for students to visit the respiratory therapy area of a clinical facility, and either observe spirometry or actually participate in this diagnostic procedure.
3. Practice obtaining throat cultures.
4. Arrange for students to visit a community or occupational health agency when the Mantoux is being performed or read.

Related Clinical Skills

1. Require students to complete a thorough respiratory assessment for each assigned patient. Discuss the relevance of this assessment with the students for patients who do not have respiratory disease.
2. Assign students to patients undergoing diagnostic tests for respiratory disorders. Arrange, if possible, for students to be with or to observe their patients while the diagnostic tests are being done.

CHAPTER 11

Nursing Interventions Common to Respiratory Disorders

LEARNING OBJECTIVES

1 Evaluate the effectiveness of deep breathing and coughing techniques in patient care.
2 Discuss the use of chest physical therapy in promoting airway clearance.
3 Identify indications for the use of artificial airways.
4 Compare artificial airways, endotracheal tubes, and tracheostomy tubes.
5 Discuss potential complications of artificial airways.
6 Develop a nursing care plan for the patient with an artificial airway.
7 Describe the key assessment criteria indicating a patient's need for oxygen therapy.
8 Discuss two methods of oxygen delivery to patients requiring long-term oxygen therapy.
9 Compare and contrast negative and positive pressure ventilators.
10 Describe commonly used negative pressure ventilators.
11 Discuss potential complications of mechanical ventilation.
12 Describe clinical tools used at the bedside to assess the level of neuromuscular blockade in the patient receiving a paralytic agent.
13 Develop a nursing care plan for the patient using mechanical ventilation.
14 Assess the function of chest tube drainage systems.

KEY TERMS

atelectasis
continuous positive airway pressure (CPAP)
controlled cough
diaphragmatic breathing
huff cough
hypoxemia
incentive spirometer (IS)
intermittent positive pressure breathing (IPPB)
metered-dose inhaler (MDI)
negative pressure ventilation
positive end-expiratory pressure (PEEP)
positive pressure ventilation
postural drainage (PD)
quad-assist cough
resisted breathing

Chapter Outline	Lecture Strategies
Breathing exercises	Ask students to describe the normal breathing pattern.
	Critical Thinking: Describe the signs and symptoms of ineffective breathing.
Incentive spirometry 　　Patient care 　　Evaluation of incentive spirometry	**Critical Thinking:** Explain the procedure for using an incentive spirometer.
	Review factors to consider in evaluating incentive spirometry.

Chapter Outline	Lecture Strategies
Intermittent positive pressure breathing	Students should be able to describe intermittent positive pressure breathing.
Directed coughing Evaluation of the cough Chest physical therapy	**Critical Thinking:** List the interventions that a nurse can perform to improve the patient's ability to cough. **Critical Thinking:** Identify the indications for chest physiotherapy.

Postural drainage
   Therapeutic percussion/vibration
   Evaluation of chest physical therapy
Suctioning
   Complications of suctioning
	Diagrams are useful in visualizing the various positions and the lung segments drained by the positions.
	
	Critical Thinking: Describe the clinical indications, procedure, and complications of suctioning a patient with and without an artificial airway.

Oxygen therapy	Students may find it difficult to think of oxygen as a drug, and it must be emphasized that exposure to high concentrations of oxygen must be limited.

Oxygen delivery systems
   Complications of oxygen therapy
   Evaluation of oxygen therapy
   Home oxygen therapy
     Delivery methods
      Reservoir devices
      Demand-flow oxygen delivery devices
      Transtracheal oxygen therapy
	Critical Thinking: Identify the indications. evaluation techniques, and complications associated with oxygen therapy.
	
	Critical Thinking: Match the oxygen delivery system with the patient's clinical condition.
	
	VIEWSTUDY image #98 shows a transtracheal catheter for oxygen administration.

Humidity therapy
Aerosol therapy
   Small-volume nebulizers
   Patient care
   Metered-dose inhalers
   Evaluation of aerosol therapy
	Critical Thinking: Describe the various types of equipment used to provide supplemental humidity to patients.
	
	Ask, "What restricted kinds of patients should be considered for metered-dose inhalers?"
	
	Critical Thinking: List the instructions that should be given to a patient to properly use a metered-dose inhaler.

Artificial airways
   Oral airways
   Nasal airways
   Endotracheal tubes
   Pharmacologic agents for intubation
	Critical Thinking: Match the types of artificial airways used in clinical practice with their indications and complications.
	
	VIEWSTUDY image #91 demonstrates an endotracheal tube.
	
	VIEWSTUDY image #92 demonstrates the technique for inflating a cuff and checking cuff pressure.
	
	VIEWSTUDY image #93 shows types of tracheostomy tubes.

Chapter Outline	Lecture Strategies
	VIEWSTUDY image #94 shows speaking tracheostomy tubes.
	VIEWSTUDY image #95 shows an Olympic tracheostomy button.
	TA 24 shows the parts of a cuffed endotracheal tube.
	Identify instances in which pharmacologic agents for intubation would be contraindicated.

Tracheostomy tubes
Complications of intubation
  Tube displacement
  Obstruction
	Various tubes may be brought to class to aid in their visualization.

Loss of cuff seal
  Retained secretions
  Bacterial colonization
	Ask students to speculate on how air leaks might be detected.

Tracheal damage
  Endolaryngeal damage
  Endosinusitis
  Aspiration
	Describe the "minimal occluding volume" technique for obtaining an adequate tracheal cuff seal.

Nursing management of the patient with an artificial airway Assessment Nursing diagnosis Planning/expected outcomes Implementation Continuity of care	Invite a member from the local chapter of the American Lung Association to discuss services that are available to these patients and their families or obtain pamphlets used for teaching.
Mechanical ventilation	**Critical Thinking:** Describe clinical indications for continuous mechanical ventilation.
Negative pressure ventilation	"Iron lungs" were closely identified with the polio epidemic of the 1950s.
Positive pressure ventilation Conventional modes of ventilation	**Critical Thinking:** Compare and contrast the various modes of positive pressure ventilation.
Other modes of ventilation Adjunctive measures Complications of ventilation	Inverse ratio ventilation (IRV) reverses the inspiratory-to-expiratory ratio (I:E) from the normal I:E of 1:2 or longer. Ask students to identify its indications.
Nursing management of patients using mechanical ventilation Assessment Nursing diagnosis Planning/expected outcomes Implementation Weaning from mechanical ventilation	

Chapter Outline	Lecture Strategies

Weaning parameters
Noninvasive monitors of weaning
   Pulse oximetry
   Exhaled carbon dioxide
Nursing management of the patient being weaned
   from mechanical ventilation
   Implementation
   Continuity of care
Chest tubes
   Definition
   Collaborative management
	Ask students to discuss use of pulse oximetry and exhaled carbon dioxide in monitoring weaning.
	
	Use a diagram to help students visualize the T-piece.
	
	VIEWSTUDY image #101 demonstrates placement of chest tubes.
	
	TA 25 illustrates a Pleur-Evac commercial drainage system.
	
	TA 26 and **VIEWSTUDY** image #102 show a three-bottle chest suction drainage system.

Nursing management of the patient with a chest tube
   Assessment
   Nursing diagnosis
   Planning/expected outcomes
   Implementation
   Evaluation/documentation
   Continuity of care
	Critical Thinking: Differentiate between the pleural disorders for which chest tubes are used.
	
	VIEWSTUDY image #99 depicts disorders of the pleura.
	
	VIEWSTUDY image #100 demonstrates flail chest, producing paradoxical respiration.
	
	Critical Thinking: Describe the operation of a modern chest tube collection system.
	
	Critical Thinking: Write nursing care plans for patients receiving incentive spirometry, oxygen therapy, chest physiotherapy, metered-dose inhalers, artificial airways, continuous mechanical ventilation, weaning trials, and chest tubes.

Related Skills

1. Working in pairs, have students practice the various coughing exercises. Provide tissues!
2. Obtain and have available various tracheostomy and endotracheal tubes so that students may examine and manipulate them. Discuss the uses for the various types of tubes.
3. Describe and demonstrate nasal and oropharyngeal suctioning and nasal and orotracheal suctioning. Have students practice this skill and provide a satisfactory return demonstration.
4. Discuss and demonstrate tracheostomy care. Have students practice this skill and provide a satisfactory return demonstration.
5. Set up chest drainage on a mannequin and discuss its function as well as general care of the patient who has a chest tube.
6. Describe and demonstrate CPT, and then have students practice the skills of percussion, vibration, and rib shaking.
7. Set up and discuss the various oxygen delivery systems. Review principles of administration and safety.

Related Clinical Skills

1. Assign students to patients with respiratory conditions who require breathing exercises, CPT, oxygen therapy, suctioning, care of chest tubes, or tracheostomy care.
2. Arrange for students to either accompany respiratory therapists or to visit that department, so that students may gain insight into the role of these health care team members.
3. Arrange for more senior students to spend time with a preceptor in an intensive care unit, assisting in the care of patients who are ventilator dependent.
4. Assign a student to a patient who will be ventilator dependent in the home setting.
5. Have the students identify 1-, 2-, 3-bottle chest tube bottles. Compare the system with a system like a Pleur-Evac. Have them trouble-shoot different situations such as bubbling in bottles, clotting in tubing, bottle breaking, and transporting a patient.
6. Assign students to a home health nurse caring for a patient with a tracheostomy. Develop a care plan to assist the family in the management of a tracheostomy.
7. Arrange for students to attend the American Cancer Society support group "I Can Cope."

12 Nursing Management of Adults with Upper Airway Disorders

LEARNING OBJECTIVES

1 Relate principles of nursing management to the care of patients with disorders of the upper airway.
2 Discuss the role of drug therapy in the management of patients with inflammatory disorders of the upper airway.
3 Identify treatment measures for the patient experiencing nasal trauma.
4 List the risk factors that contribute to the development of cancer of the larynx.
5 Identify measures to promote communication for the patient after a laryngectomy.
6 Describe the psychologic impact of laryngeal cancer and its treatment.

KEY TERMS

anosmia	pharyngitis
Caldwell-Luc procedure	radical neck dissection
coryza	rhinitis
deviated septum	rhinorrhea
epistaxis	saddle deformity
esophageal speech	sinusitis
hemilaryngectomy	submucosal resection
laryngitis	total laryngectomy
nasal septoplasty	

Chapter Outline	Lecture Strategies
Sinusitis	
Definition	
Etiology/epidemiology	
Pathophysiology	
Clinical manifestations	Because sinusitis is such a common affliction, ask the students to list symptoms of sinusitis.
Collaborative management	
Drug therapy	
Antibiotics	
Analgesics	Ask the students what the therapeutic effect of reducing edema would be.
Decongestants	
Antihistamines	
Saline	Ask, "When are intranasal steroids contraindicated?"
Intranasal steroids	
Surgical management	
Rhinitis	
Definition/etiology	
Pathophysiology	
Clinical manifestations	Ask the students to enumerate symptoms of the common cold.
Collaborative management	Ask students to find advertisements for cold remedies. Discuss the prevalence of these remedies.

Chapter Outline	Lecture Strategies

Pharyngitis
    Definition/etiology
    Pathophysiology
    Clinical manifestations
    Collaborative management
Tonsillitis
    Definition
    Etiology
    Pathophysiology
    Clinical manifestations
    Collaborative management
Laryngitis
    Definition
    Etiology
    Pathophysiology
    Clinical manifestations
    Collaborative management
Nursing management of the patient with sinusitis,
    rhinitis, pharyngitis, tonsillitis, or laryngitis
    Assessment
    Nursing diagnosis
    Planning/expected outcomes
    Implementation
    Evaluation/documentation
    Continuity of care
Vocal cord nodules
    Definition
    Etiology/epidemiology
    Clinical manifestations
    Collaborative management
Vocal cord polyps
    Definition
    Etiology/epidemiology/clinical manifestations
    Collaborative management
Nursing management of the patient with vocal cord
    nodules and polyps
Deviated septum
    Definition
    Etiology/epidemiology
    Pathophysiology
    Clinical manifestations
    Collaborative management
Nursing management of the patient with a deviated
    septum
    Assessment
    Nursing diagnosis
    Planning/expected outcomes
    Implementation
    Evaluation/documentation
Nasal polyps
    Definition
    Etiology/epidemiology
    Pathophysiology
	Ask students to prepare a list of common antihistamines, including actions, interactions, usual dosages, and side effects. Include over-the-counter medications.
	
	Critical Thinking: What nursing interventions are appropriate for a patient with inflammation of the sinuses and nasal mucosa? When are antihistamines contraindicated?
	
	Discuss the usual position of the septum and then the position of a deviated septum.
	
	Use diagrams to help students visualize the surgeries.
	
	Have students apply gauze to their noses and practice mouth-breathing and swallowing.

Chapter Outline	Lecture Strategies
Clinical manifestations	
Collaborative management	
Nursing management of the patient with nasal polyps	
Assessment	
Nursing diagnosis	
Planning/expected outcomes	
Implementation	
Evaluation/documentation	
Epistaxis	
Definition	
Etiology/epidemiology	
Collaborative management	
Pressure and positioning	
Nasal packing	
Drug therapy	
Surgical management	
Nursing management of the patient with epistaxis	**Critical Thinking:** What underlying conditions should the student assess for if epistaxis occurs, unrelated to trauma?
Assessment	
	Ask students to list signs and symptoms of hemodynamic compromise.
Nursing diagnosis	
Planning/expected outcomes	
	Critical Thinking: Describe the nursing interventions for a patient experiencing nasal trauma.
Implementation	
Evaluation/documentation	Severe epistaxis can be very frightening for the patient and family.
Continuity of care	
Nasal fractures	
Definition	
Etiology/epidemiology	
Pathophysiology	
Clinical manifestations	
Collaborative management	
Nursing management of the patient with a nasal fracture	
Assessment	Ask students to describe the assessments that they would see as necessary.
Nursing diagnosis	
Planning/expected outcomes	
Implementation	
Evaluation/documentation	
Continuity of care	
Laryngeal cancer	
Definition	
Etiology/epidemiology	
Pathophysiology	Use an anatomical model to illustrate the difference between the true and false vocal cords.
Clinical manifestations	
Collaborative management	
Staging	Summarize the criteria used in the staging of laryngeal cancer.
Radiation therapy	
Chemotherapy	
Surgical therapy	Use a diagram of the head and neck to illustrate the surgeries.
Laryngectomy	
Radical neck dissection	
Laser surgery	Ask students to explain causes of eating difficulties after radiation therapy for laryngeal cancer.
Complications	

Chapter Outline	Lecture Strategies

Nursing management of the patient with laryngeal cancer
    Assessment
    Nursing diagnosis
	The patient's and the family's psychological response and adjustment must also be assessed.

Planning/expected outcomes	**Critical Thinking:** What is the nurse's role in risk factor management to reduce the incidence of laryngeal cancer?
Implementation Preoperative care	**Critical Thinking:** Why do patients with disorders of the upper airways experience problems with nutrition?
Postoperative care Evaluation/documentation	**Critical Thinking:** What are the major elements to be included in patient teaching for individuals after a total laryngectomy and radical neck dissection?
Continuity of care	**Critical Thinking:** How can the nurse promote communication for the patient after a laryngectomy?
	If possible, invite a member of a local laryngectomy club to class, to share his or her experiences.

Related Skills

1. With the students working in pairs, ask the students to communicate with their partners without speaking. Following the exercise, discuss the experience, focusing on feelings related to voicelessness and means of communicating without a voice.
2. Review tracheostomies in detail. Demonstrate the care of tracheostomies, and after opportunity for practice, ask students to provide a successful return demonstration of tracheostomy care.

Related Clinical Skills

1. Assign students to patients who have tracheostomies and ask them to prepare the patient to be discharged with a tracheostomy.

13 Nursing Management of Adults with Lower Airway Disorders

LEARNING OBJECTIVES

1 Explain the major alterations in physiologic functioning in specific disorders of the lower respiratory tract.
2 Outline the self-care components for patients with asthma.
3 Differentiate between respiratory failure caused by oxygenation failure and by ventilatory failure, including pathophysiologic mechanisms and therapeutic interventions.
4 Discuss symptoms associated with disorders of the lower respiratory system, and describe appropriate nursing interventions.
5 Describe risk factors associated with lung cancer, chronic obstructive pulmonary disease, and lower respiratory tract infections such as pneumonia and tuberculosis.
6 Develop a teaching plan for a patient with stable chronic obstructive pulmonary disease.
7 Develop a care plan for a patient experiencing an acute asthma attack.
8 Identify parameters indicative of acute respiratory failure.
9 Describe parameters that should be monitored closely for patients with an acute exacerbation of chronic obstructive pulmonary disease, asthma, or respiratory failure.
10 Outline nursing care of patients with tuberculosis.
11 Outline nursing care of patients with pneumonia.
12 Discuss goals of therapy for patients with lung cancer.
13 Describe the nursing care required for patients who have experienced chest trauma that includes multiple rib fractures and/or pneumothorax; explain rationales.

KEY TERMS

airway clearance
asthma
chronic bronchitis
chronic obstructive pulmonary disease (COPD)
cor pulmonale
dyspnea
emphysema
flail chest
hypercapnia
hypoxemia
pneumonia
pulse oximeter
respiratory failure
shunting
status asthmaticus
tuberculosis
ventilation-perfusion mismatch

Chapter Outline	Lecture Strategies

Chronic obstructive pulmonary disease
   Definition
   Etiology/epidemiology
	TA 27 shows the effects of emphysema.
	
	Obstructing the passage of escaping air in an inflated balloon nicely illustrates this.

Chapter Outline	Lecture Strategies

Pathophysiology
    Abnormalities of gas exchange
        Ventilation-perfusion mismatch
	Critical Thinking: What are the three pathophysiologic alterations that impair gas exchange in the patient with COPD?

Shunting of pulmonary capillary blood Impaired gas diffusion Complications Clinical manifestations	**VIEWSTUDY** image #107 illustrates the pathophysiology of chronic bronchitis and emphysema.
	VIEWSTUDY image #108 illustrates morphologic types of emphysema
	VIEWSTUDY image #109 shows pulmonary blebs and bullae.
	VIEWSTUDY image #110 illustrates mechanisms involved in the pathophysiology of cor pulmonale secondary to COPD.
	VIEWSTUDY image #111 demonstrates the progression of cystic fibrosis.
History	**TA 28** depicts a patient with severe COPD.
	A useful analogy is to compare bullae to holes in bread and dough.
Physical examination Laboratory findings	Question: On the basis of the pathophysiological symptoms that have been discussed, what would you expect during a physical examination of a patient with COPD?
Collaborative management	Three major classes of bronchodilators are used for COPD patients: anticholinergics, beta-adrenergic agonists, and methylxanthines.
Nursing management of the patient with chronic obstructive pulmonary disease (COPD)	**VIDEO** volume 2 presents nursing care of the patient with COPD, including assessment, interventions, and home care.
Assessment Nursing diagnosis Planning/expected outcomes Implementation	Before discussing the assessment, have students identify assessment priorities either individually or in groups.

Drug therapy
    Airway clearance
    Oxygen therapy
    Rest and activity
    Nutrition
	Ask students to research drugs and bring this information to class to share with classmates.

Breathing exercises	Practice pursed-lip breathing with students. Demonstrate instruction of a patient in this technique.
Evaluation/documentation	**Critical Thinking:** List specific nursing interventions for the patient with COPD related to drug therapy, airway clearance, rest, nutrition, oxygen therapy, and breathing exercises.

Chapter Outline	Lecture Strategies

Continuity of care
  Impaired gas exchange
  Dyspnea
  Airway clearance
  Exercise tolerance
  Psychosocial adjustment
Asthma
  Definition
  Etiology/epidemiology
  Pathophysiology
  Clinical manifestations
  Collaborative management
Nursing management of the patient with asthma
	Critical Thinking: What are the major problem areas for the COPD patient that are addressed in planning continuity of care?

	Critical Thinking: Describe the progression of an acute asthma attack in terms of triggering stimuli and clinical manifestations.
	VIEWSTUDY image #103 demonstrates early and late phase responses of asthma.
	VIEWSTUDY image #104 illustrates the early phase response in asthma.
	VIEWSTUDY image #105 shows factors causing expiratory obstruction in asthma.
	VIEWSTUDY image #106 illustrates the pathophysiology of asthma.
	Discuss the patient teaching required for the appropriate use of inhalants.
Assessment Nursing diagnosis Planning/expected outcomes Implementation Evaluation/documentation Continuity of care Inhaled medication	Before discussing differences, have students identify areas of assessment in acute and in long-term care.
	This technique is difficult for some patients, especially older patients, and these patients should be taught to use a spacer device such as the Opithaler.
Theophylline levels	Explain causes of increased blood theophylline levels (e.g., fever, liver disease, congestive heart failure, and commonly used drugs).
Home monitoring of airway obstruction Avoiding triggers Exercise Emotional triggers Restrictive lung disease Definition Etiology/epidemiology Pathophysiology	**Critical Thinking:** How does the nurse prepare the asthma patient for self-care?
	The hallmark of restrictive disorders is decreased lung volumes.
	Distribute balloons to the students. After trying to inflate the balloons, ask the students to relate the characteristics of the balloon to decreased compliance in the respiratory system.
	Critical Thinking: What is the effect of lung restriction on pulmonary function and gas exchange?

Chapter Outline	Lecture Strategies
Clinical manifestations	Question: Why would cor pulmonale occur with restrictive lung disease?
	Dyspnea is the primary manifestation.
Collaborative management	Management will vary with cause.
Nursing management of the patient with restrictive lung disease	
Assessment	
Nursing diagnosis	
Planning/expected outcomes	
Implementation	
Evaluation/documentation	
Continuity of care	
Rehabilitation and long-term care	
Home care	
Respiratory failure	
Definition	
Pathophysiology	
Combined oxygen and ventilatory failure	
Collaborative management of respiratory failure in COPD	**Critical Thinking:** Outline the primary considerations in the collaborative management of respiratory failure that influence nursing care for the patient.
Clinical manifestations	
Mechanical ventilation	
Drug therapy	
Nutrition	
Nursing management of the patient with respiratory failure	**VIEWSTUDY** image #116 shows the relationship of systemic inflammatory response, multiple organ dysfunction syndrome, and acute respiratory distress syndrome.
Assessment	
Nursing diagnosis	
Planning/expected outcomes	
Implementation	
Evaluation/documentation	**Critical Thinking:** Discuss the advantages and disadvantages of home ventilatory care for the patient with chronic respiratory failure.
Continuity of care	
Adult respiratory distress syndrome (ARDS)	
Definition	
Etiology/epidemiology	
Pathophysiology	
Collaborative management	
Gas exchange	
Tissue perfusion	
Management of underlying disease	
Nursing management of the patient with ARDS	Use **TA 29** to discuss oxygenation and ventilatory respiratory failure.
Assessment	
Nursing diagnosis	
Planning/expected outcomes	
Implementation	
Gas exchange	
Breathing patterns	
Cardiac output	

Chapter Outline	Lecture Strategies
Airway clearance	**Critical Thinking:** Develop a care plan for the patient with a nursing diagnosis of ineffective airway clearance related to increased mucous production from a pulmonary infection.
Nutrition Individual and family coping Evaluation/documentation	Life-threatening illnesses may cause previously "resolved" family conflicts to reemerge. Weigh together advantages and disadvantages of home care for the ventilator-dependent patient.

Pneumonia
  Definition
  Etiology/epidemiology
    Mode of transmission
    Risk factors
    Bacterial pneumonias
    Viral pneumonia
    Fungal infections
    Other pneumonias
  Pathophysiology
  Clinical manifestations
  Collaborative management
Nursing management of the patient with pneumonia
  Assessment
  Nursing diagnosis
  Planning /expected outcomes
  Implementation
  Evaluation /documentation
	Careful history taking is necessary to elicit specific signs and symptoms.

Tuberculosis
  Definition
  Etiology/pathophysiology
 	
  Clinical manifestations
  Collaborative management
 	
Nursing management of the patient with tuberculosis
  Assessment
  Nursing diagnosis
  Planning /expected outcomes
 	
  Implementation
  Evaluation/documentation
 	
  Continuity of care
	TA 30 outlines the clinical manifestations of active TB.
	
	Discuss risk factors among the elderly.
	
	Show chest x-ray films of patients infected with tuberculosis.
	
	VIDEO volume 10 presents nursing care of the patient with tuberculosis, including assessment, skin testing, and patient education.
	
	Community health nurses are usually involved in case finding among contacts.
	
	Prevention of transmission of *M. tuberculosis* and compliance with drug therapy are primary goals of care.
	
	Critical Thinking: What are the primary nursing interventions related to the treatment of tuberculosis and prevention of transmission of the infection?

Lung cancer
  Definition
  Etiology/epidemiology/pathophysiology
	Critical Thinking: Describe strategies useful to prevent lung cancer.

Chapter Outline	Lecture Strategies

Clinical manifestations
    Local disease
    Metastasis
    Diagnosis
Collaborative management
    Surgical treatment
    New treatments
	Critical Thinking: Classify the clinical manifestations of lung cancer according to local disease, metastasis, and systemic effects.
	
	Endoscopic surgery is a fairly new technique, so students may want an explication of this technique.

Thoracotomy for lung resection
    Radiation therapy
    Chemotherapy
    Prevention
	Describe the processes of pneumonectomy, segmental resection, and wedge section and related complications.

Nursing management of the patient with lung cancer
    Assessment
    Nursing diagnosis
    Planning/expected outcomes
    Implementation
        Airway clearance
        Dyspnea
        Pain
        Preoperative care
        Postoperative care
    Evaluation/documentation
    Continuity of care
	Students should identify where emphasis is placed in preoperative care for these patients.

Chest trauma
    Definition
    Etiology/epidemiology
    Pathophysiology/clinical manifestations
        Rib fracture
        Flail chest
        Pulmonary contusion
        Pneumothorax
        Hemothorax
    Collaborative management
	Since the paradoxical movement is different to visualize, review the normal movement of the chest, and then relate the movement of the flail chest to this.

Nursing management of the patient with chest trauma
    Assessment
    Nursing diagnosis
    Planning/expected outcomes
    Implementation
        Emergency care
        Acute care
    Evaluation/documentation
    Continuity of care
	Critical Thinking: Compare the emergency care, acute care, and long-term care for a patient with chest trauma.

Related Skills

1. Practice, in pairs, patient teaching for: deep breathing and coughing; pursed-lip breathing; Huff cough; postural drainage.
2. Role-play, in groups of three or four with one or two students as observers, the emotional support of a patient who is dyspneic.
3. Assign students to a homebound patient with asthma. Develop a teaching plan that focuses on correct use of inhalers, oxygen utilization, and breathing exercises as part of the management of asthma.

Related Clinical Skills

1. Assign students to patients requiring nursing care for respiratory problems. In a surgical area, assign students to patients who are preoperative or who are recently postoperative and at risk for developing respiratory complications, for practice in teaching and monitoring respiratory hygiene measures.

14 Nursing Assessment of the Peripheral Vascular System

LEARNING OBJECTIVES

1 Know the main structural components of the peripheral vascular system and their functions.
2 Understand the physical and physiologic principles that control blood flow and pressure.
3 Obtain a complete and concise history from a patient with a peripheral vascular disorder.
4 Accurately examine a patient with a peripheral vascular disorder in an organized manner to obtain appropriate objective data.
5 Record the history and physical findings of a patient with a peripheral vascular disorder in a concise, accurate, and logical manner.
6 Differentiate normal from abnormal history and physical findings in a patient with a peripheral vascular disorder.
7 Describe diagnostic procedures related to the vascular system.
8 Describe the preparation and care of patients undergoing diagnostic procedures for vascular disorders.

KEY TERMS

Allen's test
arterial blood pressure
arteries
capillaries
carotid phonoangiography
central venous pressure
contrast arteriography
digital vascular imaging
edema
hydrostatic pressure
hypertension
hypotension
impedance plethysmography
lymph nodes
ocular pneumoplethysmography
peripheral resistance
retrograde filling (Trendelenburg) test
spleen
thymus gland
veins

Chapter Outline	Lecture Strategies
Anatomy and physiology Blood vessels	Ask students to recall the basic elements and functions of the peripheral vascular system.
Physical principles that determine blood flow	**Critical Thinking:** Name the factors that affect peripheral resistance.
	VIEWSTUDY image #136 shows the comparative thickness of layers of the artery, vein, and capillary.
	VIEWSTUDY image #137 shows common sites for palpating arteries.
Physiologic control of blood flow and arterial pressure Capillary dynamics Lymph vessels	**Critical Thinking:** How does the sympathetic nervous system alter blood flow during a physiologic crisis?

Chapter Outline	Lecture Strategies
Assessment 　Subjective	Some of the sensations can be likened to that experienced when an extremity "falls asleep." **Critical Thinking:** Formulate at least three questions to assess the psychosocial aspects of a patient's concern about vascular alterations.
Objective 　General assessment 　Cardiovascular 　Respiratory 　Abdominal	**Critical Thinking:** Name the pertinent indicators in assessing circulation, motion, and sensation. Ask students to detail factors to be assessed from each of the following objective categories: cardiovascular, respiratory, abdominal, peripheral vascular, and neurologic. **TA 31** offers scales for grading pulses. **TA 32** shows a grading of edema.
Peripheral vascular 　Neurologic Diagnostic and laboratory tests 　Noninvasive diagnostic studies 　　Ocular pneumoplethysmography 　　　Patient preparation	**Critical Thinking:** What manifestations distinguish arterial from venous insufficiency? **Critical Thinking:** What observations should be made of a patient following OPPG? Which observation or observations would indicate complications?
Postprocedure care 　　Carotid phonangiography 　　Ultrasound imaging 　　Impedance plethysmography 　　Segmental arterial pressure monitoring 　Invasive diagnostic studies 　　Contrast venography 　　　Patient preparation 　　　Postprocedure care 　　Contrast arteriography 　　　Patient preparation 　　　Postprocedure care 　　Digital vascular imaging 　　　Patient preparation 　　　Postprocedure care	Ask students to describe the care that the patient must receive. **Critical Thinking:** For what complications would a nurse observe a patient after contrast venography? Ask students to identify complications of the procedure.

Related Skills

1. Demonstrate assessment of the peripheral vascular system. Have students practice the skill in pairs and return a satisfactory demonstration of the skill. A variation on the return demonstration is to divide the assessment into logical units and randomly select a unit for each student.
2. Tour the radiology department and have students observe an invasive and a noninvasive diagnostic study.

Related Clinical Skills

1. Ask students to focus on assessment of the peripheral vascular system in their assigned patients. Supervise when necessary.

15 Nursing Management of Adults with Arterial Disorders

LEARNING OBJECTIVES

1 Describe the pathophysiology of arterial occlusive disease.
2 Recognize clinical manifestations of arterial occlusive disease.
3 Describe risk reduction strategies in the management of arterial occlusive disease.
4 Relate nursing management principles to the care of the patient with arterial occlusive disease, including home care and conservative treatment.
5 Outline nursing management principles for the patient with an abdominal aortic aneurysm.
6 Describe comprehensive nursing care, including home care, for the patient undergoing arterial surgery.
7 Outline the pathophysiology of the patient with Raynaud's disease and thoracic outlet syndrome.
8 Describe the clinical manifestations of the patient with subclavian steal syndrome, Raynaud's disease, and thoracic outlet syndrome.
9 Relate nursing management principles to the care of the patient with subclavian steal syndrome, Raynaud's disease, and thoracic outlet syndrome.

KEY TERMS

abdominal aorta aneurysm (AAA)
acute arterial occlusion
arterial occlusive disease
aneurysm
aortofemoral bypass
atherectomy
atherosclerosis
embolectomy
endarterectomy
extraanatomic bypass
in situ vein bypass
percutaneous transluminal angioplasty (PTA)
Raynaud's disease
reversed vein bypass
subclavian steal syndrome
thoracic outlet syndrome

Chapter Outline	Lecture Strategies

Atherosclerosis
  Definition
  Etiology/epidemiology
  Pathophysiology
	TA 33 lists risk factors for atherosclerosis.

Clinical manifestations	**TA 34** presents the effects of smoking on the vascular system.
	TA 35 and **VIEWSTUDY** image #147 illustrate the progressive development of atherosclerosis.
	VIEWSTUDY image #148 shows specific types of plasma lipoprotein delivering cholesterol to cells of the blood vessel wall.

Chapter Outline	Lecture Strategies
Collaborative management	Review actions and nursing actions associated with anti-hyperlipidemic medications. Review foods that are high in cholesterol.
Nursing management of the patient with atherosclerosis	Ask students to describe areas of focus in assessment.
Assessment	
Nursing diagnosis	
Planning/expected outcomes	**Critical Thinking:** How can people modify their lifestyles to reduce risk factors for atherosclerosis?
Implementation	
Evaluation	
Chronic infrarenal arterial disease	
Definition	
Etiology/epidemiology	**TA 36** is helpful in comparing the symptoms of claudication and chest pain.
Pathophysiology	
Clinical manifestations	
Collaborative management	**Critical Thinking:** What are the implications for the patient with intermittent claudication and rest pain?
Medical management	
Drug therapy	Review actions, interactions, side effects, and nursing actions associated with pentoxifylline. Discuss the use and effect of dextran.
Percutaneous transluminal angioplasty	Ask students to explain the procedure used in atherectomy.
Atherectomy	
Laser angioplasty	
Surgical management	In situ bypasses may go to any of the infrapopliteal vessels.
Surgical procedures	
Amputation	**Critical Thinking:** What is the nursing management for the patient treated medically for chronic infrarenal arterial disease?
Nursing management of the patient with chronic arterial occlusive disease of the extremities	
Assessment	
Nursing diagnosis	
Planning/expected outcomes	
Implementation	
Risk factor management	
Pain management	
Tissue integrity	
Emotional support	
Surgical management	If students have had previous teaching or experience in abdominal bypass surgeries, ask them to describe preoperative preparation.
Aortic and aortoiliac operations	
Lower-extremity bypass	
Preoperative preparation	**Critical Thinking:** What is the postoperative care for the patient having arterial bypass surgery?
Postoperative management	
Axillobifemoral bypass	
Evaluation	**Critical Thinking:** Explain the benefit of exercise for the patient with chronic infrarenal arterial disease.
Continuity of care	
Aneurysms	**Critical Thinking:** What are the different types of abdominal aneurysms?
Abdominal aortic aneurysm	
Etiology/epidemiology	
Pathophysiology	**VIEWSTUDY** image #175 shows a true fusiform abdominal aneurysm

Chapter Outline	Lecture Strategies
	VIEWSTUDY image #176 demonstrates surgical repair of an abdominal aortic aneurysm.
	VIEWSTUDY image #177 demonstrates replacement of aortoiliac aneurysm with a bifurcated synthetic graft.
	VIEWSTUDY image #178 shows common anatomic locations of atherosclerotic lesions of the abdominal aorta and lower extremities.
Clinical manifestations Collaborative management	Rupture of an aneurysm may be dramatic and unheralded.
Nursing management of the patient with abdominal aortic aneurysm Nursing diagnosis Planning/expected outcomes Implementation Evaluation/documentation	
Acute arterial occlusion Definition/etiology Pathophysiology/clinical manifestations Collaborative management	Ask students to speculate on the signs and symptoms of occlusion.
Nursing management of the patient with acute arterial occlusion Nonatherosclerotic peripheral vascular disease Raynaud's disease Definition/etiology Pathophysiology Clinical manifestations Collaborative management	
Nursing management of the patient with Raynaud's disease Assessment Nursing diagnosis Planning/expected outcomes Implementation Evaluation	
Thoracic outlet syndrome Definition Etiology/pathophysiology Clinical manifestations	**Critical Thinking:** Describe the problems experienced by the patient with thoracic outlet syndrome.
Collaborative management	Review the actions, interactions, side effects, and nursing activities associated with the main anticoagulants.
Nursing management of the patient with thoracic outlet syndrome Assessment Nursing diagnosis Planning/expected outcomes Implementation Postoperative care Continuity of care	

Related Skills

1. Discuss and demonstrate assessment of peripheral circulation. Have students return a satisfactory demonstration of the skill.

Related Clinical Skills

1. Assign students to patients with peripheral risk factors. Stress assessment and teaching aspects of care.

16 Nursing Management of Adults with Hypertension

LEARNING OBJECTIVES

1 Describe the types and complications of hypertension.
2 Explain the national objectives for hypertension prevention.
3 Explain the multifactorial causes for hypertension.
4 Identify high-risk factors and individuals who are predisposed to developing high blood pressure.
5 Assess an individual for the detection, screening, and follow-up of hypertension.
6 List the benefits and liabilities of therapeutic regimens in controlling hypertension.
7 Apply the concept of "self-care" to the preventive and rehabilitative interventions for people who are at high risk for or who have hypertension.
8 Compare and contrast the pharmacologic and lifestyle modifications in preventing and controlling hypertension.
9 Relate rationales for carrying out lifestyle modifications vs. pharmacologic interventions in controlling hypertension.
10 Explain the teaching/learning strategies and outcome measures for educating persons who are at high risk for or who have hypertension.

KEY TERMS

adherence
home monitoring
hypertension
hypertensive crisis
isolated systolic hypertension (ISH)
population strategy
primary hypertension
resistant hypertension
secondary hypertension
stepped-down theory
target organ disease
targeted strategy
white coat hypertension

Chapter Outline	Lecture Strategies
Hypertension (high blood pressure) Definition	**Critical Thinking:** Compare white coat, resistant, and isolated systolic hypertension. **Critical Thinking:** Briefly describe the differences between primary and secondary hypertension. **TA 37** illustrates the factors contributing to hypertension. The most frequent disease conditions associated with secondary hypertension include kidney and vascular disorders, alterations in endocrine function, and acute brain lesions.

Chapter Outline	Lecture Strategies
Etiology/epidemiology	
Genetic (nonmodifiable) factors	**Critical Thinking:** Apply the results of research studies to different populations at risk for hypertension.
Family history	
Gender	
Age	
Ethnic group	
Environmental (modifiable) factors	
Stress profile	
Personality characteristics	
Genetic factors	
Occupational situations	
Socioeconomic level	The economic impact of a therapeutic regimen is an important consideration; drug therapy can be expensive.
Dietary factors	**Critical Thinking:** Describe the role of nutrition in relation to hypertension.
Weight	
Sodium	
Potassium	
Calcium	
Magnesium	
Omega-3 fatty acids	
Lifestyle habits	**Critical Thinking:** What are health protective behaviors? What health protective behaviors can a patient do to lessen risk of developing hypertension or as an adjunct to a therapeutic regimen?
Alcohol	
Smoking	
Physical activity	
Pathophysiology	**Critical Thinking:** Which type—primary or secondary—is the most common, and what are the signs and symptoms?
Primary hypertension	
Secondary hypertension	
	Critical Thinking: Describe how hypertension develops based on the formula HBP = CO $\times$ PR (or BP = CO $\times$ PVR).
Complications	**Critical Thinking:** What are the major complications of hypertension?
Clinical manifestations	**Critical Thinking:** List three specific behaviors that hypertensive patients should exhibit.
Collaborative management	**Critical Thinking:** List at least four controversies or issues that surround hypertension and its treatment.
	VIEWSTUDY image #144 depicts a treatment algorithm for hypertension.
Lifestyle modifications	**Critical Thinking:** What nonpharmacologic interventions might the nurse initiate appropriate to the patient's condition?
Weight reduction	
Sodium restriction	
Alcohol restriction	**Critical Thinking:** What is meant by the self-care, nonpharmacologic approaches to hypertension? Specify two times when these may be particularly useful.
Physical activity	
Smoking cessation	

Chapter Outline	Lecture Strategies

Other dietary guidelines
    Calcium and magnesium
    Dietary fats
Stress management techniques
Pharmacologic modalities
	Critical Thinking: Identify two classifications other than diuretic drugs used in the treatment of hypertension, and describe what they do. Why are diuretics used initially?

	VIEWSTUDY image #145 shows the site and method of action of various hypertensive drugs.

Antihypertensive agents
    Diuretics
        Thiazide diuretics
        Loop diuretics
        Potassium-sparing diuretics
    Adrenergic inhibitors
        Central agonists
        Alpha-blockers
        Beta-blockers
        Combined alpha- and beta-blockers
    Vasodilators
        Direct vasodilators
	Critical Thinking: Compare the benefits and risks of engaging in an antihypertensive regimen.
	
	Present the broad classifications of pharmacological effects, then present more specific information.
	
	Present students with several case examples of patients receiving these medications, and ask them to determine nursing interventions and possible side effects for the patients.

Angiotensin-converting enzyme inhibitors Calcium channel blockers	**Critical Thinking:** Why should diuretics be administered in the morning?

Nursing management of the patient with hypertension
    Assessment
    Nursing diagnosis
    Planning/expected outcomes
	TA 38 offers a critical thinking guide for discussing hypertension.
	
	Draw students' attention to the six criteria established by the Joint National Committee on Detection, Evaluation, and Treatment of Hypertension.
	
	Critical Thinking: What risk factors does the nurse assess when interviewing a hypertensive patient?
	
	Critical Thinking: What effect does the health care provider have on the accuracy of blood pressure measures?

Implementation	**Critical Thinking:** Through what three strategies can adherence be enhanced? **Critical Thinking:** Around which five major areas does a teaching plan for a hypertensive patient center? **Critical Thinking:** What are five questions to consider when teaching a patient about hypertension? **Critical Thinking:** What skills are important for the nurse to possess when teaching the use of nonpharmacologic approaches to blood pressure control?
Evaluation/documentation Continuity of care	**Critical Thinking:** What outcome measures are necessary for evaluating a patient with hypertension?

Related Skills

1. Review and practice blood pressure measurement. With students working in triads, have one student observe and comment on the technique of the student performing blood pressure measurement.
2. Arrange for students to receive education and skill development in stress management.

Related Clinical Skills

1. Assign students to patients who are hypertensive. With the students, discuss what factors from the patient's history might have contributed to hypertension. Help the student to develop questions that will help explore areas of the patient's history that might not have been explored (i.e. cultural, dietary habits) and to develop nursing interventions that are appropriate to the individual patient.
2. Assign students to a hypertensive screening at a local retirement home for senior citizens.
3. Arrange for students to develop a teaching plan for hypertensive prevention and present it to senior citizens.

17

Nursing Management of Adults with Venous or Lymphatic Disorders

LEARNING OBJECTIVES

1 Identify common disorders of the venous system.
2 Recognize clinical manifestations in the individual with chronic venous insufficiency.
3 Discuss nursing diagnoses commonly associated with venous insufficiency.
4 Discuss nursing interventions appropriate in venous insufficiency.
5 Describe the nursing management for a patient having medical or surgical treatment for varicose veins.
6 Identify risk factors associated with the development of deep-vein thrombosis (DVT) and/or pulmonary embolus (PE).
7 Relate principles of nursing management to the care of the patient receiving anticoagulants.
8 Recognize the signs and symptoms of complications of anticoagulation, including heparin-induced thrombocytopenia and warfarin skin necrosis.
9 Identify laboratory values appropriate for anticoagulation.
10 Discuss the clinical manifestations of DVT and PE and their sequelae.
11 Discuss the clinical manifestations of the patient with lymphatic disorders.
12 Identify patient risk factors for complications in lymphatic disorders.
13 Relate principles of nursing management to the care of patients with lymphatic disease.

KEY TERMS

chronic venous insufficiency
compression stocking
deep-vein thrombosis (DVT)
International Normalized Ration (INR)
lymphedema
pulmonary embolus (PE)
sclerotherapy
superficial thrombophlebitis
thrombophlebitis
varicose veins
vena caval interruption

Chapter Outline	Lecture Strategies

Varicose veins
   Definition
   Etiology/epidemiology
   Pathophysiology
   Clinical manifestations
	Critical Thinking: What are varicose veins? What is the nursing management after surgical removal or sclerotherapy?

Chapter Outline	Lecture Strategies

Collaborative management
    Medical management
    Surgical management
Nursing management of the patient with varicose veins
  Assessment
  Nursing diagnosis
  Planning/expected outcomes
  Implementation
  Evaluation
	Ask students to differentiate between spider veins and varicose veins.

Superficial thrombophlebitis
  Definition
  Etiology/epidemiology
	To assist in learning the definition, break the word into its combining forms (thrombo-, phleb-, -itis), and have students determine the definition from these.
	
	Critical Thinking: What is the cause and treatment of thrombophlebitis?

Clinical manifestations
Collaborative management
Nursing management of the patient with superficial
  thrombophlebitis
  Assessment
  Nursing diagnosis
  Planning/expected outcomes
  Implementation
	Ask students to recall signs of inflammation.

Deep vein thrombosis
  Definition
  Etiology/epidemiology
  Pathophysiology
	Critical Thinking: What is deep-vein thrombosis (DVT), and how does it differ from thrombophlebitis? What three factors are necessary for thrombosis to occur? How can the nurse assess for DVT?
	
	Summarize the factors in Table 17-1 to demonstrate the wide range of predisposing factors.

Clinical manifestations Collaborative management	Venography has the disadvantage of introducing a contrast medium to which the patient may be allergic.
Prevention Immobilization	Discuss use and advantages of prophylactic anticoagulant therapy for deep vein thrombosis.
Anticoagulant therapy	Many physicians initiate coumarin drugs the day following initiation of heparin therapy to achieve the therapeutic level more quickly. Effectiveness is judged by the prothrombin time (PT) or a deheparinized PT.

Thrombolytic therapy
Compression stockings
Surgical management
Nursing management of the patient with deep-vein
  thrombosis
  Assessment
	Critical Thinking: What is phlegmasia? Clinical manifestations? What is thrombolytic therapy? What is its greatest risk? Nursing implications?
	
	Review signs of pulmonary embolism. What is the emergency management?

Nursing diagnosis Planning/expected outcomes Implementation	**Critical Thinking:** What is the most serious complication of DVT, and how may the patient prevent it?

Chapter Outline	Lecture Strategies
Anticoagulant therapy Evaluation/ documentation Continuity of care	**Critical Thinking:** What should the nurse teach the patient taking oral anticoagulants? Review the assessments, patient education, and nursing care needed for a patient on anticoagulants and thrombolytic therapy.

Pulmonary embolism
   Definition
   Etiology/epidemiology
   Pathophysiology
	Ask students to outline the physiologic changes that occur after a large clot blocks a pulmonary artery.

Clinical manifestations	Ask students to differentiate among the symptoms of pulmonary embolism, tension pneumothorax, and myocardial infarction. Students should be able to explain the use of VQ scans in ruling out PE.

Collaborative management
   Anticoagulant therapy
   Thrombolytic therapy
   Surgical intervention
      Pulmonary embolectomy
      Vena cava interruption
	Critical Thinking: What are the classic signs of pulmonary embolism? What procedures are used when heparin therapy is contraindicated?
	
	VIEWSTUDY image #179 demonstrates inferior vena caval interruption techniques to prevent pulmonary embolism.
	
	Describe the use of the Kimray-Greenfield filter, the bird's-nest filter, the nitinol, and venatech filters in vena caval interruption.

Nursing management of the patient with pulmonary
   embolism
   Assessment
   Nursing diagnosis
   Planning/expected outcomes
   Implementation
Chronic venous insufficiency
   Definition/etiology
   Epidemiology
   Pathophysiology
	Review nursing diagnoses for managing the patient with pulmonary embolism.
	
	TA 39 offers a critical thinking guide for discussing pulmonary embolism.
	
	Reflect on the various theories as to the long-term effect of ankle pressure and venous ulcer development in chronic venous insufficiency.

Clinical manifestations	Summarize Table 17-3 to compare arterial and venous ulcers.

Collaborative management
   Medical management
   Surgical management
	Discuss the variety of dressings and their advantages and disadvantages.

Nursing management of the patient with chronic venous insufficiency	**Critical Thinking:** What is the nursing management for a patient with chronic venous insufficiency? Venous ulcers?

Chapter Outline	Lecture Strategies

Lymphedema
    Definition
    Pathophysiology
    Clinical manifestations
    Collaborative management
Nursing management of the patient with lymphedema
    Assessment
    Nursing diagnosis
    Planning/expected outcomes
    Implementation
    Evaluation
	Critical Thinking: What is lymphedema and how is it manifested? How does external pneumatic compression work? Nursing management?
	
	Discuss essentials in teaching a patient how to wrap the elastic compression so that it is even and tight.

Related Skills

1. Review and practice application of compression stockings and elastic wraps.

Related Clinical Skills

1. Assign students to patients who may be at risk for DVT. Have them assess the patients specifically for risk and for signs of DVT, and plan, implement, and evaluate nursing activities that will assist in prevention.
2. Assign students to patient with chronic venous insufficiency or varicose veins so that students may become involved in nursing management of therapies. Stress the patient teaching aspects of caring for these individuals.
3. Following research and discussion of the medications, have students administer anticoagulants.

18 Nursing Assessment of the Cardiac System

LEARNING OBJECTIVES

1 Describe the basic structures and functions of the cardiac system.
2 Understand the cardiac cycle.
3 Elicit a complete and concise history from a patient with a cardiac disorder.
4 Accurately examine a patient with a cardiac disorder in an organized manner to obtain appropriate objective data.
5 Record history and physical findings of a patient who has a cardiac disorder in a concise, accurate, and logical manner.
6 Differentiate normal from abnormal history and physical findings of a patient with a cardiac disorder.
7 Describe procedures and tests related to disorders of the cardiac system.
8 Describe patient care and preparation related to diagnostic tests of the cardiac system.

KEY TERMS

afterload
atrioventricular valves
blood lipids
cardiac catheterization
cardiac cycle
cardiac output
diastole
echocardiography
isovolumetric contraction
   period
isovolumetric relaxation
   period
murmurs
myocardium
pericardial sac
preload
semilunar valves
stroke volume
systole

Chapter Outline	Lecture Strategies

Anatomy and physiology
   Structural description
 	
   Action potential of the heart
	Ask students to recall as much of this information as possible from classes in anatomy.
	
	Critical Thinking: How is the heart stimulated to contract?
	
	VIEWSTUDY image #130 depicts the orientation of the heart within the thorax.
	
	VIEWSTUDY image #131 is a schematic representation of blood flow through the heart.
	
	VIEWSTUDY image #134 shows the conduction system of the heart.

Chapter Outline	Lecture Strategies
Function of heart valves	Review the function of the valves.
Cardiac cycle	**VIEWSTUDY** image #138 shows cardiac auscultatory areas.
	VIEWSTUDY image #139 shows heart sounds.

Control of stroke volume and heart rate
   Intrinsic mechanisms
   Extrinsic mechanisms
	Critical Thinking: Describe the mechanisms that control heart rate.

Heart as part of endocrine system	Describe the right atrium's function as an endocrine gland.
Assessment	Review the historical information that is useful to obtain in a cardiac assessment.
Subjective	**Critical Thinking:** Develop at least three questions to ask patients regarding risk factors for heart impairment.
	Critical Thinking: Discuss possible psychosocial concerns of patients with cardiac alterations.

Objective
   General assessment
   Integumentary
   Cardiovascular
	Emphasize that certain kinds of data demand immediate nursing action.

	TA 40 shows appropriate areas for auscultation of the heart.
	Demonstrate assessment techniques. Have students practice palpation of PMI and auscultation of the five areas of the precordium.
	Critical Thinking: Design a logical plan for assessing the precordium of a patient in cardiac distress, setting priorities of assessment to allow for immediate intervention if indicated.

Respiratory
   Gastrointestinal
   Peripheral vascular
	Ask students to outline techniques for the respiratory, gastrointestinal, and peripheral vascular assessments.

Diagnostic and laboratory tests
   Holter monitor
   Routine chest x-ray study
	Critical Thinking: Describe the relationship of electrocardiogram, cardiac cycle, and heart sounds.

	VIEWSTUDY image #140 depicts the relationship of electrocardiogram, cardiac cycle, and heart sounds.
	VIEWSTUDY image #141 demonstrates the conventional polarity of the three standard leads is indicated by + and −.
Echocardiography Computed tomography	Echocardiography is also performed using high-dose dipyridamole.

Chapter Outline	Lecture Strategies
Nuclear cardiography	The radionucleotide will be excreted from the body in 6 to 24 hours and will not affect family, visitors, or staff.
Radionuclide angiography Myocardial perfusion scan	**Critical Thinking:** Using lay terms, describe the procedure of radionuclide angiography.
Technetium 99m pyrophosphate imaging	Ask students to identify advantages and disadvantages of technetium 99m pyrophosphate imaging.
Cardiac positron emission tomography scan	Students should be able to describe the procedure for obtaining a cardiac positron emission tomography scan.
Magnetic resonance imaging	Ask, "What would you tell a patient while preparing them for magnetic resonance imaging?"

Invasive procedures
Cardiac catheterization
    Patient preparation
    Postprocedure care
Cardiac biopsy
Pericardiocentesis
    Patient preparation
    Postprocedure care
	Critical Thinking: Describe the pretest and posttest care for a patient undergoing cardiac catheterization.

Blood/serum tests Blood studies Cardiac enzymes Myoglobin	**VIEWSTUDY** image #151 shows heart muscle enzyme levels in the blood after myocardial infarction.
Blood lipids Patient preparation Measurement of drug levels	Review normal reference ranges, by gender and age groups, for total cholesterol, triglycerides, LDL cholesterol, and HDL cholesterol.

Related Skills

1. Practice cardiac assessment in the laboratory, with students in pairs. Ask students to provide a satisfactory return demonstration of cardiac assessment skills.
2. Practice taking vital signs. Require students to provide a satisfactory return demonstration of this skill.

Related Clinical Skills

1. Assign students to patients with cardiac disorders. Help the students to perform a complete cardiac assessment with patients who are not experiencing acute symptoms. If possible, arrange to have students accompany the patients to diagnostic tests.

19 Nursing Management of Adults with Common Complications of Cardiac Disease

LEARNING OBJECTIVES

1 Describe the properties of cardiac muscle and conduction tissue that influence heart rate and rhythm.
2 Identify common cardiac dysrhythmias through the assessment of the electrocardiogram.
3 Describe appropriate nursing care for the patient experiencing dysrhythmias.
4 Choose nursing interventions appropriate to the care of patients with pacemakers.
5 Describe the pathophysiologic and compensatory mechanisms of heart failure.
6 Describe the major clinical signs and symptoms of heart failure.
7 Explain the rationale for treatment options designed to restore the balance between myocardial oxygen supply and demand.
8 Discuss nursing interventions appropriate to the care of patients experiencing heart failure.
9 Explain each step involved in the application of basic life support techniques.
10 Differentiate between defibrillation and cardioversion with respect to the physiologic effects and expected clinical outcomes of each intervention.

KEY TERMS

automaticity
cardioversion
conductivity
contractility
defibrillation
depolarization
dysrhythmia
ectopic
electrocardiogram
excitability
internal cardioverter-
   defibrillator (AICD)

P wave
pacemaker syndrome
PR interval
QRS complex
QRS interval
QT interval
refractory period
repolarization
R-R interval
ST segment
T wave
u wave

Chapter Outline	Lecture Strategies

Properties of cardiac tissue
    Pathway of current flow
Phases of the action potential
    Nonautomatic or working cells
    Automatic or pacemaker cells
    Refractory periods
	Draw upon students' prior contact with this material when discussing the physiology of the cardiac system.
	
	The depolarization/repolarization sequence is called the action potential and is recorded on waveforms on the ECG.
	
	VIEWSTUDY image #162 shows absolute and relative refractory periods

Chapter Outline	Lecture Strategies
Assessing the electrocardiogram 12-lead system	**VIEWSTUDY** image #135 demonstrates the normal electrocardiogram pattern. **VIEWSTUDY** image #150 shows indicative changes recurring in leads that examine the area of infarction.

Assessment parameters
    ECG tracing
    Waveforms
	Critical Thinking: Describe the major ECG characteristics of the following cardiac rhythms:
	
	Sinus rhythm
	Sinus tachycardia
	Sinus bradycardia
	Sinus arrhythmia
	Premature atrial complexes
	Atrial tachycardia
	Paroxysmal supraventricular tachycardia
	Atrial flutter
	Atrial fibrillation
	Premature junctional complexes
	Junctional escape rhythm
	Junctional tachycardia
	Premature ventricular complexes
	Ventricular tachycardia
	Ventricular fibrillation
	Ventricular asystole

Intervals	**TA 41** shows intervals between waveforms.
Calculating heart rate Assessing the rhythm strip	**Critical Thinking:** Briefly describe three methods used to calculate heart rate using an ECG rhythm strip. Which method(s) should be used when the cardiac rhythm is irregular?
Dysrhythmias	**VIEWSTUDY** image #159 demonstrates how, when the rhythm is regular, heart rate can be determined at a glance **VIEWSTUDY** image #160 shows normal sinus rhythm in lead II. **VIEWSTUDY** image #161 demonstrates the electrocardiogram complex. Break *dysrhythmia* into word parts and ask students to define the term, using word parts.

Supraventricular dysrhythmias
    Sinus rhythm and variants
        Sinus rhythm
            ECG criteria
        Sinus tachycardia
            ECG criteria
            Collaborative management
	Ask students to speculate on the appearance of the QRS interval in the presence of supraventricular dysrhythmias.
	
	Ask students to speculate on the work required by the myocardial muscle and subsequent impact on demand for oxygen. Review and have students practice the Valsalva maneuver.

Chapter Outline	Lecture Strategies
Sinus bradycardia Collaborative management	Ask students to review the actions, side effects, and nursing activities associated with beta-adrenergic agonists and parasympathetic blocking agents.

Sinus arrhythmia
    ECG criteria
    Collaborative management
Atrial dysrhythmias
    Premature atrial complex
    ECG criteria
    Collaborative management
	Show a diagram of an ECG tracing of sinus arrhythmia.

Atrial tachycardia
    ECG criteria
    Collaborative management
	Show an example of an ECG tracing showing atrial tachycardia.

Paroxysmal supraventricular tachycardia
    AV nodal reentry
    Circus movement tachycardia
	Show examples of an ECG with CMT.

Atrial flutter
    ECG criteria
    Collaborative management
	Show examples of an ECG with atrial flutter. Use **TA 42** here.

Atrial fibrillation
    ECG criteria
    Collaborative management
	Show ECG with atrial fibrillation. **TA 43** will be helpful here.

Junctional dysrhythmias
    Premature junctional complex
        ECG criteria
        Collaborative management
	Show an ECG tracing with PJCs. Ask students to identify appropriate treatment of PJC that stems from digitalis excess.

Junctional escape rhythm
    ECG criteria
    Collaborative management	

Junctional tachycardia
    ECG criteria
    Collaborative management
	Show an ECG tracing of junctional tachycardia.

Nursing management of the patient experiencing a supraventricular dysrhythmia
    Assessment
    Nursing diagnosis
    Planning/expected outcomes
    Implementation
    Evaluation/documentation
    Continuity of care
	Critical Thinking: Describe nursing interventions appropriate to the care of patients experiencing dysrhythmias.

Ventricular dysrhythmias	Ask students to describe reasons why ventricular dysrhythmias are more dangerous than supraventricular dysrhythmias.

Chapter Outline	Lecture Strategies

Premature ventricular complex
  Characteristics
    ECG criteria
    Collaborative management
	TA 44 shows premature ventricular complexes.

Ventricular tachycardia
  ECG criteria
  Collaborative management
    Long-term management
  Torsade de pointes
	Critical Thinking: Describe the procedure for defibrillation and cardioversion.
	
	Show an ECG tracing of ventricular tachycardia.
	
	TA 45 shows an internal cardioverter defibrillator (ICD).
	
	VIEWSTUDY image #163 demonstrates paddle placement and current flow in defibrillation.

Ventricular fibrillation
  ECG criteria
  Collaborative management
	Show an ECG tracing of ventricular fibrillation.

Ventricular asystole
  ECG criteria
  Collaborative management	

Nursing management of the patient experiencing a ventricular dysrhythmia
  Assessment
  Nursing diagnosis
  Planning/expected outcomes
  Implementation
  Evaluation/documentation
  Continuity of care	

Atrioventricular blocks
  First-degree atrioventricular block
    ECG criteria
    Collaborative management
	Show an ECG tracing of first-degree AVB from the clinical setting.

Second-degree atrioventricular block
    Type I block
      ECG criteria
      Collaborative management
	Show an ECG tracing of type I block from the clinical setting.

Type II block
      ECG criteria
      Collaborative management
	Show an ECG tracing of type II block from the clinical setting.

Type III block
      ECG criteria
      Collaborative management	

Third-degree atrioventricular block
    ECG criteria
    Collaborative management
	TA 47 illustrates third-degree AVB.

Nursing management of the patient experiencing disturbed AV conduction	

Chapter Outline	Lecture Strategies
Assessment Nursing diagnosis Planning/expected outcomes Implementation Evaluation/documentation Continuity of care	**Critical Thinking:** Describe nursing interventions appropriate to the care of patients experiencing heart blocks.

Pacemakers
  Common components
    Temporary pulse generators
    Permanent pulse generators
  Insertion
  Basic pacing parameters
    Stimulus release
    Stimulus response
    Pacemaker coding
  Physiologic pacemakers
  Pacemaker malfunctions
    Sensing disturbances
    Firing disturbances
    Capturing disturbances
	Show diagrams of both pacemakers in place.
	
	VIEWSTUDY image #164 illustrates and implantable cardioverter-defibrillator pulse generator.

Nursing management of the patient with an artificial
  pacemaker
  Assessment
  Nursing diagnosis
  Planning/expected outcomes
  Implementation
  Evaluation/documentation
	Critical Thinking: Describe nursing interventions appropriate to the care of patients experiencing each pacemaker malfunction.

Continuity of care	Break students into groups and ask them to develop a discharge plan for these patients.

Heart failure
  Definition/etiology
  Pathophysiology
    Myocardial performance
      Contractility
      Heart rate
      Afterload
      Preload
    Left versus right ventricular failure
	Review signs and symptoms.

Clinical manifestations
    Cardiovascular responses
    Pulmonary responses
    Renal and endocrine responses
    Neurologic responses
	Critical Thinking: Differentiate between physiologic effects of "forward" and "backward" failure on each side of the heart. Which component reflects compromised pumping? Which reflects congestion?
	
	VIEWSTUDY image #143 shows a massively enlarged heart caused by hypertrophy of both ventricles.
	
	VIEWSTUDY image #152 demonstrates left heart failure from elevated systemic vascular resistance.

Chapter Outline	Lecture Strategies
	VIEWSTUDY image #154 shows hypertrophic cardiomyopathy.
	Critical Thinking: Discuss three cardiovascular and three pulmonary responses associated with heart failure. How are these responses assessed clinically?

Collaborative management
    Oxygen therapy
    Pharmacologic agents
    Mechanical support
    Other interventions
	Critical Thinking: Identify the most common indications for use of each of the following emergency drugs: epinephrine, atropine, lidocaine, and isoproterenol. Which of these can be given via the endotracheal route?

Nursing management of the patient with heart failure Assessment	**VIDEO** volume 4 presents nursing care of the patient with heart failure, including coverage of assessment and patient teaching.
Nursing diagnosis Planning/expected outcomes	**TA 48** offers a critical thinking guide for discussing pulmonary edema.
Implementation Evaluation/documentation Continuity of care	Ask students to supply rationales for each of the interventions.

Cardiopulmonary resuscitation
    Basic life support
        Airway
        Breathing
        Circulation
	Critical Thinking: What do the ABCs of CPR represent?
	
	VIEWSTUDY image #169 demonstrates CPR.
	
	VIEWSTUDY image #166 shows the head-tilt/chin-lift maneuver.
	
	VIEWSTUDY image #168 illustrates the finger-sweep maneuver.
	
	VIEWSTUDY image #364 demonstrates the jaw-thrust maneuver.

Airway obstruction
    Clinical manifestations
    Collaborative management
	Critical Thinking: What is the Heimlich maneuver? Why is it so effective?
	
	VIEWSTUDY image #167 shows the Heimlich maneuver administered to a conscious (standing) victim of foreign-body airway obstruction.

Nursing management of the patient requiring resuscitation	Students who are part of a code situation need opportunity to "unpack" the situation. Provide time individually or in postconference to discuss observations, reactions, and responses.

Related Skills

1. Practice basic life support in the laboratory.

Related Clinical Skills

1. Organize a hunt for emergency equipment in the unit.
2. Arrange for students to spend time in a cardiac intensive care unit, where they can assist in the care of cardiac patients.
3. Obtain an EKG strip, lead II. Have the students identify the P, QRS, ST segment, T. In addition, have the students calculate the rate and identify any abnormalities.
4. Assign students to a home care nurse. Have students develop a care plan focusing on medication administration, energy conservation techniques, ans signs and symptoms of disease processes.

20 Nursing Management of Adults with Disorders of the Coronary Arteries, Myocardium, or Pericardium

LEARNING OBJECTIVES

1 Describe the pathophysiology of coronary artery disease.
2 Discuss the alterations in lifestyle the patient should make to reduce the risk factors associated with coronary artery disease.
3 Indicate the teaching interventions for the patient with angina pectoris.
4 Describe the nursing management during the acute and rehabilitative stages for the patient who has experienced a myocardial infarction.
5 List the patient teaching objectives in preparation for discharge of the patient with myocardial infarction.
6 Differentiate pericarditis, pericardial effusion, and cardiac tamponade as to clinical manifestations and collaborative and nursing management.
7 Compare dilated, hypertrophic, and restrictive cardiomyopathy as to etiology, pathophysiology, and collaborative and nursing management.
8 Describe the types of cardiac surgery and the preoperative and postoperative nursing management for the patient undergoing cardiac surgery.

KEY TERMS

akinesis
angina pectoris
cardiac tamponade
cardiopulmonary bypass (CPB) machine
collateral circulation
dilated cardiomyopathy (DCM)
dyskinesis
hypertrophic cardiomyopathy (HCM)
hypokinesis
intra-aortic balloon pump (IABP)
myocardial infarction (MI)
pericardial effusion
pericarditis
pulsus paradoxus
restrictive cardiomyopathy
thrombolytic agents
ventricular aneurysm

Chapter Outline	Lecture Strategies

Coronary artery disease
  Definition
  Etiology/epidemiology
	Because of its insidious onset, the incidence of atherosclerosis increases with age.

Uncontrollable risk factors Controllable risk factors	Ask students to distinguish between controllable and uncontrollable risk factors for coronary artery disease.
Pathophysiology	Describe the three morphologic types of lesions seen in atherosclerosis.

Chapter Outline	Lecture Strategies
	Ask, "What is collateral circulation?"
	Identify five different types of angina.
Clinical manifestations	**VIEWSTUDY** image #149 shows location of chest pain during angina or MI.
Physical examination	
Cardiac catheterization	
Laboratory studies	Nitrates can be administered by various routes.
Collaborative management	
Pharmacologic intervention	
Nitrates	
Beta-blockers	
Calcium channel blockers	
Antilipid medications	
Aspirin	**Critical Thinking:** Describe how atherosclerosis affects the coronary arteries and what alterations in lifestyle should be made to reduce the risk factors associated with atherosclerosis.
Lifestyle modification	
	Describe four criteria for indicating PTCA for the relief of myocardial ischemia.
Percutaneous transluminal angioplasty	
	Discuss treatment innovations in the treatment of CAD.
Innovations in the treatment of CAD	
Intracoronary stents	
Laser angioplasty	
Atherectomy	
Combination interventional therapy	
Coronary artery bypass graft surgery	
Nursing management of the patient with coronary artery disease	
Assessment	
Nursing diagnosis	
Planning/expected outcomes	
Implementation	
Evaluation/documentation	Identify, with the students, issues related to patient education in planning continuity of care for the patient with coronary artery disease.
Continuity of care	
	Critical Thinking: Why are MIs in the older patient sometimes less severe than in an individual in their early 30s?
Myocardial infarction	
Definition	
Etiology/epidemiology	Discuss the pathophysiology of myocardial infarction, particularly the three zones of cellular changes (i.e., an area of injury, an area of ischemia, and an area of infarction).
Pathophysiology	
	Define: *hypokinesis, dyskinesis,* and *akinesis.* How do these terms relate to myocardial infarction?
	Use TA 49 to examine enzyme circulation at varying levels.

Chapter Outline	Lecture Strategies

Clinical manifestations
   Chest pain
   Diagnostic studies
	Critical Thinking: What clinical manifestations and diagnostic criteria would be exhibited by a patient experiencing an MI? What complications would the nurse be assessing for after an MI? What signs and symptoms would be seen for each of the complications?
	
	TA 50 depicts sequential ECG changes occurring in MI.
	
	What are the first enzymes elevated after an MI? What enzymes are elevated later?
	
	The pain associated with an MI is feared by post-MI patients.

Collaborative management
   Pharmacologic therapy
      Thrombolytic agents
   Surgical management
      Percutaneous transluminal coronary
         angioplasty (PTCA)
      Coronary artery bypass graft surgery
	Explain the use of nitroglycerin and its administration. Explain the same for beta blockers and ACE inhibitors.
	
	Critical Thinking: Compare the drug therapy used in the treatment of angina and myocardial infarction. What are the nursing implications? patient teaching implications?
	
	Ask students to review the actions and nursing activities associated with thrombolytic agents.

Complications
   Dysrhythmias
   Congestive heart failure/cardiogenic shock
   Structural changes
      Pericarditis
      Postinfarction angina
      Thromboembolic events
Nursing management of the patient with myocardial
  infarction
  Assessment
  Nursing diagnosis
  Planning/expected outcomes
  Implementation
     Emotional support
	Ask students to identify complications, especially any structural changes, associated with myocardial infarction.
	
	VIDEO volume 3 presents nursing care of the patient undergoing myocardial infarction, including assessment, patient education, discharge planning, and rehabilitation.
	
	Ask students to think about and to describe their responses and needs if a family member were admitted with an MI.

Activity Diet	**Critical Thinking:** What guidelines for progressing in activity levels are used for the patient who has had an MI?
Patient education Evaluation/documentation	**Critical Thinking:** What factors may precipitate an anginal attack? What teaching is necessary to help the patient reduce anginal attacks? slow down the disease process? prevent complications?

Continuity of care
     Cardiac rehabilitation
     Education
	Critical Thinking: What are the teaching objectives for the patient being discharged after an MI? What are the ongoing care issues?

Chapter Outline	Lecture Strategies
Counseling Activity progression Sexual activity Medical therapy Pericarditis Definition	
	Ask students to define the term by breaking it into word parts.

Etiology/epidemiology
Pathophysiology
  Complications
Clinical manifestations
  Pericardial pain
  Dyspnea
  Pericardial friction rub
  Pericardial effusion
  Cardiac tamponade
  Diagnostic tests
Collaborative management
	Critical Thinking: What are the causes of pericarditis? What clinical signs would indicate pericarditis, pericardial effusion, and cardiac tamponade?
	
	Identify a patient in the clinical area with JVD.

Nursing management of the patient with pericarditis
  Assessment
  Nursing diagnosis
  Planning
  Implementation
  Evaluation/documentation
  Continuity of care
	Critical Thinking: What is the collaborative management and nursing management for a patient with pericarditis, pericardial effusion, and cardiac tamponade?

Cardiomyopathy
  Dilated (congestive) cardiomyopathy
    Definition
    Etiology/epidemiology
    Pathophysiology
	The pathophysiology will sound familiar to students who have studied CHF.

Clinical manifestations
    Collaborative management
  Hypertrophic cardiomyopathy
    Definition
    Etiology/epidemiology
    Pathophysiology
    Clinical manifestations
    Collaborative management
	Ask students to identify signs and symptoms of dilated cardiomyopathy and to explain how these vary, depending on the progression of the disease.

Restrictive cardiomyopathy
    Definition
    Etiology/epidemiology
    Pathophysiology
    Clinical manifestations
    Collaborative management
	Critical Thinking: How do restrictive, hypertrophic, and dilated cardiomyopathy differ in etiology and pathophysiology?

Nursing management of the patient with cardiomyopathy
  Assessment
  Nursing diagnosis
  Planning/expected outcomes
  Implementation
  Evaluation/documentation
  Continuity of care
	Ask students to describe interventions appropriate to these patients.
	
	Critical Thinking: What collaborative actions are done to manage the care given to a patient with cardiomyopathy?

Chapter Outline	Lecture Strategies

Cardiac surgery
   Cardiopulmonary bypass
   Types of surgery
   Surgical preparation
   Postoperative stabilization
   Complications
Nursing management for the patient undergoing cardiac surgery
   Assessment
   Nursing diagnosis
   Planning/expected outcomes
   Implementation
      Postoperative management
         Fluids and diet
         Activity
         Comfort
   Patient education
   Cardiac transplantation
   Cardiomyoplasty
   Evaluation/documentation
   Continuity of care
      Emotions
      Discomfort and pain
      Activities
      Occupation
	Critical Thinking: What are the different types of procedures performed during cardiac surgery? What complications can occur after heart surgery?
	
	If possible, invite patients who have undergone cardiac surgery to class to describe their experiences.
	
	Critical Thinking: Describe the preoperative teaching objectives for the patient undergoing heart surgery.
	
	Critical Thinking: What are the postoperative and ongoing nursing issues for the patient undergoing heart surgery?

Related Skills

1. Review positioning to respiratory symptoms. Have students practice and then demonstrate satisfactory knowledge and performance of positioning.
2. Role-play therapeutic interventions with patients who are anxious because of chest pain or respiratory compromise. Have students form triads, with one student acting as the nurse, the second as patient, and the third as observer. At the end of 10 minutes, ask students to switch roles and again after another 10 minutes. Encourage sharing of perceptions and feedback in the triads and in debriefing as a total group.

Related Clinical Skills

1. Assign students to patients who are experiencing cardiac signs and symptoms and/or who are in the rehabilitative stage of a cardiac condition. Encourage teaching, psychological support, and knowledge of medications as well as nursing interventions.

21 Nursing Management of Adults with Endocardial Disorders

LEARNING OBJECTIVES

1 Discuss the high-risk patient population, high-risk procedures, and preventive therapy for infective endocarditis.
2 Correlate the hemodynamic alterations with the clinical manifestations and major complications of each valvular disorder.
3 Discuss the collaborative management of patients with valvular disease.
4 Describe the assessment findings, nursing diagnoses, expected outcomes, and nursing interventions for patients with valvular disorders.
5 Identify the learning needs for preventive therapy and discharge planning for patients with valvular disorders and their families.

KEY TERMS

annuloplasty
aortic regurgitation
aortic stenosis
commissurotomy
infective endocarditis
mitral regurgitation
mitral stenosis
mitral valve prolapse
Osler nodes
percutaneous balloon
   valvuloplasty
tricuspid regurgitation
tricuspid stenosis
valvuloplasty
vegetations

Chapter Outline	Lecture Strategies

Infective endocarditis
  Definition
  Etiology/epidemiology
  Pathophysiology
  Clinical manifestations
  Collaborative management
 	
Nursing management of the patient with infective
  endocarditis
 	
Assessment
Nursing diagnosis
Planning/expected outcomes
Implementation
Evaluation/documentation
	Review signs and symptoms of systemic infection with the students.
	
	Critical Thinking: Who is at risk for developing infective endocarditis? What procedures increase patients' risk of developing infective endocarditis? What are the recommendations for preventing infective endocarditis in the at-risk population?
	
	Ask students what they would focus on in a history and in a physical assessment of a patient with endocarditis.
	
	VIEWSTUDY image #170 depicts the layers of the heart.
	
	VIEWSTUDY image #171 shows bacterial endocarditis of the mitral valve (caused by *Streptococcus viridans*).

Chapter Outline	Lecture Strategies
	VIEWSTUDY image #172 demonstrates the sequence of events in infective endocarditis.
Valvular disorders	**Critical Thinking:** For each valvular disorder (mitral, aortic, and tricuspid stenosis and regurgitation) describe how changes in cardiac and pulmonary pressures are created. What signs and symptoms develop as a result of these changes?

Mitral stenosis
  Definition
  Etiology/epidemiology
  Pathophysiology
  Clinical manifestations
Mitral regurgitation
  Definition
  Etiology/epidemiology
	Ask students to define *mitral* and *stenosis,* and then to attempt definition of mitral stenosis.
	
	VIEWSTUDY image #173 shows the cross section of valves of the heart.
	
	VIEWSTUDY image #174 demonstrates how a stenosed valve leads to decreased blood flow through the valve.
	
	TA 51 illustrates the effects of mitral stenosis.

Pathophysiology
  Clinical manifestations
Mitral valve prolapse
  Definition
  Etiology/epidemiology
  Pathophysiology
  Clinical manifestations
Aortic stenosis
  Definition
  Etiology/epidemiology
  Pathophysiology
  Clinical manifestations
Aortic regurgitation
  Definition
  Etiology/epidemiology
	Critical Thinking: Differentiate between mitral regurgitation and stenosis. How does this affect cardiac output?

Pathophysiology
  Clinical manifestations
Tricuspid stenosis
  Definition
  Etiology/epidemiology
  Pathophysiology
  Clinical manifestations
Tricuspid regurgitation
  Definition
  Etiology/epidemiology
  Pathophysiology
  Clinical manifestations
  Collaborative management
    Antibiotic therapy
    Sodium restriction, diuretic therapy, and
      inotropic agents
    Activity restriction
	Ask students what would occur if volume overload occurred in the LV.
	
	Review meaning of commissural fusion.
	
	Ask students to speculate on the effects of increased pressure in the right atrium.

Chapter Outline	Lecture Strategies

Vasodilator and antianginal therapy
Antidysrhythmic therapy
Surgical management
    Mitral valve
    Aortic valve
    Tricuspid valve
    Prosthetic heart valves
Percutaneous balloon valvuloplasty (non-surgical)
	Ensure that students are aware of the definitions of xenograft and homograft.

Nursing management of the patient with valvular
    disorders
    Assessment
    Nursing diagnosis
    Planning/expected outcomes
	Critical Thinking: Describe the major nursing diagnoses, expected outcomes, and nursing interventions for the patient with valvular disease. What can the nurse do to promote cardiac output, improve gas exchange, optimize physical activities, and prevent complications?

Implementation	**Critical Thinking:** What is the medical management of the patient experiencing heart failure? What are the nursing implications of this medical management? **Critical Thinking:** Describe the surgical interventions available for patients with valvular disorders. How does postoperative nursing management of these patients differ from management of other cardiac surgery patients?
Decreased cardiac output	Ask students what nursing actions would help monitor cardiac output.
Altered cardiopulmonary, cerebral and peripheral tissue perfusion	Ask students how they would assess adequacy of peripheral tissue perfusion and what measures they could use to enhance peripheral circulation.
Impaired gas exchange Activity intolerance Anxiety Knowledge deficit Evaluation/documentation Continuity of care	Ask students how they would monitor for pulmonary congestion. **Critical Thinking:** What should the nurse include in postoperative teaching? discharge teaching?

Related Skills

1. Review and practice approaches to the patient who is anxious. Practice can be accomplished by having the students form triads, where one student plays a patient, another the nurse, and the third takes on the role of the observer. The "patient" should take on the role of a cardiac patient who is facing cardiac surgery, or who has had distressing cardiac symptoms.
2. Review and practice assessment of peripheral circulation.

Related Clinical Skills

1. Assign students to a home care nurse who is working or will be working with postoperative cardiac patients at home. Students should be alert to the types of care available to the patients, the assessments that are made of the patients and their families, and the planning and coordination necessary to bring about care of the patients.
2. Assign more senior students to buddy with nurses who are caring for postoperative cardiac patients.

CHAPTER 22

Nursing Assessment of the Hematologic System

LEARNING OBJECTIVES

1 Know the basic components of the blood and the functions of each.
2 Elicit a complete and concise history from a patient with a hematologic disorder.
3 Accurately examine a patient with a hematologic disorder in an organized manner to obtain appropriate objective data.
4 Record history and physical findings of a patient with a hematologic disorder in a concise, accurate, and logical manner.
5 Differentiate normal from abnormal history and physical findings of a patient with a hematologic disorder.
6 Describe tests related to the diagnosis and detection of disorders of the hematologic system.
7 Discuss patient preparation and care involved in administering tests that diagnose hematologic disorders.

KEY TERMS

activated partial thromboplastin time (APTT)
coagulation
coagulation factor assays
complete blood count (CBC)
erythrocyte
gastric analysis
hematocrit
leukocytes
plasma
platelets
red cell indices
Schilling test

Chapter Outline	Lecture Strategies

Anatomy and physiology
  Blood plasma
    Erythrocytes
	Critical Thinking: Compare the different types of blood cells and describe their functions.
	
	VIEWSTUDY image #118 shows the development of blood cells.

Platelets Leukocytes	**Critical Thinking:** How does the blood coagulate? What factors affect blood coagulation? **VIEWSTUDY** image #119 illustrates the coagulation mechanism.
Assessment Subjective	**Critical Thinking:** Design at least three questions to ask patients about health care habits in relation to bleeding.

Chapter Outline	Lecture Strategies

Objective
  Integumentary
  Oropharyngeal cavity
	Ask students to identify oral symptoms associated with acute myelomonocytic or monocytic leukemia. What might they see in a patient receiving warfarin therapy?

Lymphatic
  Cardiovascular
  Respiratory
	Too much pressure on palpation could possibly prevent determination of the presence of lymphadenopathy.

Abdominal
  Musculoskeletal
  Urinary
  Neurologic
	Critical Thinking: Describe an effective approach in examining a painful joint.

Diagnostic and laboratory tests
  Complete blood count
    Red blood cell count
    Hemoglobin
    Hematocrit
    Red cell indices
    White blood cell count
    Differential WBC count
	Critical Thinking: What laboratory determinations are usually considered part of the complete blood count?

Peripheral smear
  Laboratory tests for leukemias and anemias
    Bone marrow aspiration
      Patient preparation
      Procedure
	Critical Thinking: What laboratory tests are useful in the detection and diagnosis of leukemia?

Objective
  Integumentary
  Oropharyngeal cavity

  Lymphatic
  Cardiovascular
  Respiratory
  Abdominal
  Musculoskeletal
  Urinary
  Neurologic
Diagnostic and laboratory tests
  Complete blood count
    Red blood cell count
    Hemoglobin
    Hematocrit
    Red cell indices
    White blood cell count
    Differential WBC count
    Peripheral smear
  Laboratory tests for leukemias and anemias
    Bone marrow aspiration
      Patient preparation
      Procedure
      Postprocedural care
    Schilling test
      Patient preparation
      Procedure
    Gastric analysis
      Patient preparation
      Postprocedural care
  Laboratory tests for hemolytic disorders
  Laboratory tests for bleeding disorders
  Laboratory tests for gammopathies
  Erythrocyte sedimentation rate
  C-reactive protein (CRP)

Related Skills

1. Demonstrate and then have students practice assessment of the hematological system.

Related Clinical Skills

1. Assign students to patients who are undergoing bone marrow biopsy. Have students prepare the patients, accompany them during the test, and finally, carry out postprocedural care.
2. Tour a pathology laboratory and have a laboratory technician explain diagnostic tests.
3. Explain procedures for drawing blood for different laboratory tests that prevent damage to cells.

23
Nursing Management of Adults with Hematologic Disorders

LEARNING OBJECTIVES

1 Correlate the pathophysiology of patients with common hematologic disorders with their typical clinical manifestations.
2 Discuss the options for collaborative management of patients with disorders of the hematologic system.
3 Apply the nursing process to the care of patients with disorders of the hematologic system.
4 Discuss the nursing implications associated with medications used to treat hematologic disorders.
5 Develop patient education guides for patients with common disorders of the hematologic system.
6 Discuss the psychosocial implications of the symptoms associated with hematologic disorders.
7 Identify potential complications of hematologic disorders, and describe appropriate nursing assessment and intervention strategies.
8 Discuss nursing implications for continuity of care for patients with hematologic disorders.

KEY TERMS

allogeneic transplant
anemia
apheresis
autologous transplant
erythrocytopenia
erythrocytosis
hemarthrosis
hypochromic
leukemia
leukocytosis
leukopenia
macrocytic
microcytic
neutropenia
normochromic
normocytic
pernicious anemia
sickle cell anemia
thrombocytopenia
thrombocytosis
tumor lysis syndrome

Chapter Outline	Lecture Strategies
Disorders of red blood cells	Review terms. Present summarized content from Table 23-1.
Aplastic anemia	
Definition	
Etiology/epidemiology	
Pathophysiology	
Clinical manifestations	
Collaborative management	
Iron deficiency anemia	
Definition	
Etiology/epidemiology	
Pathophysiology	Question: What effect would iron deficiency have on RBCs?
Clinical manifestations	Clearly differentiate those symptoms that are general and those that are specific.

Chapter Outline	Lecture Strategies
Collaborative management	**Critical Thinking:** What patient teaching is appropriate for patients receiving iron therapy?
Anemia associated with chronic disease	
Definition	
Etiology/epidemiology	**Critical Thinking:** What components should be included in a nursing history and assessment for anemia? Why are people who have had surgery for peptic ulcer disease at risk for anemia?
Pathophysiology	
Clinical manifestations	
Collaborative management	
Hemolytic anemia	
Definition	
Etiology/epidemiology	
Pathophysiology	
Clinical manifestations/collaborative management	
Sickle cell anemia	**VIEWSTUDY** image #123 shows inheritance patterns of sickle cell disease.
Definition/etiology	
Pathophysiology	
Clinical manifestations	**VIEWSTUDY** image #124 illustrates sickle cell hemoglobin.
Collaborative management	**VIEWSTUDY** image #125 demonstrates clinical manifestations of sickle cell disease.
Blood loss anemia	
Definition	
Pathophysiology	
Clinical manifestations	
Collaborative management	
Megaloblastic anemia	
Definition/etiology	
Pathophysiology	
Clinical manifestations	
Collaborative management	
Thalassemias	
Definition/etiology	
Pathophysiology	
Clinical manifestations	
Collaborative management	
Polycythemia vera	**VIEWSTUDY** image #126 shows the differentiation between primary and secondary polycythemia.
Definition/etiology	
Pathophysiology/clinical manifestations	**VIEWSTUDY** image #127 demonstrates the sequence of events that occurs during disseminated intravascular coagulation.
Collaborative management	
Nursing management of the patient with a red blood cell disorder	
Assessment	
Nursing diagnosis	**Critical Thinking:** List two common nursing diagnoses appropriate for most patients with anemia.
Planning/expected outcomes	
Implementation	
Evaluation/documentation	
Continuity of care	**Critical Thinking:** Explain the nursing implications for continuity of care for the patient with anemia.
Disorders of white blood cells	**Critical Thinking:** List three common nursing diagnoses associated with WBC disorders.
Leukemias	Students should become familiar with the four clinical types of the disease.

Chapter Outline	Lecture Strategies
	Carefully review the terms *remission, consolidation,* and *intensification.*
	Discuss the ethical issues involved in treatment.
Acute myelogenous leukemia	
Definition	
Etiology/epidemiology	
Pathophysiology	
Clinical manifestations	
Collaborative management	
Acute lymphocytic leukemia	
Definition/etiology	
Pathophysiology	
Clinical manifestations	
Collaborative management	
Chronic myelogenous leukemia	Chronic myelogenous leukemia is unique from the other leukemias in that it may occur in three phases. Onset tends to be much more insidious than that of the acute leukemias.
Definition/etiology	
Pathophysiology	
Clinical manifestations	
Collaborative management	
Chronic lymphocytic leukemia	Ask students to describe patients who are most susceptible to chronic lymphocytic leukemia.
Definition/etiology	
Pathophysiology	
Clinical manifestations	
Collaborative management	
Neutropenia	Point out the wide range of causes of neutropenia: leukemia and lymphoma disease; cancer treatment; and certain drugs.
Definition/etiology	
Clinical manifestations	
Collaborative management	**Critical Thinking:** How does the leukemia disease process lead to problems of anemia, thrombocytopenia, and leukopenia?
Lymphomas	
Hodgkin's disease	
Definition	
Etiology/epidemiology	
Pathophysiology	Summarize the classification system.
Clinical manifestations	Summarize the stages.
Collaborative management	Summarize the MOPP protocol.
Non-Hodgkin's lymphoma	Difficult to define. Most NHLs are derived from B lymphocytes.
Definition	
Etiology/epidemiology	
Pathophysiology	
Clinical manifestations	
Collaborative management	Review the CHOP protocol.
Multiple myeloma	
Definition	
Etiology/epidemiology	
Pathophysiology	
Clinical manifestations	
Collaborative management	

Chapter Outline	Lecture Strategies
Nursing management of the patient with a white blood cell disorder Assessment Nursing diagnosis	**Critical Thinking:** What components should be included in a nursing history and assessment with a white blood cell disorder?
Planning/expected outcomes	**Critical Thinking:** What nursing strategies should be used to decrease incidence of infection in patients with white blood cell disorders?
	Critical Thinking: Why won't the leukopenic patient necessarily exhibit the classic signs and symptoms of infection?
Implementation Evaluation/documentation	**Critical Thinking:** Discuss nursing implications in the care of the patient with multiple myeloma.
Continuity of care	**Critical Thinking:** What teaching is appropriate for the patient with a white blood cell disorder?
Disorders of coagulation	
Thrombocytopenia Definition/etiology	Have students break this word down into its separate parts and attempt definition.
Pathophysiology Clinical manifestations Collaborative management	Summarize the drugs implicated in thrombocytopenia.
Thrombocytosis Definition/etiology Clinical manifestations Collaborative management	
Hemophilia Definition Etiology/epidemiology Clinical manifestations	Formerly, half of those born with hemophilia died by the age of 5 years.
Collaborative management	**Critical Thinking:** What supportive care measures could be used to improve comfort for the hemophiliac patient (and family)?
Disseminated intravascular coagulation Definition Etiology/epidemiology Pathophysiology Clinical manifestations	**TA 52** illustrates the clinical manifestations of disseminated intravascular coagulation.
	VIEWSTUDY image #122 demonstrates the sequence of events in extravascular hemolysis.
	VIEWSTUDY image #128 shows intended sites of action for therapies in disseminated intravascular coagulation.

Chapter Outline	Lecture Strategies
Collaborative management	Discuss the interpretation to be made if schistocytes are detected when a complete blood count is done. Relate this to the newer diagnostic test, D dimer.

Vitamin K deficiency
    Definition
    Etiology
    Pathophysiology
    Clinical manifestations
    Collaborative management
Nursing management of the patient with coagulation
    disorder
    Assessment
	Ask students to recall foods rich in Vitamin K.
	
	Critical Thinking: What components should be included in a nursing history and assessment with a coagulation disorder?

Nursing diagnosis Planning/expected outcomes	**Critical Thinking:** List three potential nursing diagnoses associated with coagulation disorders.
Implementation	**Critical Thinking:** List five nursing interventions included in bleeding precautions. **Critical Thinking:** What nursing strategies could be used to improve patient comfort in the presence of active bleeding?
Evaluation/documentation	**Critical Thinking:** How would you evaluate the effectiveness of the care for patients who are at risk for bleeding?
Continuity of care	**Critical Thinking:** What are measures that promote continuity of care for the patient (and family) with a coagulation disorder?
Special treatment considerations	

Transfusion therapy
    Donors and donation
    Processing
	Review the four blood groups with the students.

Administration Transfusion reactions	Discuss with students the procedure for administration of blood components in your clinical agency.

Infection risk
    Plasmapheresis
    Documentation
	Students may have concerns about the screening of blood. Address these concerns in light of precautions and risks associated with hepatitis and HIV.

Bone marrow transplant
    Definition/etiology
    Collaborative management
Nursing management of the patient with bone marrow
    transplant
	Critical Thinking: How is bone marrow obtained for transplant?
	
	Critical Thinking: Discuss nursing management of the person receiving a bone marrow transplant.
	
	Review nursing diagnoses associated with bone marrow transplantation.

Related Skills

1. Establish setups for the administration of blood components so that the students can see the setups and work with them. Have the students walk through the procedure for administration of blood components. Set up situations in which transfusion reactions have occurred, and ask students to verbalize the cause of the reaction and the associated nursing actions.
2. Review principles of hand washing and protective or reverse isolation with students. Ask students to return a satisfactory demonstration of these procedures.

Related Clinical Skills

1. Assign students to patients with disorders covered in this chapter. Assist students as necessary to carry out specific assessments and interventions related to the care of patients with hematologic disorders.
2. Assign the student to a homebound patient with sickle cell disease. Develop a teaching plan to prevent sickle cell crisis and to use nonpharmacologic interventions in the relief of pain or discomfort.

24 Nursing Assessment of the Immune System

LEARNING OBJECTIVES

1 Identify the essential components of the immune system.
2 Describe the role of antigens in differentiating "self" from "nonself" in immune responses.
3 Compare and contrast the functions of tissues and cells in the immune system.
4 Identify agents and events that can stimulate immune activity.
5 Differentiate between the nonspecific and specific immune response in terms of the purpose and cells involved.
6 Describe the phases in the nonspecific immune response.
7 Describe the role of CD4/helper T cells as coordinators of the specific immune response.
8 Identify factors that alter the function of the immune system.
9 State measures appropriate for use in assessing a patient's immune function.

KEY TERMS

antibodies
antigens
B cells
cell-mediated immunity (CMI)
cytokines
granuloma
histocompatibility antigens
immune surveillance
immunocompetence
immunoglobulin
inflammation
interferons
interleukins
lymphocytes
macrophages
memory cells
natural killer cells
neutrophils
nonspecific immune response
opsonin
phagocytosis
plasma cells
specific immune response
T cells

Chapter Outline	Lecture Strategies

The body's defenses
  Antigens
    Histocompatibility antigens
    White blood cell response to antigens
 	
  Physical barriers to infection
    Skin and mucous membranes
    Normal flora
 	
Tissues of the immune system
	Critical Thinking: What are the essential components of the immune system?
	
	TA 53 shows the mechanisms involved in inflammation.
	
	To illustrate the concepts of phagocytosis and chemotaxis, use the analogy of inspecting the new kid on the block.
	
	Critical Thinking: How do the various tissues and cells of the immune system provide protection against non-self?
	
	VIEWSTUDY image #26 shows the organs of the immune system.

Chapter Outline	Lecture Strategies
	VIEWSTUDY image #27 demonstrates cellular events involved in T-cell activation.
Bone marrow	Diagram the relationship of parent cells and WBCs as a tree.
Granulocytes	
Neutrophils	
Eosinophils	
Basophils	
Mast cells	
Monocytes/macrophages	
Lymphocytes	
Lymphoid tissue	
Thymus	
Spleen	
Lymphatic system	
Mucosal lymphoid system	
Stimulation of immune activity	**Critical Thinking:** Give examples of different agents and events that can stimulate an immune response.
	Before discussing ischemia, ask students why cells would be injured as a result of decreased stimulation.
Nonspecific immune response	**Critical Thinking:** What is the sequence of events in a nonspecific immune response?
	VIEWSTUDY image #30 demonstrates the mechanism of action of interferon.
	VIEWSTUDY image #35 shows mass production of interferon.
Purpose	Relate these signs to ones that the students may have experienced themselves.
Cardinal signs	
Vascular activity	
Vasodilation	
Increased vascular permeability	
Cellular activity	
Chemical mediators and cytokines	
Systemic effects of inflammation	Fever is a *normal* response to inflammation.
Specific immune response	**Critical Thinking:** What are the primary differences between a nonspecific and a specific immune response?
Lymphocyte activation	
T cell–mediated immunity	**VIEWSTUDY** image #28 illustrates the relationships and functions of macrophages, B lymphocytes, and T lymphocytes in an immune response.
	VIEWSTUDY image #29 demonstrates primary and secondary immune responses
CD4 T lymphocytes	Stress the terms *humoral immunity* and *cellular immunity* because these are used frequently in other discussions.
Interleukin 2	
Gamma interferon	

Chapter Outline	Lecture Strategies
CD8 lymphocytes Natural killer cells B cell–mediated/humoral immunity Immunoglobulin activity Transplant rejection	**VIEWSTUDY** image #33 shows patterns of HLA inheritance. **VIEWSTUDY** image #34 shows monoclonal antibodies.
Assessment of immune responses	Ask students to identify factors to be considered in assessing immune responses.
Factors that influence immune function 　Age 　Sex 　Nutritional status 　Stressors 　Therapeutic modalities	**Critical Thinking:** How do age and nutritional status affect the function of the immune system?

Related Skills

1. Review and practice the various methods of temperature measurement. Ask students to provide a satisfactory return demonstration of the methods commonly employed in their clinical setting.
2. Review standard patient precautions.

Related Clinical Skills

1. Assign students to patients with fevers. With the students, review all clinical, laboratory, and assessment data pertinent to the fever response and appropriate nursing management for each patient.

25 Nursing Management of Adults with Immune Disorders

LEARNING OBJECTIVES

1 Identify common causes of immunodeficient states.
2 Develop a nursing care plan for the neutropenic patient.
3 Describe common theories underlying immunologic tolerance and autoimmune disorders.
4 Identify the nursing needs of patients with systemic lupus erythematosus.
5 Differentiate among type I, type II, type III, and type IV hypersensitivity reactions.
6 State the precautions needed in providing blood products and new drugs to patients with a history of allergic reactions.
7 Explain the possible influence of social mores on the nursing care of patients infected with human immunodeficiency virus (HIV).
8 Describe the source and significance of opportunistic infections in the patient with acquired immunodeficiency syndrome (AIDS).
9 Identify available resources for individuals with HIV disease.
10 Implement the nursing process for patients with HIV or AIDS.

KEY TERMS

acquired immune deficiency syndrome (AIDS)
AIDS-related complex (ARC)
anaphylaxis
antinuclear antibodies (ANAs)
autoantibodies (AABs)
autoantigens (AAgs)
biologic response modifiers
human immunodeficiency virus (HIV)
hypersensitivity
immunomodulators
Kaposi's sarcoma
neutropenic
retroviruses
serum sickness
systemic lupus erythematosus

Chapter Outline	Lecture Strategies
Immunodeficient status 　Etiology/pathophysiology 　　Chemotherapy and radiation 　　Diseases and infections 　　Protein calorie malnutrition 　Clinical manifestations 　Collaborative management Nursing management of the immunodeficient patient 　Assessment 　Nursing diagnosis 　Planning/expected outcomes	This term is easily defined by breaking it into two parts: *immuno-* and *-deficient*.

Chapter Outline	Lecture Strategies

Implementation
    Reducing risk of infection
    Oral hygiene
    Skin care
    Nutrition
    Psychosocial needs
    Patient education
Evaluation/documentation
Continuity of care

Critical Thinking: Explain the key nursing interventions for a patient who is immunodeficient.

Autoimmune disorders
    Definition
        Tolerance of self-antigens
    Theories of autoimmunity
    Mimicry/changes in self-antigens
    Genetic susceptibility
    Sequestered antigens

Critical Thinking: How does an autoimmune disorder develop?

Systemic lupus erythematosus
    Definition
    Etiology/epidemiology
    Pathophysiology
    Clinical manifestations
    Collaborative management

Critical Thinking: What are the clinical manifestations associated with SLE?

Nursing management of the patient with systemic
    lupus erythematosus
    Assessment
        Fatigue
        Pain
        Personal appearance
    Nursing diagnosis
    Planning/expected outcomes
    Implementation
        Acute care
        Community settings
        Patient education
    Evaluation/documentation

Allergic immune reactions
    Definition
    Etiology/pathophysiology
        Type I hypersensitivity: immediate reactions
            Localized reactions

            Systemic reactions
        Type II hypersensitivity: cytotoxic reactions
        Type III hypersensitivity: immune-complex
        reactions
        Type IV hypersensitivity: cell-mediated reactions
Nursing management of the patient with allergic
    immune reactions
    Assessment
    Nursing diagnosis

Critical Thinking: Give an example of each of the four types of hypersensitivity reactions.

VIEWSTUDY image #31 depicts the steps in an allergic type I reaction.

VIEWSTUDY image #32 illustrates the clinical manifestations of systemic anaphylactic reactions.

Critical Thinking: What is the emergency management for anaphylactic response?

Chapter Outline	Lecture Strategies
Planning/expected outcomes Implementation 　Transfusion reactions 　Drug reactions 　Health-seeking behaviors Continuity of care Evaluation/documentation	**Critical Thinking:** What teaching is required for a patient with an allergic reaction?
Human immunodeficiency virus disease 　Definition 　Etiology/epidemiology	**Critical Thinking:** Compare and contrast the following stages of HIV disease: primary or acute HIV infection, asymptomatic HIV infection, mild symptomatic HIV disease, and advanced HIV disease.
Pathophysiology	**TA 54** presents the spectrum of HIV disease. Ask students to explain how retroviruses replicate. **VIEWSTUDY** image #36 shows how HIV is surrounded by an envelope of proteins. **VIEWSTUDY** image #37 shows how HIV has gp120 proteins that attach to the CD4 receptors on the surface of CD4+ lymphocytes. **VIEWSTUDY** image #38 demonstrates the viral load in the blood and CD4+ lymphocyte counts over the spectrum of HIV infection. **VIEWSTUDY** image #39 depicts the timeline for the spectrum of HIV infection.
Clinical manifestations 　Collaborative management	**Critical Thinking:** Describe the clinical manifestations of advanced HIV disease.
Specific opportunistic infections and malignancies 　　Protozoal infections 　　　*Pneumocystis carinii* pneumonia 　　　Toxoplasmosis 　　　Cryptosporidiosis 　　Fungal infections 　　　Candidiasis 　　　Cryptococcosis 　　　Histoplasmosis 　　Bacterial infections 　　　*Mycobacterium avium-intracellulare* complex 　　　*Mycobacterium tuberculosis* 　　Viral infections 　　　Herpes simplex virus 　　　Varicella-zoster virus 　　　Cytomegalovirus 　　Malignancies 　　　Kaposi's sarcoma	Point out that toxoplasmosis is one of the leading causes of encephalitis. **Critical Thinking:** Why are patients with HIV disease at risk for opportunistic infections? Because about 50% of persons with advanced HIV disease experience this infection, it is important for nurses involved with these patients to be aware of the signs and symptoms.

Chapter Outline	Lecture Strategies
Nursing management of the patient with HIV disease 　Assessment 　Nursing diagnosis 　Planning/expected outcomes 　Implementation 　Evaluation/documentation 　Continuity of care	**Critical Thinking:** Discuss the psychologic factors that might complicate your care of a patient with HIV disease. **Critical Thinking:** Describe the important patient care needs that should be addressed in a care plan for a patient with HIV disease.

Related Skills

1. In the laboratory ask students to identify and assess for opportunistic infections for a patient with AIDS.

Related Clinical Skills

1. Assign a student to a patient with AIDS. Have the student, together with the patient, identify possible community resources and sources of support for the patient.
2. Arrange for students to follow a nurse while he or she tends to a dying AIDS patient. Develop a teaching plan regarding safety and standard precautions as well as care for a dying patient.

26 Nursing Assessment of the Renal and Urinary Systems

LEARNING OBJECTIVES

1 Understand the basic structures and functions of the renal and urinary systems.
2 Elicit a complete and concise history from a patient with a renal or urinary disorder.
3 Accurately examine a patient with a renal or urinary disorder in an organized manner to obtain appropriate objective data.
4 Record history and physical findings for a patient with a renal or urinary disorder in a concise, accurate, and logical manner.
5 Differentiate normal from abnormal history and physical findings of a patient with a renal or urinary disorder.
6 Describe tests and procedures used in the diagnosis of renal and urinary disorders.
7 Describe patient preparation and care related to diagnostic tests of the renal and urinary system.

KEY TERMS

Bowman's capsule
colloid osmotic pressure
composite urine specimen
cystoscopy
distal convoluted tubule
electrolytes
glomerular filtration rate (GFR)
hematuria
loop of Henle
nephrons
proximal convoluted tubule
retrograde pyelography
renal plasma clearance
urea
ureters
urethra
urethritis
urinalysis
urodynamic studies

Chapter Outline	Lecture Strategies

Anatomy and physiology
  Renal system
    Structural description
	Diagrams of the kidneys are useful in helping students visualize their structure and function.
	
	VIEWSTUDY image #229 illustrates a longitudinal section of the kidney.
	
	VIEWSTUDY image #230 shows a nephron of the kidney.
	
	VIEWSTUDY image #231 illustrates the blood supply of the nephron.

Chapter Outline	Lecture Strategies
Functions of nephrons and collecting ducts	The transport maximum can be visualized by comparing it to the work productivity of each worker in a factory. Each worker has his individual capacity for work in an 8-hour period.
Bowman's capsule	**Critical Thinking:** What is the glomerular filtration rate and what factors influence the production of glomerular filtrate? **VIEWSTUDY** image #232 demonstrates reabsorption and secretion in the tubules.
Proximal convoluted tubule Loop of Henle Distal convoluted tubule Collecting ducts Control of renal function Homeostasis of water Homeostasis of electrolytes Homeostasis of blood acidity (pH) Other renal functions	Outline the renin-angiotensin system. **VIEWSTUDY** image #233 demonstrates the renin-angiotensin mechanism.
Changes in renal function in the older adult	Ask students to suggest changes in renal function in the older adult.
Urinary system Structural description Assessment Subjective assessment Objective assessment	**VIEWSTUDY** image #228 shows the organs of the urinary system. Specific data related to the various signs and symptoms will help in differentiating disorders of the renal system from disorders in other systems.
General assessment Integumentary system Cardiovascular system Respiratory system Abdomen Male genitalia Female genitalia Diagnostic and laboratory tests Urinalysis Urine culture Patient preparation Composite urine collections Creatinine clearance Patient preparation Use of radioisotopes for renal clearance Serum collections Diagnostic imaging Routine x-ray studies of kidneys, ureters, and bladder Excretory urogram	**Critical Thinking:** Design at least three questions to discreetly ask patients about voiding symptoms. **Critical Thinking:** Distinguish between the meaning of dull versus tympanic sounds elicited by percussion over the urinary bladder area. **Critical Thinking:** Explain the procedure for collecting composite urine specimens, as it might be explained to a patient. **Critical Thinking:** Discuss patient preparation and post-test care for intravenous pyelography, retrograde pyelography, and cystoscopy.

Chapter Outline	Lecture Strategies

Patient preparation
Renal angiography
    Patient preparation
    Postprocedure care
Renal scans
    Patient preparation
Computed tomography for evaluation of kidneys
Renal ultrasonography
Special procedures
    Cytoscopy
        Patient preparation
        Postprocedure care
    Renal biopsy
        Patient preparation
        Postprocedure care
    Urodynamic studies
	Obtain and show actual examples of imaging results.

Differentiate what takes place in each of the following procedures: cystometry, uroflowmetry, electromyography, and urethral pressure profile.

VIEWSTUDY image #234 shows a cystoscopic examination of the bladder in a man.

VIEWSTUDY image #237 shows a normal intravenous pyelogram.

Related Skills

1. Have students practice and return a satisfactory demonstration of assessment of the renal/urinary system.
2. Demonstrate the handling of materials for a urine culture and urinalysis.

Related Clinical Skills

1. Supervise students in the collection and storage of urine specimens. Ensure that they are aware of where the specimens are kept and/or taken.
2. Assign students to patients awaiting definitive diagnosis of suspected urinary tract disorders. Ask students to focus on assessment and teaching with these patients, and if possible, arrange for them to observe diagnostic imaging procedures of the renal/urinary tracts.
3. Have students develop a teaching plan to prepare a patient for a special urinary procedure.

27 Nursing Management of Adults with Renal Disorders

LEARNING OBJECTIVES

1 Apply the nursing process to the management of patients with renal disorders.
2 Discuss continuing health maintenance for patients with renal disorders.
3 Identify factors that may contribute to the development of renal disorders.
4 Compare acute and chronic renal failure.
5 Compare the etiology and clinical presentation of prerenal, intrarenal, and postrenal acute renal failure.
6 Compare the oliguric and diuretic phases of acute renal failure.
7 List effects of renal dysfunction on the major body systems.
8 Explain the uremic syndrome.
9 Differentiate among hemodialysis, peritoneal dialysis, and hemofiltration.
10 Describe nursing interventions for patients undergoing hemodialysis, peritoneal dialysis, and hemofiltration.

KEY TERMS

acute renal failure
anuria
azotemia
chronic renal failure (CRF)
dialysis
end-stage renal disease
hemodialysis
hemofiltration
hydronephrosis
nephrolithiasis
nephrotic syndrome
oliguria
uremic frost
uremic syndrome

Chapter Outline	Lecture Strategies

Renal vascular disorders
  Definition
  Etiology/epidemiology
  Pathophysiology
  Clinical manifestations
  Collaborative management
Nursing management of the patient with renal vascular disorders
  Assessment
  Nursing diagnosis
  Planning/expected outcomes
  Implementation
	Unless students have studied hypertensive diseases, review the renin-angiotensin-aldosterone system with them.
	
	Ask students to delineate appropriate areas of assessment.
	
	Critical Thinking: List at least five possible causes of prerenal disease, and develop at least two nursing interventions specific to each.

Chapter Outline	Lecture Strategies
Evaluation/documentation Continuity of care	Ask students to delineate reasons for monitoring weight.
Inflammatory, infectious, and congenital renal disorders	

Polycystic kidney disease
  Definition
  Etiology/epidemiology
  Pathophysiology
  Clinical manifestations
  Collaborative management
	VIEWSTUDY image #240 shows polycystic kidneys.

Interstitial nephritis Definition	Break term into its separate word parts and have students attempt its definition.

Etiology/epidemiology
  Pathophysiology
  Clinical manifestations
  Collaborative management
	Critical Thinking: List eight drugs that can be nephrotoxic.

Glomerulonephritis
  Definition
  Etiology/epidemiology
  Pathophysiology
  Clinical manifestations
  Collaborative management
	Ask students to speculate as to the size of the kidney in chronic disease.

Pyelonephritis
  Definition
  Etiology/epidemiology
  Pathophysiology
  Clinical manifestations
  Collaborative management
	Critical Thinking: Ask students to explain why patients with chronic renal disease may be anemic.
	
	Critical Thinking: Identify five signs or symptoms of pyelonephritis, and describe appropriate nursing interventions for each.

Nephrotic syndrome
  Definition
  Etiology/epidemiology
  Pathophysiology
  Clinical manifestations
  Collaborative management
	Ask students to discuss the basis for the primary symptoms.

Renal tuberculosis
  Definition
  Etiology/epidemiology
  Pathophysiology
  Clinical manifestations
  Collaborative management	

Renal abscess
  Definition
  Etiology/epidemiology
  Pathophysiology
  Clinical manifestations
  Collaborative management
	Ensure that students know what is meant by *septic*.

Chapter Outline	Lecture Strategies

Nursing management of the patient with inflammatory, infectious, and congenital renal disorders
  Assessment
  Nursing diagnosis
  Planning/expected outcomes
  Implementation
  Evaluation/documentation
  Continuity of care
    Rehabilitation
    Long-term care
    Home care
	Critical Thinking: Develop a patient teaching plan specific to the prevention of recurrent urinary tract infections.

Renal obstruction	

Hydronephrosis
  Etiology/epidemiology
  Pathophysiology
  Clinical manifestations
  Collaborative management
	Ask students to define *hydronephrosis* from the word parts.

Renal calculi
  Etiology/epidemiology
  Pathophysiology
  Clinical manifestations
	VIEWSTUDY image #238 illustrates location of calculi in the urinary tract.
	
	VIEWSTUDY image #239 shows an x-ray image of a staghorn calculus.

Collaborative management	**Critical Thinking:** Develop a low-purine meal plan appropriate to patients who form uric acid renal calculi.

Renal neoplasm
  Etiology/epidemiology
  Pathophysiology
  Clinical manifestations
  Collaborative management
Nursing management of the patient with renal obstruction
  Assessment
  Nursing diagnosis
  Planning/expected outcomes
  Implementation
    Postoperative care
  Evaluation/documentation
  Continuity of care
	Critical Thinking: How would you evaluate your nursing interventions for a patient with renal neoplasm?

Renal failure	**VIEWSTUDY** image #245 shows primary renal disease leading to end-stage renal failure.

Definition
  Etiology/epidemiology
Acute renal failure
  Definition
    Prerenal conditions
    Intrarenal conditions
    Postrenal conditions
  Pathophysiology
  Phases of acute renal failure
	Ask students to describe the physiologic impact of renin.

Chapter Outline	Lecture Strategies
Clinical manifestations Oliguric phase Diuretic phase Recovering phase Collaborative management Oliguric phase Diuretic phase	**Critical Thinking:** Compare and contrast the oliguric and diuretic phases of acute renal failure on at least five criteria. Break students into small groups and ask the groups to delineate the physiologic bases for specific signs and symptoms. **Critical Thinking:** Describe at least five clinical manifestations of the uremic syndrome, and develop two nursing interventions appropriate to each.
Chronic renal failure Definition/etiology Clinical manifestations	**Critical Thinking:** Discuss at least one systemic effect that chronic renal failure has on each of the following systems: cardiovascular, respiratory, genitourinary, gastrointestinal, neurologic, integumentary, and hematopoietic. **VIEWSTUDY** image #244 demonstrates clinical manifestations of chronic uremia **VIEWSTUDY** image #246 shows mechanisms of renal osteodystrophy.
Collaborative management	Ask students to describe reasons for the various interventions.
Dialysis	**VIEWSTUDY** image #247 illustrates osmosis and diffusion across a semipermeable membrane.
Hemodialysis Continuous hemofiltration	**VIEWSTUDY** image #249 demonstrates methods of vascular access for hemodialysis. **VIEWSTUDY** image #250 shows components of a hemodialysis system. It can be helpful for students if they can hear first-hand the experiences of a patient who undergoes or has undergone dialysis.
Peritoneal dialysis	**Critical Thinking:** What would be an appropriate home care plan for a patient on continuous ambulatory peritoneal dialysis? **VIEWSTUDY** image #251 demonstrates continuous arteriovenous hemofiltration. **VIEWSTUDY** image #248 shows the Tenckhoff catheter used in peritoneal dialysis. **Critical Thinking:** Compare and contrast hemodialysis and peritoneal dialysis by at least five criteria. **TA 55** shows internal arteriovenous fluids.

Chapter Outline	Lecture Strategies
Transplantation	The need for organs exceeds supply. Public education supports the need for organ donation. What are the legal issues involved in donor/recipient organ transplant?
	VIEWSTUDY image #252 demonstrates the mechanism of action of T-cytotoxic lymphocyte activation and attack of renal transplanted tissue.
	VIEWSTUDY image #253 demonstrates the surgical placement of transplanted kidney.
Nursing management of the patient with renal failure	**VIDEO** volume 12 presents nursing care of the patient with chronic renal failure, including causes and effects, multisystem assessment, dialysis, patient teaching, and home care.

Assessment
Nursing diagnosis
Planning/expected outcomes
Implementation
    Fluid intake
    Dietary intake
    Comfort/rest
    Prevention of infection and injury
    Psychologic care
    Patient teaching
    Preoperative care
    Postoperative care
	Ask students to delineate areas of assessment.
	
	Critical Thinking: What community resources are available to help family members and patients with CRF?

Evaluation/documentation
Continuity of care
    Rehabilitation
    Long-term care
    Home care	

Related Skills

1. In the laboratory setting have students set up a peritoneal dialysis.
2. Have the students debate the pros and cons of organ transplants.

Related Clinical Skills

1. Assign a student to a patient undergoing peritoneal or hemodialysis. In post-conference have the student describe the procedure and nursing care.
2. In the clinical setting, assign students to care of a patient with renal disease. Assess each student's ability to plan nursing care using a team approach, especially in relation to discharge planning, dietary needs, and long-term care.
3. Assign the students to a patient receiving continuous ambulatory peritoneal dialysis. Have students observe the patient administering his or her own treatment.

28 Nursing Management of Adults with Urinary Tract Disorders

LEARNING OBJECTIVES

1 Describe the pathophysiology, clinical manifestations, and collaborative management of the different types of incontinence.
2 Develop a nursing care plan for the incontinent patient.
3 Identify nursing interventions to promote urinary continence in the older adult.
4 State the pathophysiology and clinical manifestations associated with urinary retention.
5 Outline the nursing management required for urinary retention.
6 Discuss the common causes and management of urinary tract infections.
7 Identify the clinical manifestations of urinary tract infections in the older adult.
8 Develop a teaching plan that would help prevent a recurrence of a urinary tract infection.
9 Identify the major causes of urinary obstruction.
10 Describe the pathophysiology, clinical manifestations, and collaborative management of urinary tract trauma.
11 Describe the nursing management of the patient with bladder or urethral trauma.
12 Discuss the collaborative management of tumors of the bladder.
13 Outline the nursing management of the patient with either continent or incontinent urinary diversions.

KEY TERMS

bacteriuria
continent urinary
   diversions
cystectomy
cystitis
dysuria
functional incontinence
hematuria
ileal conduit
intermittent
   self-catheterization
overflow incontinence
reflex incontinence
suprapubic
   catheterization
stress incontinence
total incontinence
urethral catheterization
urethritis
urethrovesical reflux
urge incontinence
urinary incontinence
urinary retention
urinary tract infection
   (UTI)
urolithiasis
urosepsis

Chapter Outline	Lecture Strategies
Urinary incontinence 　Definition 　Etiology/epidemiology 　Pathophysiology 　　Acute (transient) incontinence 　　Persistent (established/chronic) incontinence	**Critical Thinking:** What are the four types of urinary incontinence? Review the classifications in Table 28-1 while discussing causes.

Chapter Outline	Lecture Strategies

Clinical manifestations
   Geriatric considerations
Collaborative management
   Surgical interventions
      Artificial urinary sphincter
      Vesicourethral suspension
      Pubovaginal sling
      Periurethral bulking injection therapy
Pharmacologic interventions
Nursing management of the patient with urinary
incontinence
Assessment
Nursing diagnosis
Planning/expected outcomes
	Have students suggest some of the most important geriatric considerations in treating incontinence.
	
	Review the classification, actions, interactions, and side effects and nursing actions of the drugs utilized in management of incontinence.

Implementation Supportive measures	**Critical Thinking:** Develop a bladder training program for an incontinent patient.
Pelvic floor exercises (Kegel)	Explain the Kegel exercises and have students practice them.

Bladder training
   Biofeedback
   Mechanical devices
	Ask students to discuss bladder retraining for the patient with urge incontinence.

Containing (incontinence) garments	Bring some of these garments to class. Bring devices to class.

Urinary drainage devices
   Psychologic support
   Patient education
Evaluation/documentation
Continuity of care
   Rehabilitation
   Long-term care
   Home care
Urinary retention
Definition
Etiology/epidemiology
Pathophysiology
Clinical manifestations
Collaborative management
	Use **TA 56** to illustrate a closed drainage system with three-way catheter.
	
	Ask the students to describe intervention for the elderly "forgetful" incontinent patient.
	
	Critical Thinking: List the clinical manifestations of acute urinary retention.

Catheterization	Ask students to differentiate the use and purpose of ureteral catheters, nephrostomy tubes, urethral catheters, and indwelling catheters with double inflatable balloons. Bring samples of each device for discussing administration. **VIEWSTUDY** image #241 illustrates different types of commonly used catheters. **VIEWSTUDY** image #242 depicts methods of urinary diversion.

Chapter Outline	Lecture Strategies
	VIEWSTUDY image #243 demonstrates creation of a Kock pouch.
Pharmacologic interventions	Review actions, interactions, side effects, and nursing actions associated with cholinergics.
Surgical interventions	
Nursing management of the patient with urinary retention	
Assessment	
Nursing diagnosis	
Planning/expected outcomes	**Critical Thinking:** What interventions should be taken to establish urinary drainage in a patient with urinary retention?
Implementation	
Evaluation/documentation	
Continuity of care	
Urinary tract infections	
Definitions	**Critical Thinking:** Describe the common causes of a UTI.
Etiology/epidemiology	
Pathophysiology	
	VIEWSTUDY image #235 illustrates sites of infectious processes in the urinary tract.
Clinical manifestations	
	Review the actions, interactions, side effects, and nursing actions associated with phenazopyridine.
Collaborative management	
Nursing management of the patient with a urinary tract infection	
Assessment	Discuss why contraceptive methods, sexual activity, and bubble baths contribute to UTIs.
Nursing diagnosis	
Planning/expected outcomes	
Implementation	
Evaluation/documentation	
Continuity of care	**Critical Thinking:** What behaviors are necessary to prevent recurrence of a UTI?
Urinary tract obstruction	
Definition	**Critical Thinking:** How do strictures and cancer of the bladder contribute to a urinary obstruction?
Etiology/epidemiology	
Pathophysiology	
Clinical manifestations	**VIEWSTUDY** image #236 demonstrates common causes of urinary tract obstruction.
Collaborative management	
Nursing management of the patient with urinary tract obstruction	
Assessment	
Nursing diagnosis	
Planning/expected outcomes	
Implementation	
Evaluation/documentation	
Bladder/urethra trauma	
Definition	
Etiology/epidemiology	Explain the sources of most bladder or urethral trauma injuries. Ask, "Why is a full bladder more susceptible to injury?"
Pathophysiology	
Clinical manifestations	
Collaborative management	
Nursing management of the patient with bladder or urethral trauma	

Chapter Outline	Lecture Strategies

Assessment
Nursing diagnosis
Planning/expected outcomes
Implementation
Evaluation/documentation
Continuity of care
Tumors of the bladder
  Definition
  Etiology/epidemiology
  Pathophysiology
  Clinical manifestations
  Collaborative management
    Chemotherapy
    Radiation therapy
    Photodynamic therapy
    Surgical management
      Urinary diversions
      Incontinent diversions
      Continent diversions
Nursing management of the patient with bladder
  cancer
  Assessment
  Nursing diagnosis
    Preoperative
    Postoperative
  Planning/expected outcomes
  Implementation
    Preoperative
    Postoperative
    After chemotherapy
    After radiation therapy
  Evaluation/documentation
  Continuity of care
	Point out that meticulous catheter care is needed with these patients.
	
	Ask, "How can these particular patients get the optimal benefits of radiation therapy?"
	
	TA 57 illustrates incontinent urinary diversions.
	
	Compare administration and use of a Kock's pouch, the Mainze reservoir, the Indiana reservoir, and the Camey procedure.
	
	Ask students to plan for care of the patient with a tumor of the bladder, including both pre- and postoperative interventions.

Related Skills

1. Discuss and demonstrate urinary catheterization. Have students practice urinary catheterization and return a satisfactory demonstration of the procedure.
2. Discuss and demonstrate care of the urinary drainage septum. Demonstrate urine sampling from a urinary drainage septum. Have students practice and demonstrate these skills.

Related Clinical Skills

1. Assign students to patients with urinary tract problems. Where possible, provide opportunity for students to catheterize patients or to work with patients on bladder training regimens.
2. Assign a student to a home health patient and develop a teaching plan to prevent urinary tract infections. Provide catheter care as needed.

Nursing Assessment of the Neurologic System

LEARNING OBJECTIVES

1 Understand the basic anatomic structure of the neurologic system.
2 Outline the manner in which information is carried to and relayed from the central nervous system.
3 Describe the difference between stereotyped and voluntary responses.
4 Obtain relevant subjective information from the patient who has a neurologic alteration.
5 Using correct technique, examine the patient to obtain appropriate objective information about the neurologic system.
6 Differentiate abnormal from normal subjective and objective findings related to the neurologic system.
7 Describe procedures and tests used in the diagnosis and detection of disorders of the neurologic system.
8 Discuss the preparation and care of patients undergoing diagnostic tests of the neurologic system.

KEY TERMS

acetylcholine
adaptation
autonomic nervous system
brain scan
brainstem
cerebellum
cerebrospinal fluid
cerebrum
computed tomography
cranial nerves
diencephalon
echoencephalography
electroencephalography
electromyography
evoked potential studies
ganglia
graphesthesia
limbic system
lumbar puncture
magnetic resonance imaging
medulla oblongata
meninges
myelography
nerve impulse
neurons
neurotransmitter
norepinephrine
receptors
reflex
resting potential
reticular activating system
spinal cord
spinal nerves
stereognosis
ventricles

Chapter Outline	Lecture Strategies

Anatomy and physiology
  Detecting changes in internal and external
  environment
	Ask students, "Which body structure contains more receptors: the brain or the skin?"
	
	Critical Thinking: Describe the path a nerve impulse takes in the following situations:
	  a. Bringing about a simple rectus femoris stretch reflex
	  b. Smelling and identifying a smoky odor
	
	VIEWSTUDY image #290 shows the structural features of neurons.

Chapter Outline	Lecture Strategies

Chapter Outline

Carrying sensory information to and motor
   information from central nervous system
   Structure of neurons
   Function of neurons

Structure and function of spinal nerves, cranial
   nerves, and nerve tracts
Planning a response to sensory stimulation
Planning and integrating involuntary, stereotyped
   responses
   Spinal cord
      Structure
      Functions
   Brainstem, cerebellum, and diencephalon
      Structure
      Functions
Planning and integrating voluntary, unpredictable
   responses
   Cerebrum
      Structure
      Functions

Language and speech
Sensory perception and interpretation

Muscle control
Emotion
Consciousness of self
Analysis and thought
Memory
Assessment
   Subjective

Lecture Strategies

VIEWSTUDY image #291 demonstrates resting membrane potential.

VIEWSTUDY image #292 depicts saltatory conduction in a myelinated nerve fiber.

VIEWSTUDY image #293 illustrates a synapse.

The efferent and afferent neurons might be envisioned as an assembly line of workers, with the afferent neurons carrying raw materials to the big industrial plant and efferent neurons carrying away finished product.

Summarize the numbers and origins of the spinal nerves and the functions of the cranial nerves.

VIEWSTUDY image #294 is a schematic cross-section of spinal cord.

VIEWSTUDY image #295 shows a basic diagram of a reflex arc.

Summarize the functions of the brain stem, cerebellum and diencephalon.

VIEWSTUDY image #296 shows the right hemisphere of the cerebrum, lateral surface.

VIEWSTUDY image #297 shows the major divisions of the central nervous system.

VIEWSTUDY image #298 shows the diencephalon (thalamus and hypothalamus).

VIEWSTUDY image #299 illustrates the limbic system.

Cut an orange in half lengthwise to illustrate the two hemispheres, the corpus callosum, and meninges.

The growth of an infant demonstrates the development of the secondary sensory areas.

Critical Thinking: Discuss potential etiologic factors to consider when a patient reports severe headache.

Chapter Outline	Lecture Strategies
Objective Cerebral function	Use the box outlining neurologic screening examination for an overview of the steps used in assessing cerebral function, cranial nerve function, cerebellar function, motor function, sensory function, and reflexes.
Cranial nerve function Cerebellar function Motor function Sensory function Reflexes	**Critical Thinking:** Design at least three pertinent questions to ask a witness to an accident regarding an unconscious patient brought into the emergency room. **Critical Thinking:** Describe an effective approach to examining the pupils of a restless, disoriented patient with brain damage. Use **TA 58** to discuss recording reflexes. Have students practice with a reflex hammer. **TA 59** shows testing for Babinski's reflex.

Diagnostic and laboratory tests
  Lumbar puncture
    Patient preparation
    Procedure
    Postprocedure care
  Queckenstedt's test
  Neuroradiologic examinations
    Skull and spinal roentgenograms
    Computed tomography
      Patient preparation
      Procedure
      Postprocedure care
    Myelography
      Patient preparation
      Procedure
      Postprocedure care
    Pneumoencephalography
    Cerebral angiography
      Patient preparation
      Postprocedure care
    Digital subtraction angiography
      Patient preparation
      Postprocedure care
    Brain scan
      Patient preparation
    Magnetic resonance imaging
      Patient preparation
    Electroencephalography
      Procedure
      Evoked potential studies
    Electromyography
      Patient preparation
      Procedure
	Critical Thinking: Differentiate between CT and a brain scan.
	
	Ask students to identify patients or situations that call for digital subtraction angiography.
	
	Critical Thinking: Explain electroencephalography as it might be explained to a patient.
	
	The appearance of a patient having an EEG may bring thoughts of Frankenstein to the minds of students or patients. Emphasize that the test is painless.

Chapter Outline	Lecture Strategies

Nerve conduction velocities
Cerebrovascular flow tests
    Oculoplethysmography and oculopneumo-
plethysmography
    Carotid phonangiography
    Ultrasound arteriography	

Related Skills

1. Demonstrate and then ask students, in pairs, to practice assessment of the neurological system.

Related Clinical Skills

1. Assign students to patients who have undiagnosed neurological problems and who are undergoing the process of diagnostic evaluation of these problems. Students can focus especially on the assessment of these patients, as well as on their psychological and educational requirements.
2. Have the student prepare a teaching plan for a patient undergoing a diagnostic neurologic test. The teaching plan should cover both pre- and postprocedure aspects.

30 Nursing Management of Adults with Common Neurologic Problems

LEARNING OBJECTIVES

1 Define the relevant terms associated with the common neurologic problems of altered level of consciousness, increased intracranial pressure, seizure, and headache.
2 Describe the etiologic factors for, pathophysiologic conditions of, clinical manifestations associated with, and collaborative management for common neurologic problems.
3 Describe the types of seizures and the types of headache.
4 Discuss the nursing management, including assessment, nursing diagnosis, planning and expected outcomes, implementation, evaluation, and documentation for common neurologic problems.
5 Discuss the continuing nursing management related to long-term care, home care, or rehabilitation for common neurologic problems.

KEY TERMS

clonic phase
coma
convulsion
decerebration
decortication
epilepsy
headache
herniation syndrome
increased intracranial pressure (ICP)
oculocephalic reflexes (doll's eyes)
seizure
status epilepticus
stupor
tonic-clonic seizures
tonic phase

Chapter Outline	Lecture Strategies

Altered levels of consciousness
   Definition
   Etiology/epidemiology
	Ask students to discuss whether a confused and rambling patient with Alzheimer's disease is "conscious."

Pathophysiology	Ask students to recall the function of the ARAS.
Clinical manifestations Level of consciousness	**Critical Thinking:** Describe the clinical features of the various levels of consciousness.
	Critical Thinking: How do breathing patterns, pupillary and motor responses, and ocular positioning and reflexes relate to levels of brain function?
	VIEWSTUDY image #303 illustrates the components of the brain.
	VIEWSTUDY image #312 shows how each area of the brain controls a particular activity.

Chapter Outline	Lecture Strategies
Pattern of breathing	Have students demonstrate patterns of breathing.
Pupillary changes	
Oculomotor responses	
Motor responses	
Collaborative management	
Emergency management	
Surgical management	
Nursing management of adults with altered level of consciousness	
Assessment	
Nursing diagnosis	Point out that patients in a coma usually experience decreased cardiac output and are at risk for altered body temperature.
Planning/expected outcomes	Ask students to draw up a preliminary nursing plan for a patient experiencing coma.
Implementation	**Critical Thinking:** How does the nurse prevent deconditioning and promote safety for the patient with an altered level of consciousness?
Evaluation/documentation	
Continuity of care	
Rehabilitation	
Long-term care	Involving the family members helps alleviate their sense of powerlessness.
Home care	
Increased intracranial pressure	**TA 60** is a schematic representation of the different causes of increased intracranial pressure.
Definition	
Etiology/epidemiology	
Pathophysiology	Ask students to envision a tightly closed pan with rising dough inside. Ask them to speculate on the fate of the dough.
	TA 61 depicts clinical correlates of compensated and uncompensated phases of intracranial hypertension.
Cerebral edema and brain swelling	Explain that brain swelling is an increase in cerebral blood volume.
Herniation syndrome	
Clinical manifestations	**Critical Thinking:** What is the progression of clinical manifestations as intracranial pressure increases?
	VIEWSTUDY image #304 shows the intracranial volume-pressure curve.
	VIEWSTUDY image #305 depicts progression of increased intracranial pressure.
	VIEWSTUDY image #307 shows decorticate and decerebrate posturing.
	VIEWSTUDY image #308 demonstrates a pupillary check for size and response.
	VIEWSTUDY image #309 shows abnormal respiratory patterns associated with coma.

Chapter Outline	Lecture Strategies
	VIEWSTUDY image #310 depicts raccoon eyes and rhinorrhea.
Collaborative management	Review the action, interactions, side effects, and nursing activities associated with mannitol.
Nursing management of the patient with increased intracranial pressure	
Assessment	
Nursing diagnosis	**Critical Thinking:** Relate the compensatory mechanisms for increased intracranial pressure to the therapeutic interventions used to decrease intracranial pressure.
Planning/expected outcomes	
Implementation	**Critical Thinking:** Describe the nursing interventions to reduce intracranial pressure.
	Ask students to explain <it>why<eit> the nurse should dim the lights and prevent any isometric activity, including posturing or pushing against a footboard.
	Students should be able to identify risk factors associated with ICP monitor-related infections.
Evaluation/documentation	
Continuity of care	
Rehabilitation	
Long-term care	
Home care	Ask students to envision themselves taking home a loved one with unresolved intracranial pressure. Ask them to prepare lists as to what they'd like to know and to compare these lists.
Seizures	
Definition	
Etiology/epidemiology	
Causes	
Classification	
Pathophysiology	
Tonic phase	
Clonic phase	
Metabolic changes	
Status epilepticus	**Critical Thinking:** Why is status epilepticus a medical emergency?
Clinical manifestations	**Critical Thinking:** Compare the clinical manifestations of generalized seizures and partial seizures.
	Auras can serve a protective function in that they can afford an individual the opportunity to seek a more protected environment.
Collaborative management	Have students review the anticonvulsants with regard to interactions and nursing activities that are associated with the drugs.
Nursing management of the patient with seizures	
Assessment	
Nursing diagnosis	
Planning/expected outcomes	
Implementation	
Seizure care	

Chapter Outline	Lecture Strategies
Status epilepticus Seizure precautions Patient and family education	**Critical Thinking:** What is included in a teaching plan for a patient with seizures?

Evaluation/documentation
Continuity of care
    Long-term care
    Home care
    Rehabilitation
	Ask students to differentiate between short-term and long-term outcome criteria.

Seizures in elders
Headache
    Definition
    Etiology/epidemiology
        Migraine
        Tension headache
        Cluster headache
        Other types of headaches
    Pathophysiology
    Clinical manifestations
    Collaborative management
	Use Table 30-8 in examining the classifications or types of headaches.
	
	Critical Thinking: How do etiologic mechanisms that produce headaches relate to the collaborative management strategies prescribed?

Nursing management of the patient with headaches
    Assessment
    Nursing diagnosis
    Planning/expected outcomes
    Implementation
    Evaluation/documentation
    Continuity of care
        Long-term care
        Home care
        Rehabilitation
Headache in elders
	Critical Thinking: What is included in the nursing assessment of a patient with a headache?
	
	Together, outline criteria used to evaluate evidence of pain control.

Related Skills

1. Demonstrate and then ask students to practice pupil examinations.

Related Clinical Skills

1. Assign students to patients with seizure activity or mild intracranial pressure.
2. Assign students to a patient in a coma. Arrange for them to use the Glasgow neurologic assessment tool as a part of their assessment.
3. Have students develop a teaching plan for a patient with a migraine headache.

31 Nursing Management of Adults with Degenerative Disorders

LEARNING OBJECTIVES

1 Identify the physiologic and psychosocial principles underlying the medical and nursing regimens for the patient with a degenerative neurologic disorder.

2 Intervene effectively to support positive coping mechanisms used by the patient and family.

3 Provide patient and family education on diet, exercise, medications, and complications associated with degenerative diseases.

4 Support the patient's need for independence and safety.

5 Implement the nursing process for a patient and family with a degenerative neurologic disorder.

6 Identify changes in nursing interventions that occur as the patient moves from the initial to late stages of a degenerative disease.

7 Provide information about local and national resources for patients and families.

KEY TERMS

agnosia
Alzheimer's disease
amyotrophic lateral sclerosis (ALS)
apraxia
bradykinesia
chorea
dementia
dyskinesia
Huntington's disease
Parkinson's disease
rigidity

Chapter Outline	Lecture Strategies
Degenerative disorders of the cerebrum	

Alzheimer's disease
    Definition
    Etiology/epidemiology
    Pathophysiology
	Students may have heard of concerns related to the use of aluminum cookware and the incidence of Alzheimer's disease.

Clinical manifestations Collaborative management	Ask students to imagine that they are expressing the early stages of Alzheimer's disease and to describe their feelings related to the experience. Discuss how these feelings relate to the experience. Discuss how these feelings might affect care of the patient with the disease.

Nursing management of the patient with Alzheimer's
    disease
    Assessment
    Nursing diagnosis	

Chapter Outline	Lecture Strategies
Planning/expected outcomes Implementation Evaluation/documentation Continuity of care	**Critical Thinking:** Identify interventions aimed at preventing common complications, including contractures, thrombophlebitis, atelectasis, decubitus ulcers, and constipation.
Home care	**Critical Thinking:** Construct guidelines for home care after hospitalization, including diet, activities of daily living, exercise, and medications for patients and families coping with each of the degenerative diseases.
Degenerative diseases of the basal ganglia	
Parkinson's disease 　Definition 　Etiology/epidemiology	**VIEWSTUDY** image #318 shows the characteristic appearance of a patient with Parkinson's disease.
Pathophysiology	**VIEWSTUDY** image #319 demonstrates pathogenesis of amyotrophic lateral sclerosis.
Clinical manifestations	**TA 62** illustrates stages of parkinsonism.
Collaborative management 　　Protective drug therapy 　　Symptomatic drug therapy 　　Supportive care Nursing management of the patient with Parkinson's 　disease 　Assessment 　Nursing diagnosis 　Planning/expected outcomes	The use of brain cells from anencephalic infants for transplantation has been intensely debated because of ethical considerations.
Implementation 　Evaluation/documentation 　Continuity of care	Ask students to practice the communication techniques, such as diaphragmatic breathing, that a patient with parkinsonism might find useful.
Huntington's disease 　Definition 　Etiology/epidemiology 　Pathophysiology 　Clinical manifestations 　Collaborative management	**Critical Thinking:** State guidelines for determining the need for genetic counseling for patients and families coping with a degenerative disorder.
Nursing management of the patient with Huntington's 　disease *Degenerative disorders of the spinal cord*	**Critical Thinking:** Describe circumstances under which the patient should be permitted independence and those under which the nurse should intervene to maintain patient safety.
Amyotrophic lateral sclerosis 　Definition 　Etiology/epidemiology 　Pathophysiology 　Clinical manifestations 　Collaborative management Nursing management of the patient with amyotrophic 　lateral sclerosis 　Assessment	**Critical Thinking:** List three nursing assessments essential to the care of the patient with degenerative diseases.

Chapter Outline	Lecture Strategies
Nursing diagnosis Planning/expected outcomes	**Critical Thinking:** List four nursing diagnoses common to all patients with degenerative neurologic diseases.
Implementation Evaluation/documentation Continuity of care	**Critical Thinking:** Describe the characteristics of successful patient and family adjustment to degenerative neurologic disease.

Related Clinical Skills

1. Assign students to patients with diseases that were discussed in the chapter. Provide support and close supervision of students who are feeding patients with swallowing difficulties, since this can be frightening, especially for beginning students.
2. Arrange for students to accompany home care nurses on visits to patients with degenerative disorders. Ask students to direct their attention to how the patient performs self care and functions at home.
3. Assign students to a nursing home that has patients with Alzheimer's disease. Develop a care plan to meet the patients' needs.

32 Nursing Management of Adults with Infectious, Inflammatory, or Autoimmune Disorders

LEARNING OBJECTIVES

1 Apply principles of nursing management to the care of the patient with infectious and autoimmune disorders of the nervous system.
2 Describe the medical and nursing treatment for the patient with infectious and autoimmune disorders of the nervous system and the physiologic principles underlying these treatment modalities.
3 Identify the common complications of infectious and autoimmune disorders of the nervous system.
4 Evaluate the needs of the patient's family for information, emotional support, and planning/ expected outcomes.
5 Evaluate the home care needs of patients with chronic nervous system disease.

KEY TERMS

brain abscess
bulbar weakness
encephalitis
epidural abscess
Guillain-Barré syndrome (GBS)
meningitis
multiple sclerosis (MS)
myasthenia gravis (MG)
nuchal rigidity
optic neuritis
parameningeal infections
subdural empyema
thymectomy

Chapter Outline	Lecture Strategies
Infectious and inflammatory diseases	
Meningitis	Break the word *meningitis* down into its parts and ask students to work through its definition in this way.
Definition	
Etiology/epidemiology	
Pathophysiology	Ask students to speculate on the reason for headache, nuchal rigidity, fever, and altered levels of consciousness.
Complications	
Clinical manifestations	
Collaborative management	
	Review the classifications, actions, side effects, interactions, and nursing activities associated with commonly used antimicrobials.
Drug therapy	
	Critical Thinking: Name the chemoprophylactic drugs and vaccines available to prevent common forms of meningitis.
Symptomatic and preventive care	
Nursing management of the patient with meningitis	**Critical Thinking:** List the assessment priorities for the acutely ill patient with an infection of the nervous system.
Assessment	
Nursing diagnosis	

Chapter Outline	Lecture Strategies
Planning/expected outcomes	**VIEWSTUDY** image #300 demonstrates cerebrospinal fluid circulation.
Implementation	Ask students to describe nursing interventions appropriate to preventing complications and maintaining comfort.
Preventing complications	
Maintaining comfort	
Drug therapy	
Evaluation/documentation	
Continuity of care	
Parameningeal infections	
Definition	
Etiology/epidemiology	
Pathophysiology	
Complications	
Clinical manifestations	
Collaborative management	
Nursing management of the patient with parameningeal infections	
Assessment	
Implementation	
Encephalitis	
Definition	
Etiology/epidemiology	
Pathophysiology	
Clinical manifestations	
Collaborative management	**Critical Thinking:** State how therapeutic regimen priorities differ for meningitis, parameningeal infections, and encephalitis.
Nursing management of the patient with encephalitis	
Assessment	
Nursing diagnosis	Review the side effects, interactions, and nursing activities associated with vidarabine and acyclovir.
Implementation	
Other infectious diseases	
Autoimmune disorders	
Multiple sclerosis	
Definition	
Etiology/epidemiology	Ask a representative from the Multiple Sclerosis Society to discuss the disease, current research impact on the disease, and services of the society.
Pathophysiology	
Clinical manifestations	
Collaborative management	
Drug therapy	
Symptomatic management	
Nursing management of the patient with multiple sclerosis	
Assessment	
Nursing diagnosis	
Planning/expected outcomes	Involvement of the family is critical since the onset of disease commonly occurs during peak child-bearing years and during the peak of career development and progress.
Implementation	
Evaluation/documentation	

Chapter Outline	Lecture Strategies
Continuity of care	**Critical Thinking:** Discuss ways in which the nurse can involve the family in the care of the patient with an infectious or autoimmune disease of the nervous system.
Guillain-Barré syndrome	
Definition/etiology	
Pathophysiology	
Clinical manifestations	Ask students to visualize themselves as rapidly becoming flaccid and unable to move.
Collaborative management	
Nursing management of the patient with Guillain-Barré syndrome	**Critical Thinking:** Describe the common techniques used to assess pulmonary status in the patient with Guillain-Barré syndrome or myasthenia gravis.
Myasthenia gravis	
Definition/etiology	
Pathophysiology	
Clinical manifestations	**Critical Thinking:** State interventions aimed at preventing common complications of Guillain-Barré syndrome.
Collaborative management	**TA 63** shows anticholinesterase drugs in myasthenia gravis.
Drug therapy	**Critical Thinking:** List the purpose and side effects of immunosuppressive drugs used to treat autoimmune disorders.
Surgical therapy	
Plasma exchange	
Crisis management	
Nursing management of the patient with myasthenia gravis	
Assessment	
Nursing diagnosis	
Planning/expected outcomes	
Implementation	Ask students what area of preoperative and postoperative care would be of most concern with these patients.
Crisis management	
Drug therapy	
Thymectomy	
Plasma exchange	
Evaluation/documentation	
Continuity of care	**Critical Thinking:** Construct a care plan for home care following discharge of a patient with a chronic autoimmune or infectious disease of the nervous system.

Related Skills

1. Review and demonstrate tests for meningeal irritation. Ask students to practice the tests and return a satisfactory demonstration of these assessments.
2. Set up a Hickman central line on a mannequin and demonstrate its care.
3. Review care of IV sites and lines. Require students to practice and then demonstrate the changing of an IV dressing, line, and solution.

Related Clinical Skills

1. Assign students to patients with infectious or autoimmune neurological disorders. Ask students to focus on patient teaching, psychosocial support, and involvement of families as well as on other aspects of care.
2. Assign students to a home care nurse and develop a teaching plan for a patient with multiple sclerosis.

33 Nursing Management of Adults with Cerebrovascular Disorders

---

LEARNING OBJECTIVES

1 Describe the incidence and social impact of cerebrovascular disorders.
2 Identify the major risk factors for developing cerebrovascular disorders.
3 Differentiate the pathophysiology and clinical manifestations of transient ischemic attack, completed stroke, and subarachnoid hemorrhage.
4 Differentiate the signs and symptoms of persons with right and left hemispheric stroke.
5 Discuss major medications and surgical procedures that may be used to treat cerebrovascular disorders.
6 Relate principles of nursing management to the care of a patient in the acute stage of stroke.
7 Relate principles of nursing management to the care of the stroke patient in the rehabilitative stage.
8 Differentiate the traditional and neurodevelopmental (Bobath) approaches in the care and retraining of stroke patients.
9 Identify essential elements for family teaching and preparation for home care of the stroke patient.
10 Identify long-term needs in the rehabilitation of the elderly stroke patient.

KEY TERMS

aneurysm
anosognosia
aphasia
apraxia
arteriovenous malformation (AVM)
Bobath technique
lacunar brain infarction
nonprogressing stroke
progressing stroke
reversible ischemic neurologic deficit (RIND)
stroke
subarachnoid hemorrhage (SAH)
transient ischemic attack (TIA)

Chapter Outline	Lecture Strategies
Cerebrovascular disorders Definition	**TA 64** outlines impairments with cerebrovascular accidents. **Critical Thinking:** Discuss the major causes of stroke, using Table 33-1 to relate these causes to categorization.
Etiology/epidemiology Pathophysiology	**VIEWSTUDY** image #301 shows the arteries at the base of the brain. **VIEWSTUDY** image #313 demonstrates the circle of Willis and vertebrobasilar circulation.

Chapter Outline	Lecture Strategies
Ischemic cerebrovascular accident	Ask, "What is lacunar brain infarction?"

Hemorrhagic cerebrovascular accident
    Intracerebral hemorrhage
    Subarachnoid hemorrhage
	Identify signs of increased intracranial pressure.
	
	Critical Thinking: What are the three major complications that threaten the recovery of the patient with SAH?

Clinical manifestations
    Transient ischemic attack
    Reversible ischemic neurologic deficit
    Stroke in evolution
    Completed stroke
	Distinguish among the three classifications of CVAs.
	
	Critical Thinking: During what period after SAH is vasospasm most likely to occur?
	
	Ensure that students are comfortable with terms such as *ipsilateral, contralateral, apraxia, hemianopsia,* and other neurologic terms.

Right and left cerebrovascular accident	Can students define the term *anosognosia*?
Aphasia	Invite a speech therapist to class to discuss the types of aphasia and approaches to treatment.
Visual changes Arterial occlusion	Use Table 33-3 to correspond the major cerebral arteries to related signs and symptoms of occlusion.
Cerebral aneurysms Diagnosis of cerebrovascular accident	Table 33-4 outlines the clinical grading of aneurysms.
Collaborative management Drug therapy	**Critical Thinking:** Why is close monitoring of the patient with SAH so important when antihypertensive agents are used?
Surgical management	**Critical Thinking:** Discuss the role of surgery in treatment of SAH, discussing both types and timing. **VIEWSTUDY** image #360 demonstrates effects of independent changes in arterial blood pressure, oxygen, or carbon dioxide on cerebral blood flow. Ask students to define embolectomy or thrombectomy.
Nursing management of the patient with acute cerebrovascular disorders Assessment	**VIDEO** volume 8 presents nursing care of the patient with an acute cerebrovascular disorder, including assessment and rehabilitation.
Nursing diagnosis	**Critical Thinking:** What are four priority nursing diagnoses essential during the acute stage of care of the stroke patient?

Chapter Outline	Lecture Strategies
Planning/expected outcomes	**Critical Thinking:** Develop a standard nursing care plan for an adult patient with a completed stroke with severe residual effects after either a right or left CVA.
Implementation Airway clearance	**VIEWSTUDY** image #315 illustrates manifestations of right-sided and left- sided stroke.

Cerebral perfusion
  Altered physical mobility
  Fluid balance
  Ineffective coping
  Risk for injury
  Impaired verbal communication
  Knowledge deficit
Evaluation/documentation
	Ask students to describe nursing activities that would prevent alterations in cerebral blood flow.

Continuity of care	**Critical Thinking:** Discuss the major teaching required by the family in preparation for the transition to the home.
Bobath techniques	**Critical Thinking:** Differentiate the traditional and Bobath approaches in the care and retraining of stroke patients.
	Demonstrate the typical gait of a stroke patient. Demonstrate a transfer using the traditional and Bobath methods.

Self-care
  Urinary elimination
  Bowel elimination
  Cognitive function
  Sensory-perceptual function
  Impaired swallowing
  Activity intolerance
  Coping
  Discharge planning
	Bring aids for self-care to class.
	
	Critical Thinking: How would you respond to a person saying that the older patient who has had a stroke should not participate in a comprehensive rehabilitation program because it would not be cost effective?

Related Skills

1. Arrange for students to visit an occupational therapy department to gain a first-hand look at therapies and assistive devices for stroke patients.
2. Have students practice the roles of stroke patient and caregiver, working in pairs. Direct students in the patient role to "try on" neurological dysfunctions such as anosognosia, hemiparesis, and expressive aphasia. At the conclusion of the exercise, discuss feelings and experiences related to the roles.

Related Clinical Skills

1. Assign students to patients with strokes, either in the acute or rehabilitative phases. Encourage students to discuss care of the patients with other members of the multidisciplinary team.
2. Assign a student to a patient in the home care setting. Develop a teaching plan designed to help the patient and family cope with the patient's disabilities as well as safety measures in the home.

Nursing Management of Adults with Intracranial Disorders

LEARNING OBJECTIVES

1 Differentiate among mild, moderate, and severe head injury.
2 Describe the potential complications after a head injury, including cerebral edema, intracranial bleeding, syndrome of inappropriate secretion of antidiuretic hormone, diabetes insipidus, convulsive disorders, carotid-cavernous fistula, meningitis, and hyperthermia/hypothermia.
3 Discuss the techniques needed to assess level of consciousness in the head-injured patient.
4 Implement a plan of care for the head-injured patient and family.
5 Discuss the necessary components of the discharge plan for the head- injured patient.
6 Identify symptoms associated with the specific location of a brain tumor.
7 Describe the nursing care for a patient after a craniotomy.
8 Describe the nursing care required when the patient is undergoing radiation therapy or chemotherapy for the treatment of a brain tumor.

KEY TERMS

acceleration-deceleration injuries
burr holes
cerebral edema
closed injuries
concussion
contusion
coup/contrecoup injury
craniectomy
cranioplasty
craniotomy
epidural hematoma
intracerebral hematoma
open injuries
rotation injuries
skull fracture
stereotaxic surgery
subdural hematomas

Chapter Outline	Lecture Strategies
Head injury	
Definition	
Etiology	
Classifications	Summarize classifications.
Pathophysiology	Use your hands to illustrate the injuries.
Mechanisms of injury	
Skull fractures	**TA 65** illustrates types of hematomas
Primary and secondary injuries	As children, some of the students may have experienced concussion.
Progression of tissue injury	
Potential complications	
Cerebral edema	

Chapter Outline	Lecture Strategies
Syndrome of inappropriate secretion of antidiuretic hormone and diabetes insipidus	**Critical Thinking:** What symptoms help the nurse in differentiating between diabetes insipidus and syndrome of inappropriate secretion of ADH?
	Ask students to list functions of the hypothalamus.
	Summarize the causes of DI and SIADH and the clinical manifestations.
Stress ulcers Convulsive disorders Carotid-cavernous fistula Meningitis Hyperthermia/hypothermia Clinical manifestations Collaborative management Medical treatment Surgical treatment Drug therapy Nutritional therapy Investigational therapies Nursing management of the patient with a head injury	Use a diagram to illustrate the location and nature of the fistula. Review actions, interactions, side effects, and nursing activities associated with key drugs listed here. **Critical Thinking:** What are the nursing priorities in the care of the patient with a severe head injury? **VIEWSTUDY** image #311 shows an epidural hematoma in the temporal fossa. **VIEWSTUDY** image #359 shows an intracranial volume-pressure curve.
Assessment Nursing diagnoses Planning/expected outcomes Implementation Vital signs and neurologic signs Respiratory control Intracranial pressure Cardiovascular functioning Intake and output Pain and restlessness Seizure activity Infection Family interaction Evaluation/documentation Continuity of care	**Critical Thinking:** How would you interpret a patient's Glasgow Coma Scale score of 7? Ask students to speculate as to the cause of cardiac dysrhythmias in patients with head injuries. Current research suggests that the family of a head-injured patient experiences stress, regardless of the degree of injury. Ask students to recall some of the physical manifestations of this stress.
Rehabilitation	Ask students to consider when they think rehabilitation should begin and why it should begin at the stage they specify.
Discharge planning	**Critical Thinking:** What information should be available to the family before the patient is discharged?

Chapter Outline	Lecture Strategies

Long-term care
Home care
Brain tumors
  Definition
  Etiology
  Headache
  Pathophysiology
  Clinical manifestations
    Headache
    Vomiting
    Level of consciousness
    Motor and sensory losses
    Seizures
    Autonomic and vasomotor changes
    Visual changes
  Collaborative management
    Surgical intervention
 	
    Craniotomy
 	
    Radiosurgery
    Transsphenoidal surgery
  Drug therapy
    Chemotherapy
      Methods of administration
    Radiation therapy
    Interstitial brachytherapy
    Volumetric interstitial hyperthermia
    Dietary therapy
    Other therapy
Nursing management of the patient with a brain
  tumor
  Assessment
  Nursing diagnosis
  Planning/expected outcomes
  Implementation
    Vital signs
    Seizure activity
    Preoperative nursing care
    Intraoperative care
    Postoperative care
    Support during chemotherapy or radiation
      therapy
  Evaluation/documentation
  Continuity of care
    Rehabilitation
    Long-term care
    Home care
	If possible, invite a member of the National Head Injury Foundation to discuss support groups for long-term care patients and their families.
	
	Critical Thinking: What symptoms would be expected from a frontal lobe tumor? parietal lobe? temporal lobe? occipital lobe?
	
	Critical Thinking: Which diagnostic study is most specific for tumors?
	
	Use diagrams to illustrate supratentorial, infratentorial, and stereotaxic approaches.
	
	Critical Thinking: What are the major concerns of a patient who is to undergo a craniotomy?
	
	Discuss the two types of radiosurgical techniques.
	
	Ask a specialist to discuss interstitial brachytherapy and volumetric interstitial hyperthermia.
	
	Critical Thinking: What specific nursing interventions are appropriate for the patient following a supratentorial procedure?

Related Skills

1. Discuss and role-play supportive and educative interventions that are appropriate for a family with a member who is experiencing a life-threatening crisis. A nurse clinician or a family therapist, especially skilled in family intervention, may be invited to assist with this discussion.
2. Review seizure precautions.

Related Clinical Skills

1. Assign students to patients with mild head injuries or to those recovering from head injuries or brain tumors. Ask students to follow their patients through various therapies. Involve the students in discharge planning, when possible.
2. Assign students to a hospice nurse who is caring for a patient with a brain tumor. Have the students develop a care plan focusing on signs and symptoms of the disease process as well as pain management techniques.

35

Nursing Management of Adults with Spinal Cord Disorders

LEARNING OBJECTIVES

1 Identify the areas of the spinal cord that are most prone to trauma and explain why.
2 Describe the four major mechanisms of spinal cord trauma.
3 Define the classifications of spinal cord injury and the associated manifestations.
4 Discuss the syndromes of spinal shock and autonomic dysreflexia, and identify the medical and nursing interventions related to these syndromes.
5 Identify five nursing diagnoses associated with spinal cord injury.
6 Identify the major complications of spinal cord injury.
7 List the goals of rehabilitation for the patient with paraplegia and the patient with quadriplegia.
8 Describe the types and clinical manifestations of spinal cord tumors.
9 Describe the various types of medical interventions for spinal cord tumor.
10 Discuss the cause of intervertebral disk disease and the current treatment modalities, including preoperative and postoperative care.
11 Develop a care plan for the patient with a spinal cord disorder related to trauma, tumor, or intervertebral disk disease.

KEY TERMS

anterior cord syndrome
autonomic dysreflexia
Brown-Séquard's syndrome
cauda equina lesion
central cord syndrome
extradural tumors
extramedullary tumors
heterotropic ossification
hyperesthesia
intervertebral disk disease
intradural tumors
intramedullary tumors
neurogenic shock
paraplegia
quadriplegia
spinal shock
Stryker frame

Chapter Outline	Lecture Strategies
Spinal cord injury Definition	Differentiate among Brown-Séquard's syndrome, anterior cord syndrome, central cord syndrome, and a cauda equina lesion. **VIEWSTUDY** image #324 illustrates three syndromes associated with incomplete cord lesions.
Etiology/epidemiology	The "typical" patient is particularly devastated by spinal cord injury because of the loss of an active lifestyle and the disruption of career and education.

Chapter Outline	Lecture Strategies
	Critical Thinking: Describe the "typical victim" of spinal cord injury.
	VIEWSTUDY image #322 illustrates the mechanisms of spinal injury.

Pathophysiology
Clinical manifestations
Collaborative management
   Prehospital and emergency management
   Immobilization
	Critical Thinking: What is the cause of complete spinal cord dissolution in severe trauma?

	Explain the use of the Stryker frame, demonstrating with the actual device, if possible.
	VIEWSTUDY image #326 shows a kinetic therapy treatment table (Rotorest bed).
	TA 66 illustrates a Halo vest.
	Bring a halo traction vest to class during discussion of its application and care
	VIEWSTUDY image #325 shows Vinke tongs for cervical immobilization..

Pharmacologic therapy
   Complications
Nursing management of the patient with spinal cord
   injury: Acute phase
	Ask students to present a nursing care plan for the patient taking methylprednisolone.

	TA 67 offers a critical thinking guide for the patient with autonomic dysreflexia.
Assessment Nursing diagnosis	The patient's emotional and psychological responses to alterations in function are also important.
	Use the box on motor score grades to discuss assessment of voluntary motor movement.
Planning/expected outcomes	Ask students to identify specific outcome criteria for the acute phase plan of care.

Implementation
   Evaluation/documentation
   Documentation
   Continuity of care
      Rehabilitation
      Long-term care
Nursing management of the patient with spinal cord
   injury: Rehabilitation phase
	Discuss nutrition considerations for the patient with a spinal cord injury. patient.

	VIDEO volume 11 presents nursing care of the patient with spinal injury, including bowel and bladder management, skin care, and rehabilitation.
	Ask, "What is heterotropic ossification?"
Assessment Nursing diagnosis	**Critical Thinking:** What is the major nursing responsibility related to prevention of low back pain?
Planning/expected outcomes	How does the specific outcome criteria for the rehabilitation phase differ from the acute phase?

Chapter Outline	Lecture Strategies
Implementation	**Critical Thinking:** Name three physiologic complications of spinal cord injury, and identify nursing measures aimed at their prevention.
	VIEWSTUDY image #323 demonstrates that symptoms, degree of paralysis, and potential for rehabilitation depend on the level of the lesion.
	Refer students to the box on care of the patient in a halo brace for this discussion.
	Critical Thinking: Describe the nursing interventions for the patient exhibiting symptoms of autonomic dysreflexia.
Spinal cord tumors	**Critical Thinking:** How does the growth rate of spinal cord tumors affect the development of related symptoms?
Definition/etiology	
Clinical manifestations	
Collaborative management	
Nursing management of the patient with spinal cord tumors	**VIEWSTUDY** image #327 depicts types of spinal cord tumors.
Assessment	
Nursing diagnosis	
Planning/expected outcomes	
Implementation	
Evaluation/documentation	
Continuity of care	
Rehabilitation	
Home care	
Intervertebral disk disease	**VIEWSTUDY** image #348 shows compression of the spinal cord caused by herniation of a nucleus pulposus into the spinal cord.
Definition	
Etiology/epidemiology	
Pathophysiology	
Clinical manifestations	
Collaborative management	Review the actions, side effects, interactions, and nursing activities associated with NSAIDs.
Nursing management of the patient with intervertebral disk disease	
Assessment	
Nursing diagnosis	
Planning/expected outcomes	
Implementation	**Critical Thinking:** What is the importance of a postoperative exercise program for the patient with disk disease?
Continuity of care	
Rehabilitation	
Home care	

Related Skills

1. Demonstrate and require students to practice placing a patient with a potential spinal cord injury in a neutral position. Demonstrate and instruct students to practice the jaw-thrust maneuver.
2. Require students to practice and return a satisfactory demonstration of assessment of motor and sensory functioning.

Related Clinical Skills

1. Assign students to patients who are recovering from a spinal cord injury or back surgery. Where possible, have students accompany their patients to physiotherapy and occupational therapy to gain a more comprehensive view of the interdisciplinary team approach.

36

Nursing Management of Adults with Peripheral or Cranial Nerve Disorders

LEARNING OBJECTIVES

1 Define the three types of degenerative processes seen in peripheral nerve disease.
2 Describe the six common signs of peripheral nerve disease.
3 Outline the nursing management for patients with trauma of the peripheral nerves.
4 Describe the pathophysiology and clinical manifestations of nutritional polyneuropathies.
5 Discuss the nursing management for patients with nutritional polyneuropathies.
6 Describe the symptoms of neuropathy caused by toxins.
7 Identify the components of a nursing assessment for a patient with toxic neuropathy.
8 Describe the clinical manifestations of Charcot-Marie-Tooth disease.
9 Compare the pathophysiology and clinical manifestations of trigeminal neuralgia and facial nerve paralysis.
10 Discuss the collaborative management for patients with cranial nerve disorders.

KEY TERMS

anhidrosis
axonal degeneration
Bell's palsy
carpal tunnel syndrome
Charcot-Marie-Tooth disease
microvascular decompression
nutritional deficiency neuropathy
percutaneous chemoneurolysis with glycerol
percutaneous radiofrequency thermal lesioning
Phalen's sign
polyneuropathy
segmental demyelination
tarsal tunnel syndrome
Tinel's sign
trigeminal neuralgia
wallerian degeneration

Chapter Outline	Lecture Strategies
Peripheral nerve disorders	Ask students to recall their concepts of the peripheral nervous system.
Pathophysiology	**Critical Thinking:** What are the three pathophysiologic processes that occur in peripheral nerve disease?
Clinical manifestations	**Critical Thinking:** Jane Smith is assessed for peripheral nerve disease and is found to have reflex changes, anhidrosis, and sensory impairment. What other three signs of peripheral nerve disease should be included in the assessment?

<table>
<tr><td>

Chapter Outline

Median nerve injury
  Definition
  Etiology

  Pathophysiology
  Clinical manifestations
  Collaborative management
    Conservative management
    Surgical management

Ulnar nerve injury
  Definition
  Etiology/pathophysiology
  Clinical manifestations
Radial nerve injury
  Definition
  Etiology/pathophysiology
  Clinical manifestations
Femoral nerve injury
  Definition
  Etiology/pathophysiology
  Clinical manifestations
Sciatic nerve injury
  Definition
  Etiology/pathophysiology
  Clinical manifestations
Common peroneal nerve injury
  Definition
  Etiology/pathophysiology
  Clinical manifestations
Tarsal tunnel syndrome
  Definition/pathophysiology
  Collaborative management of peripheral nerve
  injury
Nursing management of the patient with peripheral
  nerve disorder
  Assessment
  Nursing diagnosis

  Planning/expected outcomes
  Implementation
  Evaluation/documentation
  Continuity of care
Nutritional deficiency neuropathy
  Definition/etiology
  Pathophysiology/clinical manifestations
  Collaborative management

</td><td>

Lecture Strategies

Use **TA 68** to help students understand the nature of carpal tunnel syndrome.

VIEWSTUDY image #334 illustrates the wrist structures involved in carpal tunnel syndrome.

Critical Thinking: Audrey Jones is diagnosed with ulnar nerve injury. Name two appropriate nursing diagnoses.

Critical Thinking: Explain the reason for proper intramuscular technique to prevent peripheral nerve disease.

Ask students to name foods rich in B vitamins.

</td></tr>
</table>

Chapter Outline	Lecture Strategies

Toxic neuropathy
    Definition/etiology
    Pathophysiology/clinical manifestations
    Collaborative management
Nursing management of the patient with toxic
    neuropathy
    Assessment
    Nursing diagnosis
    Planning/expected outcomes
    Evaluation/documentation
    Continuity of care
Neuropathies associated with malignancy
    Definition
    Pathophysiology
    Clinical manifestations
    Collaborative management
Charcot-Marie-Tooth disease (peroneal muscular
    atrophy)
    Definition
    Etiology/pathophysiology
    Clinical manifestations
Nursing management of the patient with Charcot-
    Marie-Tooth disease
    Assessment
    Nursing diagnosis
    Planning/expected outcomes
    Evaluation/documentation
    Continuity of care
 	
Cranial nerve disorders
 	
Trigeminal neuralgia
    Definition
    Etiology/pathophysiology
    Clinical manifestations
    Collaborative management
 	
    Medical therapy
    Surgical management
Nursing management of the patient with trigeminal
    neuralgia
    Assessment
    Nursing diagnosis
	Critical Thinking: List three causes of toxic neuropathy.
	
	VIEWSTUDY image #320 shows the trigeminal nerve and its three main divisions.
	
	Critical Thinking: Describe the symptoms of trigeminal neuralgia.
	
	Critical Thinking: The patient is being treated with carbamazepine for trigeminal neuralgia. He is experiencing ataxia and drowsiness. What other side effects can he expect with this drug?
	
	Critical Thinking: What medications are often prescribed for patients with trigeminal neuralgia?
	
	Critical Thinking: What are the minor and major surgical interventions for trigeminal neuralgia?
	
	Critical Thinking: Discuss the nursing assessment for trigeminal neuralgia.

Chapter Outline	Lecture Strategies

Planning/expected outcomes
Implementation
  Preoperative care
  Postoperative care
Evaluation/documentation
Continuity of care
Facial nerve paralysis
  Definition
  Etiology/epidemiology
  Pathophysiology
  Clinical manifestations
	Critical Thinking: What factors should be included in the preoperative and postoperative care of patients undergoing surgery for trigeminal neuralgia?
	
	Critical Thinking: Describe the condition of facial nerve paralysis.
	
	VIEWSTUDY image #321 demonstrates facial characteristics in Bell's palsy:

Collaborative management
Nursing management of the patient with facial nerve
  paralysis
  Assessment
  Nursing diagnosis
  Planning/implementation
  Evaluation/documentation
  Continuity of care
	Critical Thinking: Why is prednisone the drug of choice to treat facial nerve paralysis?

Related Skills

1. Require students to review and practice the application of moist heat.
2. Review and ask students to practice assessment of gait and reflexes.

Related Clinical Skills

1. Assign students to patients who are experiencing peripheral nerve disorders.
2. In postconference, review medical and nursing activities that may produce iatrogenesis (such as improper cast application, improper injection techniques, and improper positioning). Discuss what can be done to reduce the incidence of iatrogenic disease.

37

Nursing Assessment of the Eye

LEARNING OBJECTIVES

1 Know the anatomy of the eye's internal and external structures.

2 Understand the physiologic processes by which visual accommodation, binocular vision, and color perception occur.

3 Elicit a complete and concise history from a patient with an eye disorder.

4 Accurately examine a patient with an eye disorder in an organized manner to obtain appropriate objective data.

5 Record history and physical findings of a patient with an eye disorder in a concise, accurate, and logical manner.

6 Differentiate normal from abnormal history and physical findings of a patient with an eye disorder

7 Describe procedures related to the detection and diagnosis of ocular disorders.

8 Describe patient preparation and care for diagnostic tests of the eye.

KEY TERMS

accommodation	nystagmus
aqueous humor	palpebral fissure
canal of Schlemm	PERRLA
ciliary body	phoria
choroid	ptosis
cones	retina
conjunctiva	rods
electroretinography	sclera
fluorescein angiography	tonometry
iris	tropia
lens	vitreous humor

Chapter Outline	Lecture Strategies
Accessory structures of the eye	**Critical Thinking:** How do the accessory structures of the eye serve to protect it?
Anatomy and physiology	**Critical Thinking:** Describe the three layers of the eye and the functions they serve. **VIEWSTUDY** image #56 illustrates the human eye. **VIEWSTUDY** image #57 shows a close-up view of the ciliary body, zonules, lens, and anterior and posterior chambers.
The eyeball	During discussion, use an anatomical model of the various structures of the eyeball.

Chapter Outline	Lecture Strategies
Visual acuity Visual accommodation	**VIEWSTUDY** image #59 demonstrates the visual pathway.
Physiology of binocular vision Assessment	**Critical Thinking:** What are the photoreceptor cells, and how do they enable the perception of color?
Subjective	Ask students what vitamin is associated with good vision. Many may have been advised to eat carrots as a child to improve or maintain vision.
	Critical Thinking: Design at least three questions to ask patients about eye health care habits.
	TA 69 shows the Snellen chart for assessment of visual acuity.
Objective	Anxiety and apprehension may accompany eye examination and may affect the patient's ability to cooperate.
	Critical Thinking: Describe an effective approach to examining a painful, edematous, tightly closed eye just after injury.
	Critical Thinking: Discuss psychologic factors to consider when a patient must wear an eye prosthesis.
	Critical Thinking: Discuss special considerations in regard to eye integrity in adults with chronic systemic conditions, such as diabetes mellitus and cerebral vascular accident.
Diagnostic and laboratory tests Electroretinography Patient preparation Tonometry Patient preparation	**Critical Thinking:** Describe the procedure for intravenous fluorescein angiography as it might be explained to a patient.
Procedure Schiøtz' tonometer Applanation tonometer Intravenous fluorescein angiography Patient preparation Procedure Postprocedure care Ocular ultrasonography Patient preparation Procedure Computed tomography Patient preparation Magnetic resonance imaging	**Critical Thinking:** Discuss tonometry relative to purpose, contraindications, and procedure.

Related Skills

1. Ask students working in pairs to complete an objective and subjective assessment of the eyes.

Related Clinical Skills

1. Assign students to patients who are undergoing diagnostic tests for eye disorders. Ask students to prepare patients and accompany the patients during the diagnostic testing.
2. Assign students to an outpatient eye clinic to observe diagnostic procedures used in evaluating eye disorders.

38 Nursing Management of Adults with Eye Disorders

LEARNING OBJECTIVES

1 Outline the nursing plan and intervention for management for the following eye disorders: glaucoma, cataract, retinal degeneration, ocular emergency, retinal detachment, hordeolum, conjunctivitis, blindness, and diabetic retinopathy.
2 Describe pathophysiology, etiology, incidence, symptoms, and collaborative management for each of the common eye disorders.
3 Develop a nursing care plan for postoperative care of a patient having cataract surgery.
4 Recognize pertinent observations to document for patients with eye disorders.
5 Identify actions, indications for use, and side effects of medications having mydriatic and miotic properties.
6 Write a teaching plan for a patient with chronic glaucoma.
7 Discuss nursing responsibilities to society for prevention of blindness and adaptation to living with chronic eye disorders.

KEY TERMS

astigmatism
cataract
chalazion
closed-angle glaucoma
conjunctivitis
glaucoma
hordeolum
hyperopia
keratoplasty
lacrimation
legal blindness

macular degeneration
myopia
nyctalopia
photophobia
presbyopia
primary open-angle
   glaucoma (POAG)
refraction
scotoma
uveitis

Chapter Outline	Lecture Strategies
Disorders of refraction	Use diagrams of the eye to illustrate the refractive errors.
	Critical Thinking: Describe the visual changes associated with common errors of eye refraction.
	VIEWSTUDY image #58 illustrates refraction disorders.
	VIEWSTUDY image #62 shows emmetropic, myopic, and hyperopic eyes with corrected and uncorrected vision.
Glaucoma	
Primary open-angle glaucoma Etiology/epidemiology	

Chapter Outline	Lecture Strategies

Pathophysiology
Clinical manifestations

Critical Thinking: Differentiate among the presenting symptoms of primary open-angle and primary closed-angle glaucoma and detached retina.

Collaborative management
Closed-angle glaucoma
    Definition/etiology
    Pathophysiology
    Clinical manifestations
    Collaborative management
Secondary glaucoma
Nursing management of the patient with glaucoma
    Assessment
    Nursing diagnosis
    Planning/expected outcomes
    Implementation
    Evaluation/documentation
    Continuity of care

Degenerative disorders of the eye—changes with aging

Cataract
    Definition
    Etiology/pathophysiology
    Clinical manifestations
    Collaborative management

    Postoperative complications
    Preoperative teaching
    Postoperative care
Nursing management of the patient with cataracts
    Assessment
    Nursing diagnosis
    Planning/expected outcomes
    Implementation
        Preoperative teaching
        Postoperative care
    Evaluation/documentation

    Continuity of care
Retinal degeneration
    Etiology/pathophysiology
    Clinical manifestations/collaborative management
Nursing management of the patient with macular retinal degeneration
    Assessment
    Nursing diagnosis
    Planning/expected outcomes
    Implementation
Vascular occlusive disease
    Definition/etiology
    Collaborative management

Review the actions, main side effects, and nursing responsibilities associated with miotics, adrenergic agents, and carbonic anhydrase inhibitors.

Critical Thinking: What signs and symptoms in primary closed-angle glaucoma indicate an ophthalmic emergency?

Ask students to describe the rationale for bed rest.

Critical Thinking: What activities increase intraocular pressure?

Use a diagram of the eye to illustrate location of changes.

Review actions, side effects, and nursing activities associated with mydriatics and cycloplegics.

TA 70 offers a critical thinking guide for postoperative cataract hemorrhage.

Critical Thinking: What discharge teaching is necessary for the patient after cataract removal?

Ask students how they would assess color vision.

Differentiate among the six most common occlusive ocular disorders.

Chapter Outline	Lecture Strategies
Diabetic retinopathy	Who is more likely to get diabetic retinopathy?
Definition	
Epidemiology	Describe the three stages of diabetic retinopathy.
Pathophysiology	
Clinical manifestations/collaborative management	Ask, "How often should diabetic patients have a comprehensive eye exam through dilated pupils? Why?" (Answer: Because there are usually no early symptoms with diabetic retinopathy, these patients should have a comprehensive exam at least once a year.)
Nursing management of the patient with diabetic retinopathy	
Assessment	
Nursing diagnosis	
Planning/expected outcomes	
Implementation	
Evaluation/documentation	
Ocular emergencies	
Etiology/epidemiology	
Collaborative management	
First aid and emergency management	**Critical Thinking:** How should a foreign body be removed from the eye?
Management of injury from foreign bodies	
Complications of corneal foreign bodies	Anyone who has contacts and who has suffered corneal abrasion will identify with this complication.
Management of chemical injury	**Critical Thinking:** Describe the emergency management of chemical injury to the eye caused by alkaline and acid substances.
Nursing management of the patient with an ocular emergency	**VIEWSTUDY** image #63 illustrates surgical repair of retinal break with detachment by use of the scleral buckling technique.
Retinal detachment	
Etiology/epidemiology/pathophysiology	
Clinical manifestations	
Collaborative management	Discuss the relatively new use of pneumatic retinopexy.
Nursing management of the patient with retinal detachment	
Preoperative care	
Postoperative care	Ask students to discuss the reasons for administration of mydriatics and cycloplegics.
Special surgical procedures	
Keratoplasty	
Nursing management of the keratoplasty patient	
Preoperative care	
Postoperative care	
Removal of an eye	
Indications for surgery	
Nursing management of the patient undergoing eye removal	
Inflammatory and infectious diseases	
Chalazion	
Definition/etiology	
Clinical manifestations	
Collaborative management	

Chapter Outline	Lecture Strategies

Hordeolum
    Etiology/clinical manifestations
    Collaborative management
Conjunctivitis
    Definition
    Etiology/clinical manifestations
    Collaborative management
Trachoma
    Definition/etiology
    Collaborative management
Uveitis
    Definition/etiology
    Clinical manifestations
    Collaborative management

Critical Thinking: What are the patient teaching implications for the various eye medications used in the Collaborative management of eye disorders?

Critical Thinking: What are the implications for nursing management of the patient with an eye infection?

Blindness
    Definition

Point out the 20/200 line on the Snellen's chart.

    Sensory deprivation

Obtain various aids so that students may manipulate and use them.

    Emotional response
Special considerations for patients with HIV
    Ocular effects of AIDS

Critical Thinking: How can the nurse help the patient cope physically and psychologically with blindness? Discuss role changes that may be needed for the blind patient and family.

Related Skills

1. Discuss and demonstrate administration of eye ointment and drops.
2. Demonstrate proper application of eye patches and pressure dressings.
3. Break group into pairs and blindfold one person in each pair. With the second member of the pair acting as a guide, have the pairs walk into other areas of the academic setting. Discuss the proper way to walk with a visually impaired individual.
4. Have the students assess one another's vision, using a Snellen's chart.

Related Clinical Skills

1. Assign students to patients who are undergoing surgery for cataracts or glaucoma.
2. Assign students to a patient undergoing outpatient cataract surgery and follow the postoperative period through to the home setting. Develop a teaching plan that focusses on medication administration and patient safety.

39 Nursing Assessment of the Ear

LEARNING OBJECTIVES

1 Identify the anatomic structure and general functions of the ear.
2 Understand the process by which the ears sense sound and changes in body position.
3 Elicit a complete and concise history from a patient with an ear disorder.
4 Accurately examine a patient with an ear disorder in an organized manner to obtain appropriate objective data.
5 Differentiate normal from abnormal history and physical findings of a patient with an ear disorder.
6 Describe tests related to the diagnoses of otologic disorders.
7 Describe patient care for procedures by which ear disorders are diagnosed.

KEY TERMS

audiometry
caloric test
cochlea
dynamic equilibrium
electronystagmography
eustachian tube
external ear
inner ear
middle ear
past-point test

presbycusis
Rinne test
Romberg test
spondee threshold test
static equilibrium
tinnitus
tympanocentesis
vertigo
vestibular apparatus
Weber test

Chapter Outline	Lecture Strategies

Anatomy and physiology
    Structure and functions of external and middle ear
    Structure and functions of inner ear
	Critical Thinking: Describe the roles that the external ear, middle ear, and inner ear play in hearing sounds of different frequencies.

Cochlea Vestibular apparatus	**VIEWSTUDY** image #60 shows the external, middle, and inner ear.
Assessment	**VIEWSTUDY** image #61 shows normal landmarks of the right tympanic membrane.
Subjective	**Critical Thinking:** Design at least three questions to ask patients about health care habits in relation to the ears.
Objective	Have students practice Weber and Rinne tests with tuning forks.
	TA 71 is helpful in discussing interpretation of tuning fork tests.
Ears	**TA 72** shows structural landmarks of the tympanic membrane.

Chapter Outline	Lecture Strategies
	Critical Thinking: Describe an effective approach to examining a painful ear.
	Critical Thinking: Discuss psychologic factors to consider when a patient has an ear deformity.
	Critical Thinking: Discuss the nursing implications in examining a patient's ear with the otoscope.
	Critical Thinking: Describe how Rinne and Weber tests are performed. What is the difference between the tests in terms of hearing assessment?

Mouth, throat, and temporomandibular joint
    Neck and nodes
Diagnostic and laboratory tests
  Audiometric testing
    Screening audiometry
    Impedance audiometry
    Tympanometry
	Describe examination techniques for a patient with an ear complaint.

Spondee threshold test
  Word recognition tests
  Romberg test
  Past-point test
  Caloric test
    Patient preparation
    Procedure
	Ask students to describe each of the following tests as they would to a patient about to undergo each procedure: Spondee threshold test; word recognition tests; Romberg test; past-point test; caloric test.

Electronystagmography test
  X-ray examination
  Culture
  Tympanocentesis
    Patient preparation
    Postprocedure care
	Have students suggest conditions or situations which would indicate each of the following procedures: electronystagmography test; X-ray examination; culture; tympanocentesis.

Related Skills

1. Ask students to practice assessment of the ear, working in pairs.

Related Clinical Skills

1. Assign students to patients with disorders of the ear.
2. Assign students to a geriatric clinic in which senior citizens are receiving ear examinations as part of a screening. Have them observe the placement of hearing aids in the elderly.

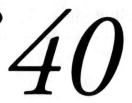

40 Nursing Management of Adults with Ear Disorders

LEARNING OBJECTIVES

1 Summarize various ways to decrease noise pollution in the home and community.
2 Describe individuals who would benefit from a hearing aid and the importance of choosing and maintaining the aid.
3 Describe the degenerative changes in the ear caused by aging.
4 Describe the various aural hygienic methods used to reduce hearing loss.
5 Describe procedures to keep the ear clean and free of wax or foreign objects.
6 Describe clinical findings and nursing interventions for cholesteatoma and otitis media.
7 Recognize the importance of the symptom of vertigo in inner ear problems.
8 Describe the progress of Ménière's disease and nursing care during the acute and remission stages.
9 Compare the differences in assessing the tympanic membrane and mastoid process and the outer, middle, and inner ears.

KEY TERMS

acoustic neuroma
actinic keratosis
cerumen
cholesteatoma
cochlear implant
conductive hearing loss
external otitis
labyrinthitis
Ménière's disease
myringitis

myringoplasty
otitis media
otomycosis
otosclerosis
presbycusis
sensorineural hearing loss
swimmer's ear
tinnitus
tympanosclerosis
vestibular neuronitis

Chapter Outline	Lecture Strategies
Hearing loss	Loud music may cause hearing loss.
Definition/etiology	
Hearing loss from noise	**Critical Thinking:** You have been asked to teach a class on ways to decrease noise pollution in the home, hospital, and community. What would you include?
Etiology/pathophysiology/clinical manifestations	
Collaborative management	
Conductive hearing loss	Give students earplugs and ask them to experience communicating with a partner while plugs are in place.
Sensorineural hearing loss	
	Critical Thinking: As a person ages, hearing quality changes. Describe these changes and what, if anything, can be done about them.
Presbycusis	Bring examples of the various hearing aids to class.

Chapter Outline	Lecture Strategies

Etiology/pathophysiology
Collaborative management
Other types of hearing loss
 	
Collaborative management
  Hearing aids
Nursing management of the patient with a hearing
  aid
Cochlear implants
Nursing management of the patient with a cochlear
  implant
Continuity of care
Nursing management of the person with hearing loss
  Assessment
  Nursing diagnosis
  Planning/expected outcomes
  Implementation
  Evaluation/documentation
 	
External ear disorders
 	
Infection
  Definition/etiology
  Pathophysiology
  Clinical manifestations
  Collaborative management
Neoplastic changes
  Definition
  Pathophysiology
  Clinical manifestations
  Collaborative management
Trauma
  Etiology
  Clinical manifestations
  Collaborative management
Nursing management of the patient with external ear
  disorders
  Assessment
  Nursing diagnosis
  Planning/expected outcomes
  Implementation
  Evaluation/documentation
  Continuity of care
	It is useful to have samples of the aids that are available so that students may more easily visualize placement and care during this discussion.
	
	Utilize diagrams during discussion to aid in visualization of the implant.
	
	Critical Thinking: What type of hearing-impaired individuals may be helped by a hearing aid? a cochlear implant? How would you teach a patient to keep his or her hearing aid in working order?
	
	Ask students to rate the impact of hearing loss in their lives on a scale of 1 to 10 and discuss their ratings with a partner.
	
	Review proper application of ear drops.
	
	Prepare a short questionnaire for the students that allows them to assess their general knowledge of ear care. Administer questionnaire before discussion of ear care.
	
	Critical Thinking: What procedure or procedures might the nurse use to remove hardened earwax? to remove a foreign body from the ear?
	
	Critical Thinking: What procedure might the nurse use to keep the ear clean (routine cleaning)?
	
	TA 73 demonstrates removal of cerumen.

Chapter Outline	Lecture Strategies
Middle ear, tympanic membrane, and mastoid disorders	**Critical Thinking:** What similar problems occur in the inner, middle, and outer ear? List various problems that occur only in one particular area of the ear.
Infection	
Definition/etiology/pathophysiology	
Clinical manifestations	**VIEWSTUDY** image #64 shows three common tympanic perforations.
Collaborative management	
Congenital disorders	
Definition/etiology	
Clinical manifestations	
Collaborative management	
Neoplastic changes	
Definition/etiology	
Pathophysiology	
Clinical manifestations	
Collaborative management	
Degenerative changes	
Definition/etiology	
Pathophysiology	
Clinical manifestations	
Collaborative management	
Trauma	
Definition/etiology	
Collaborative management	
Nursing management of the patient with disorders of the middle ear, tympanic membrane, and mastoid	
Assessment	
Nursing diagnosis	
Planning/expected outcomes	
Implementation	**Critical Thinking:** What clinical findings and nursing interventions would be used with a patient with a diagnosis of otitis media? otitis media with effusion? otitis media without effusion? acute otitis media?
Evaluation	
Inner ear disorders	
Infection	
Definition/etiology	
Pathophysiology	
Clinical manifestations	**Critical Thinking:** What clinical findings and nursing interventions would be used with a patient with a diagnosis of cholesteatoma?
Collaborative management	
Neoplastic disorders	
Definition/etiology	
Pathophysiology/clinical manifestations	
Collaborative management	
Motion sickness	
Definition/etiology/pathophysiology	
Clinical manifestations	
Collaborative management	Review the classifications, interactions, side effects, and nursing activities associated with the medications.
Barotrauma	
Definition/etiology/pathophysiology	
Clinical manifestations	
Collaborative management	
Ménière's disease	**Critical Thinking:** Why is vertigo commonly a symptom of an inner ear problem?
Definition/etiology	

Chapter Outline	Lecture Strategies

Pathophysiology
Clinical manifestations
Collaborative management
Nursing management of the patient with disorders of
  the inner ear
Assessment
Nursing diagnosis
Planning/expected outcomes
Implementation
Evaluation

Critical Thinking: What would you teach a patient newly diagnosed with Ménière's disease about home care?

Related Skills

1. Demonstrate use of an ear syringe and the application of eardrops. Ask students to practice and demonstrate competence in these skills.

Related Clinical Skills

1. Assign students to patients with hearing deficits and ask them to develop care plans that specifically address the communication needs of these patients. Supervise the insertions and care of hearing aids as necessary.

41

Nursing Assessment of the Musculoskeletal System

LEARNING OBJECTIVES

1 Know the main structural components of the musculoskeletal system and their functions.
2 Understand the sequence of events that produces muscle contraction and relaxation.
3 Elicit a complete and concise history from a patient with a musculoskeletal disorder.
4 Accurately examine a patient with a musculoskeletal disorder in an organized manner to obtain appropriate objective data.
5 Record history and physical findings of a patient with a musculoskeletal disorder in a concise, accurate, and logical manner.
6 Differentiate normal from abnormal history and physical findings of a patient with a musculoskeletal disorder.
7 Describe tests and procedures used in the diagnosis of musculoskeletal disorders.
8 Describe the patient care that is necessary for each of the tests used to diagnose musculoskeletal disorders.

KEY TERMS

anti-DNA binding antibody (anti-DNA)
appendicular skeleton
arthroscopy
axial skeleton
cancellous bone
complement fixation
contraction
crepitus
dense bone

fasciculations
joints
kyphosis
lordosis
muscle fibers
muscle spindles
scoliosis
synovial biopsy
synovial fluid
tremors

Chapter Outline	Lecture Strategies

Anatomy and physiology
  Bones
    Structure and function of a typical long bone
    Structure and function of the skeleton
	Use diagrams of the long bone to illustrate the discussion of the composition of bone.

Joints	Use a diagram to assist students in visualizing the components of a synovial joint.

Muscles
  Structure of muscle fibers
  Muscle contraction
  Energy sources of contraction
  Isolated single muscle fibers and complete
    muscles
	Critical Thinking: Explain the process by which muscle contraction occurs.

Chapter Outline	Lecture Strategies
Muscles in the intact individual	Summarize the types of contractions, the factors involved in the strength of contraction, and the muscle groups.
	Critical Thinking: Describe the different types of normal skeletal muscle contractions.
Assessment Subjective	**Critical Thinking:** Design three questions to discreetly assess the psychosocial ramifications of musculoskeletal disorders.
	Critical Thinking: Describe musculoskeletal changes related to aging.
Objective	**Critical Thinking:** In what ways might musculoskeletal alterations affect a patient's self-care abilities and independent functioning?

General assessment
    Integumentary
    Musculoskeletal
	TA 74 presents muscle strength grading.

Musculoskeletal special tests	Ask students to identify the purpose of the following tests: McMurray's sign, the drawer test, Lachmann's test, Patrick's (FABER) test, Tinel's sign.
Diagnostic and laboratory tests Radiography	X-ray studies are commonly associated with fractures and other disorders.

Standard radiography
      Patient preparation
    Myelography
      Patient preparation	

Arthrography
      Patient preparation
      Procedure
      Postprocedure care
	Obtain x-ray films that have been taken during arthrography.

Bone scan
      Patient preparation
      Procedure
	Critical Thinking: Your patient seems concerned about having a radioactive substance injected as part of a bone scan. What information can you give the patient about the safety of the radioactive substance?

Computed tomography
      Patient preparation
    Magnetic resonance imaging
      Patient preparation	

Biopsy
      Patient preparation
      Postprocedure care
	Ask students to suggest appropriate indications for each of the following procedures: Biopsy; synovial fluid analysis; arthroscopy; electromyography.

Synovial fluid analysis
      Patient preparation
      Postprocedure care	

Arthroscopy
      Patient preparation
      Postprocedure care
	Critical Thinking: Describe the patient care required before and after arthroscopy.

Electromyography Laboratory tests	

Related Skills

1. Discuss and demonstrate assessment of the musculoskeletal system. With students working in pairs, require them to practice and return a satisfactory demonstration of this area of assessment.

Related Clinical Skills

1. Assign students to patients who are awaiting diagnosis of musculoskeletal disorders. Emphasize the need for thorough assessment and for teaching related to diagnostic measures. When possible, arrange for students to accompany patients while they are undergoing diagnostic procedures.
2. Assign students to observe diagnostic tests used to evaluate musculoskeletal disorders.
3. Have students prepare a teaching plan that covers the periods both before and after a procedure.

42 Nursing Management of Adults with Musculoskeletal Trauma

LEARNING OBJECTIVES

1 Explain the nursing management for patients with contusions, strains, sprains, bursitis, epicondylitis, and dislocations

2 Discuss nursing management of the patient with sports injuries or repetitive syndrome.

3 Describe principles of treatment, nursing interventions, and rationales for patients with fractures.

4 Compare the nursing management for a patient with traction to that of a patient with a cast.

5 Discuss the stages of fracture healing, nonunion, and delayed healing.

6 Identify potential hazards of immobility and complications of musculoskeletal trauma on a patient's health status.

7 Develop a care plan for a patient with an internal fixation device.

8 Identify the collaborative and nursing management for a patient with a traumatic amputation.

9 Relate the psychologic and physiologic effects of a traumatic amputation and surgical amputation.

KEY TERMS

anterior cruciate ligament (ACL) tear
avascular necrosis
Buck's traction
cervical traction
closed fracture
compartment syndrome
delayed union
external fixation device
fat embolism syndrome (FES)
gas gangrene
nonunion
open fracture
open reduction internal fixation (ORIF)
osteomyelitis
phantom pain
rhabdomyolysis
rotator cuff tear
Russell's traction

Chapter Outline	Lecture Strategies
Soft tissue trauma	
Contusion	Ask students to describe the color changes that accompany bruises.
Definition	
Etiology	
Pathophysiology	
Clinical manifestations	
Strain	Ask students to define strain.
Definition	
Etiology	
Pathophysiology	
Clinical manifestations	
Sprain	
Definition	
Etiology	
Pathophysiology	

Chapter Outline	Lecture Strategies

Clinical manifestations
Collaborative management
Nursing management of the patient with soft tissue
    trauma
    Assessment
    Nursing diagnosis
    Planning/expected outcomes

Critical Thinking: Describe nursing management for contusions, strains, sprains, bursitis, epicondylitis, and dislocations.

VIEWSTUDY image #333 shows soft-tissue injury of the hip.

    Implementation
    Evaluation/documentation
    Continuity of care
Sports injuries and repetitive stress injury

What should the nurse teach the patient and family about taking muscle relaxants?

Critical Thinking: Explain the basis of sports injuries and repetitive stress injury.

Ask students to identify four possible causes of repetitive stress injury.

Bursitis and epicondylitis
    Definition
    Etiology/pathophysiology

What is the difference between bursitis and epicondylitis? How are they similar and different in their clinical manifestations?

    Clinical manifestations
    Collaborative management

VIEWSTUDY image #332 illustrates bursae of the shoulder joint.

Nursing management of the patient with bursitis and
    epicondylitis
    Assessment
    Nursing diagnosis
    Planning/expected outcomes
    Implementation
    Evaluation/documentation
    Continuity of care

Ask students to suggest appropriate interventions.

Skeletal trauma

Dislocations
    Definition
    Etiology
    Pathophysiology
    Clinical manifestations
    Collaborative management

Discuss the scope of the pathophysiology of dislocations in adults.

Nursing management of the patient with a dislocation
    Assessment
    Nursing diagnosis
    Planning/expected outcomes
    Implementation
    Evaluation/documentation
    Continuity of care

Fractures
    Definition
    Etiology

Ask, "Can you identify three types of stress to the bone? Four bases for identifying a specific fracture?"

Chapter Outline	Lecture Strategies
Pathophysiology 　Classification	**VIEWSTUDY** image #337 shows fracture classification according to communication.
Types of fracture 　Location 　Alignment status	**VIEWSTUDY** image #336 shows types of fractures **VIEWSTUDY** image #342 shows a femur with the location of various types of fractures.
Bone healing	**VIEWSTUDY** image #338 depicts fracture classification according to location.
Clinical manifestations	**VIEWSTUDY** image #339 demonstrates bone healing. **Critical Thinking:** Describe the eight signs and symptoms of a fracture and explain the pathologic basis of each sign or symptom.
Collaborative management 　Prehospital care	Ask students to describe materials that they might use at the scene of an accident to splint a fracture. If possible, obtain various internal fixation devices to show to the students. **Critical Thinking:** Summarize the three treatment methods and rationales for a patient with a fracture.
Fracture complications 　　Tetanus	**Critical Thinking:** Explain the pathologic basis of complications of fractures, including avascular necrosis, compartment syndrome, gas gangrene, osteomyelitis, and fat embolus. **Critical Thinking:** Explain the basis of nonunion and delayed healing. What are two of the most likely fractures associated with compartment syndrome? **TA 76** offers a critical thinking guide for discussing compartment syndrome. Explain how osteomyelitis is classified. Identify leading features of FES.
Traction 　Lower extremity traction 　Upper extremity traction 　Skeletal traction 　Cervical traction 　Pelvic traction 　External fixation devices	**TA 77** shows balanced suspension traction (skeletal).

Chapter Outline	Lecture Strategies
Nursing management of the fracture patient immobilized by traction	**VIDEO** volume 1 presents nursing care of the patient with a hip fracture, with emphasis on assessment and pre- and postoperative care.
	Critical Thinking: What are the stages of fracture healing?
	TA 75 outlines these stages.
	Critical Thinking: What are the hazards of immobility on body systems?
Assessment Nursing diagnosis Planning/expected outcomes Implementation Neurovascular	**Critical Thinking:** What actions should the nurse implement to prevent hazards of immobility?
Neurologic Perfusion Pain Infection Altered mobility Traction Skin Knowledge deficit Sensory/perceptual alterations Coping Bowel elimination Bladder elimination Sleep Nutrition Self-care deficit	Ask, "Why should the nurse wrapping an elastic bandage for skin traction avoid putting pressure on the outer aspect of the calf just below the knee?" Discuss appropriate nursing interventions related to pain, infection, altered mobility, and skin breakdown. **Critical Thinking:** Compare the nursing management for a patient in traction to that for a patient with a cast.
Evaluation/documentation Continuity of care	Ask students to outline evaluation criteria for the patient in traction.
Casting Cast materials	**VIEWSTUDY** image #340 illustrates common casts used in treatment of disorders of the musculoskeletal system.
Variations in cast application	Review variations of technique or strategy in applying a cast.
	VIEWSTUDY image #341 demonstrates finishing edges of a cast with waterproof adhesive strips.
	VIEWSTUDY image #344 shows the halo apparatus attached to a body cast.
Nursing management of the patient in a cast Assessment	**Critical Thinking:** Identify the five Ps and summarize questions and observations for each one.

Chapter Outline	Lecture Strategies
Nursing diagnosis Planning/expected outcomes	Stress the five Ps of neurovascular checks. With students in pairs, have them perform neurovascular checks on each other's fingers.

Implementation
   Circulation
   Safety
   Comfort
   Skin care
   Self-care deficit
   Emotional support
   Altered mobility
   Patient and family teaching
   Ambulatory aids
Evaluation/documentation
Continuity of care
   Cast removal
   Rehabilitation
	Ask students to speculate on the appearance of a casted limb.

Internal fixation Hip fractures	TA 78 is helpful in discussing the types of hip fractures.
Etiology Pathophysiology Clinical manifestation Collaborative management	Ask students to write a description of the causes and treatment of hip fractures as if they were writing it for patients.

Nursing management of the patient with open reduction and internal fixation
   Preoperative assessment
   Nursing diagnosis
   Planning/expected outcomes
   Implementation
   Evaluation/documentation
   Continuity of care
      Physical therapy
      Cold and heat applications
      Massage
      Exercise
         Isometric exercises
         Range-of-motion exercises
         Isotonic exercises
         Isokinetic exercises
	Critical Thinking: Describe nursing diagnoses, interventions, and rationales for a patient with an internal fixation (hip pinning).
	
	Outline together a preliminary nursing care plan for the patient with open reduction and internal fixation.
	
	Differentiate among isometric, range-of-motion, isotonic, and isokinetic exercises.

Amputation
   Definition
   Etiology
   Pathophysiology
   Clinical manifestations
   Collaborative management
      Amputated stump
      Replantation
	VIEWSTUDY image #346 shows the location and description of amputation sites of upper and lower extremities.

Nursing management of the patient with replantation Assessment	Guide students in forming a nursing management plan for the patient with replantation.

Chapter Outline	Lecture Strategies

Nursing diagnosis
Planning/expected outcomes
Implementation
  Leech therapy
Evaluation/documentation
Continuity of care

Nursing management of the patient with amputation
  Assessment
  Nursing diagnosis
  Planning/expected outcomes
  Implementation
  Evaluation/documentation
  Continuity of care

Critical Thinking: Identify the collaborative management of amputations, digit replantation, and leech therapy.

Critical Thinking: What are the nursing actions for a patient with a an amputation? Include both physiologic and psychologic actions.

VIEWSTUDY image #347 illustrates stump bandaging for an above-the- knee stump.

Related Skills

1. Arrange for students to visit a prosthetist to observe a fitting for a prosthesis and the types of prostheses that are available.
2. Demonstrate and ask students to practice the correct technique for wrapping a stump.
3. Demonstrate the setup for Buck's traction and skeletal traction, and have students, in teams, set up the necessary systems.
4. Ask a physiotherapist to demonstrate the use of crutches, and then ask students to practice the various gaits and walking up and down stairs.

Related Clinical Skills

1. Assign students to a patient with either a fracture or an amputation.
2. Assign students to patients in traction or to those with casts. Assess students' abilities to provide skin care, promote mobilization, and petal cast edges.
3. Assign students to a home-bound patient with an amputation. Develop a teaching plan, including safety measures, to help the patient and family adjust to the home environment after an amputation.
4. Arrange for students to observe physical therapy training for patients with casts or amputations.

43 Nursing Management of Adults with Degenerative, Inflammatory, or Autoimmune Musculoskeletal Disorders

LEARNING OBJECTIVES

1 Identify the two classifications of arthritis, giving examples of each type.
2 Identify the effects of at least four major medication groups used to treat arthritis.
3 List five factors contributing to the development of osteoporosis.
4 State the pathophysiology of arthritis, gout, osteoporosis, osteomalacia, Paget's disease, and muscular dystrophy.
5 State at least two nursing interventions for chronic musculoskeletal disorders in regard to home care management.
6 Identify at least three musculoskeletal disorders significantly affecting the morbidity of the aged adult.
7 Formulate nursing care plans for patients with arthritis, gout, osteoporosis, osteomalacia, Paget's disease, and muscular dystrophy.
8 Formulate a nursing care plan for an arthritic patient with a total hip replacement.
9 Apply knowledge of pathophysiology to the nursing care of a patient who has osteomyelitis.
10 Identify appropriate nursing care for the patient with low back pain.
11 Outline nursing care for the patient who has hallux valgus.

KEY TERMS

arthritis
Bouchard's nodes
boutonniere deformity
bunion
degenerative joint disease (DJD)
distal interphalangeal (DIP) joint
gout
Heberden's nodes
herniated nucleus pulposus (HNP)
muscular dystrophy
osteoarthritis (OA)
osteomalacia
osteomyelitis
osteoporosis
Paget's disease
proximal interphalangeal (PIP) joint
radiculopathy
rheumatoid arthritis (RA)
sciatica
swan-neck deformity
ulnar drift

Chapter Outline	Lecture Strategies
Arthritis	**Critical Thinking:** Discuss at least two classifications of arthritis and give examples of each classification.
Osteoarthritis	**VIEWSTUDY** image #349 shows joints most frequently involved in osteoarthritis
Definition	
Etiology/epidemiology	**VIEWSTUDY** image #350 demonstrates typical deformities of rheumatoid arthritis.

Chapter Outline	Lecture Strategies
	VIEWSTUDY image #351 depicts common extraarticular manifestations of rheumatoid arthritis.
Pathophysiology	**TA 79** shows Bouchard node.
Clinical manifestations	Ask, "What are Heberden's nodes and Bouchard's nodes?"
Collaborative management	**Critical Thinking:** Discuss four major medication groups used to treat arthritis.

Surgical management
Nursing management of the patient with osteoarthritis
  Assessment
  Nursing diagnosis
  Planning/expected outcomes
  Implementation
  Evaluation/documentation
  Continuity of care
Rheumatoid arthritis
  Definition
  Etiology/epidemiology
  Pathophysiology
  Clinical manifestations
  Collaborative management
	Describe the five categories of surgical procedures which may alleviate pain or correct deformities and restore function.

Surgical management Nursing management of the patient with rheumatoid arthritis	Refer to Table 43-5 to differentiate the processes and purposes of synovectomy, arthrodesis, osteotomy, and implant arthroplasty.

Assessment
  Nursing diagnosis
  Planning/expected outcomes
  Implementation
  Evaluation/documentation
  Continuity of care
Nursing management of the patient with joint replacement
  Assessment
  Nursing diagnosis
	Critical Thinking: What are the special implications for the aged adult with rheumatoid arthritis?
	
	Ask students to suggest signs of dislocation of a joint prosthesis. Ask them to identify the five Ps of neurovascular assessment.

Planning/expected outcomes	**Critical Thinking:** Formulate a nursing care plan for a patient with a total hip replacement.

Implementation
  Evaluation/documentation
  Continuity of care
	Ask, "What purpose does a pneumatic sequential compression device (SCD) serve?"
	
	TA 80 illustrates correct and incorrect hip flexion after total hip replacement.

Gout
  Definition
  Etiology/epidemiology
  Pathophysiology
	VIEWSTUDY image #352 shows tophaceous gout.

Chapter Outline	Lecture Strategies

Clinical manifestations
Collaborative management
Nursing management of the patient with gout
  Assessment
  Nursing diagnosis
  Planning/expected outcomes
  Implementation
  Evaluation/documentation
  Continuity of care
Osteoporosis
  Definition
  Etiology/epidemiology
  Pathophysiology
  Clinical manifestations
  Collaborative management
Nursing management of the patient with osteoporosis
  Assessment
  Nursing diagnosis
  Planning/expected outcomes
  Implementation
  Evaluation/documentation
  Continuity of care
Osteomalacia
  Definition
  Etiology/epidemiology
  Clinical manifestations
  Collaborative management
Nursing management of the patient with osteomalacia
  Assessment
  Nursing diagnosis
  Planning/expected outcomes
  Implementation
  Evaluation/documentation
Osteomyelitis
  Definition
  Etiology/epidemiology
  Pathophysiology
  Clinical manifestations
  Collaborative management
Nursing management of the patient with osteomyelitis
  Assessment
  Nursing diagnosis
  Planning/expected outcomes
  Implementation
  Evaluation/documentation
  Continuity of care
Paget's disease
  Definition
  Etiology/epidemiology
  Pathophysiology
  Clinical manifestations
  Collaborative management
	Critical Thinking: What are the five factors that contribute to the development of osteoporosis?
	
	TA 81 illustrates structural deformity of kyphosis.
	
	Critical Thinking: Discuss in detail the pathophysiology of any of the following musculoskeletal disorders: arthritis, osteoporosis, osteomalacia, Paget's disease, and muscular dystrophy.
	
	Ask students to explain why an increased availability of vitamin D and calcium are necessary.
	
	Critical Thinking: Discuss the effects of osteomyelitis on the skeletal system.
	
	VIEWSTUDY image #345 demonstrates development of osteomyelitis infection.
	
	Critical Thinking: What are the nursing interventions for patients with chronic musculoskeletal disorders specific to home care management?

Chapter Outline	Lecture Strategies

Nursing management of the patient with Paget's disease
    Assessment
    Nursing diagnosis
    Planning/expected outcomes
    Implementation
    Evaluation/documentation
    Continuity of care
Low back pain
    Definition
    Etiology/epidemiology
    Pathophysiology
 	
    Clinical manifestations
    Collaborative management
Nursing management of the patient with low back pain
    Assessment
    Nursing diagnosis
    Planning/expected outcomes
    Implementation
    Evaluation/documentation
    Continuity of care
Hallux valgus
    Definition
    Etiology
    Pathophysiology
    Clinical manifestations
    Collaborative management
Nursing management of the patient with hallux valgus
    Assessment
    Nursing diagnosis
    Planning/expected outcomes
    Implementation
    Evaluation/documentation
 	
Degenerative muscle disease
 	
Muscular dystrophy
    Definition
    Etiology/epidemiology
    Pathophysiology
    Clinical manifestations
    Collaborative management
Nursing management of the patient with muscular dystrophy
    Assessment
    Nursing diagnosis
    Planning/expected outcomes
    Implementation
    Evaluation/documentation
    Continuity of care
	Outline both activities and abnormalities that may contribute to low back pain.
	
	Identify the slightly different functions of the MRI and the CT scan in evaluating low back pain.
	
	Critical Thinking: Describe nursing measures for the patient with low back pain.
	
	Critical Thinking: Identify a teaching plan for the patient with hallux valgus.
	
	Critical Thinking: Describe the types of muscular dystrophy.

Related Skills

1. Discuss and demonstrate the use of proper body mechanics in lifting, especially in relation to the movement and transfer of patients.
2. Arrange for a physiotherapist to discuss and demonstrate the use of TENS.

Related Clinical Skills

1. Ask students to assess their elderly patients for clinical manifestations of arthritis and to develop specific interventions for the relief of symptoms.
2. Assign the students to home health patients with a diagnosis of osteoarthritis or rheumatoid arthritis. Develop a teaching plan with specific interventions for the relief of symptoms.
3. Develop a teaching plan for a homebound patient with osteoporosis.
4. Assign students to health care facilities that focus on women's health needs and inform participants of prevention of osteoporosis.

44 Nursing Assessment of the Endocrine System

LEARNING OBJECTIVES

1 Know the basic anatomic components of the endocrine system.
2 Describe the manner in which the hormones secreted by the endocrine glands regulate body functions.
3 Elicit a complete and concise history from a patient with an endocrine disorder.
4 Accurately examine a patient with an endocrine disorder in an organized manner to obtain appropriate objective data
5 Record history and physical findings of a patient with an endocrine disorder in a concise, accurate, and logical manner.
6 Differentiate normal from abnormal history and physical findings of a patient with an endocrine disorder.
7 Describe tests and procedures that are used in the diagnosis of endocrine system disorders.
8 Describe the patient care that is required for each of the tests and procedures used to diagnose endocrine system dysfunction.

KEY TERMS

corticotropin (ACTH)
corticotropin-releasing hormone (ACTH-RH)
cortisol
exophthalmos
glucagon
glucocorticoid
glycosylated hemoglobin
growth hormone
insulin
melatonin
parathyroid hormone (PTH)
thyrotropin (TSH)
thyrotropin-releasing hormone (TSH-RH)

Chapter Outline	Lecture Strategies

Anatomy and physiology
  Mechanism of hormone action
  Hormones secreted by nervous system
    Melatonin
  Hormones indirectly controlled by nervous system
    Growth hormone
      Control of growth hormone
	Critical Thinking: What are the categories of hormones secreted by the endocrine system? On what basis are they categorized?
	
	VIEWSTUDY image #255 shows the locations of the major endocrine glands.
	
	VIEWSTUDY image #256 demonstrates hormone-receptor action: steroid hormones.
	
	VIEWSTUDY image #257 demonstrates hormone-receptor action: peptide hormones and catecholamines.

Chapter Outline	Lecture Strategies
	VIEWSTUDY image #258 illustrates simple negative feedback: calcium and parathyroid hormone.
	VIEWSTUDY image #259 demonstrates the hypothalamic- pituitary<en>target gland feedback loop.
	VIEWSTUDY image #260 shows the general relationship between the hypothalamus, the pituitary, and target tissues.
Mechanism of growth hormone action	GH, without the presence of somatomedin, can be likened to the old saying of "all dressed up and no place to go."
Cortisol Control of cortisol	**Critical Thinking:** Explain the process of negative feedback and give examples of it.
Mechanism of cortisol action Thyroid hormones Control of thyroid hormones Mechanism of thyroid hormone action Hormones controlled by chemical concentration Hormones controlled by calcium concentration Hormones controlled by glucose concentration Assessment Subjective	**Critical Thinking:** Name three effects of cortisol.
	It may be useful to review physiological responses to stress to place the responses of the endocrine system in perspective.
Objective General assessment Skin, hair, and nails	**Critical Thinking:** Design at least three questions to ask patients about risk factors in relation to the endocrine system.
Head and face	Ask students to define *exophthalmos*. **TA 82** shows the posterior approach to thyroid examination.
Neck Heart Extremities Neurologic Diagnostic and laboratory tests Thyroid function tests Laboratory tests Thyroid scan	**Critical Thinking:** Describe an effective approach to examining a painful thyroid gland.
Patient preparation Thyroid ultrasonography Thyroid biopsy	Obtain thyroid scans and point out areas of hyperactivity and hypoactivity. Ask students to suggest three uses of the thyroid biopsy test.
Parathyroid function tests Laboratory tests Skeletal roentgenograms	Ask students to review the tests in Tables 44-1, 44-2, and 44-3 for an informal quiz in class.

173

Chapter Outline	Lecture Strategies

Adrenal function tests
    Clinical laboratory tests
    Computed tomography
    Adrenal arteriography
    Adrenal venography
        Patient preparation
        Aftercare
    Scintigraphy
        Patient preparation
Pituitary function tests
    Serum studies
    Roentgenogram of hand and wrist
    Roentgenogram of sella turcica
Assessment of hypoglycemia
    Serum insulin
    C-peptide
    Prolonged fast
Diagnostic tests for diabetes mellitus
    Fasting blood glucose
    Two-hour postprandial glucose test
    Glycosylated hemoglobin test
    Serum fructosamine
    Glucose tolerance test
        Patient preparation
	Critical Thinking: Outline what you would tell a patient who is undergoing adrenal venography, a thyroid scan, or a test for plasma renin activity.
	
	Review insulin degradation.
	
	Critical Thinking: Describe each of the tests that are used in the diagnosis of diabetes mellitus.

Related Skills

1. With students working in pairs, have them practice assessment of the thyroid gland.
2. Discuss collection of 24-hour urine specimens.

Related Clinical Skills

1. Assign students to patients awaiting diagnosis of suspected endocrine disorders. Instruct students to focus particularly on physical assessment and on preparation of patients for diagnostic procedures. Where possible, have students accompany patients while they are undergoing diagnostic procedures.
2. Arrange for students to develop a pre- and postprocedure teaching plan for a patient undergoing a diagnostic test for endocrine disorders.

45 Nursing Management of Adults with Hypothalamus, Pituitary, or Adrenal Disorders

LEARNING OBJECTIVES

1 Describe the effects of excess glucocorticoids on adipose tissue distribution, protein and carbohydrate metabolism, the immune system, and the inflammatory response.
2 Explain the physiologic effects of deficiencies of cortisol, aldosterone, and gonadotropins.
3 Differentiate the signs and symptoms of mineralocorticoid and glucocorticoid deficiencies.
4 Explain the general treatment principles of diseases caused by hormone deficiency or excess.
5 Differentiate between normal adrenal function and dysfunction.
6 Relate the pathophysiology of adrenal and pituitary diseases to the nursing management of patients with the diseases.
7 State the possible consequences of long-term steroid therapy.
8 Identify potential family pattern alterations and learning needs of patients experiencing Cushing's syndrome, acromegaly, hypopituitarism, and Addison's disease.
9 Develop a nursing care plan for the patient experiencing adrenal or pituitary dysfunction.

KEY TERMS

acromegaly
addisonian crisis
Addison's disease
central diabetes insipidus
Cushing's syndrome
diabetes insipidus (DI)
hypopituitarism
nephrogenic diabetes insipidus
pheochromocytomas
primary hyperaldosteronism
secondary hyperaldosteronism
syndrome of inappropriate secretion of antidiuretic hormone (SIADH)

Chapter Outline	Lecture Strategies

Hypothalamic dysfunction
    Definition/etiology
    Pathophysiology
    Clinical manifestations
Nursing management of the patient with
    hypothalamic dysfunction
    Assessment
	
	Ask students to describe disruptions that would occur if the homeostatic or endocrine functions were disrupted.

Chapter Outline	Lecture Strategies

Planning/implementation
Continuity of care
 	
Disorders of the Anterior Pituitary Gland
 	
Hypopituitarism
   Definition
   Etiology/epidemiology
   Pathophysiology
	Critical Thinking: Describe the pathophysiologic changes associated with hypopituitarism, diabetes insipidus, SIADH, Cushing's syndrome, and Addison's disease.
	
	VIEWSTUDY image #266 demonstrates the pathophysiology of the syndrome of inappropriate antidiuretic hormone.
	
	VIEWSTUDY image #274 illustrates the hypothalamic-pituitary-gonadal axis.

Clinical manifestations Diagnostic tests	**Critical Thinking:** Why are the signs and symptoms of mineralocorticoid deficiency different from those of glucocorticoid deficiency? Ask students what they would expect a patient to exhibit if the patient were experiencing acromegaly.

Collaborative management
      Hormone replacement therapy
      Emergency treatment
Nursing management of the patient with
   hypopituitarism
   Assessment
   Nursing diagnosis
   Planning/expected outcomes
   Implementation
   Evaluation/documentation
   Continuity of care
Hyperpituitarism: acromegaly
   Definition
   Etiology/epidemiology
   Pathophysiology
   Clinical manifestations
      Diagnostic tests
   Collaborative management
      Surgery
      Radiotherapy
      Pharmacotherapy
Nursing management of the patient with acromegaly
   Assessment
   Nursing diagnosis
   Planning/expected outcomes
   Implementation
   Evaluation/documentation
   Continuity of care
	Review interactions, side effects, and nursing activities associated with mineralocorticoids and glucosteroids.

Chapter Outline	Lecture Strategies

Posterior Pituitary Dysfunction

Diabetes insipidus
   Definition
   Etiology/epidemiology
   Pathophysiology
   Clinical manifestations
      Diagnostic tests
   Collaborative management
Nursing management of the patient with diabetes
   insipidus
   Assessment
   Nursing diagnosis
   Planning/expected outcomes
   Implementation
   Evaluation/documentation
   Continuity of care
Syndrome of inappropriate secretion of antidiuretic
   hormone
   Definition
   Etiology/pathophysiology
   Clinical manifestations
   Collaborative management
Nursing management of the patient with SIADH
   Assessment
   Nursing diagnosis
   Planning/expected outcomes
   Implementation
   Evaluation/documentation
   Continuity of care

Adrenal Gland Dysfunction

Addison's disease
   Definition
   Etiology/epidemiology
   Pathophysiology
   Clinical manifestations
      Diagnostic tests
   Collaborative management
   Management of addisonian crisis
Nursing management of the patient with Addison's
   disease
   Assessment
   Nursing diagnosis
   Planning/expected outcomes
   Implementation
   Evaluation/documentation
   Continuity of care

Cushing's syndrome
   Definition
   Etiology/epidemiology

VIEWSTUDY image #265 demonstrates the physiology of release or restriction of antidiuretic hormone.

Ask students to speculate as to the signs and symptoms that the patient will display.

Ask students to generate appropriate nursing diagnoses.

Review interactions and nursing activities associated with the drugs in Table 45-2.

Ask students to recall the signs and symptoms of hyponatremia.

Ask students to describe the types of assessment they would make for this patient.

Critical Thinking: Explain the hormonal and physiologic differences between diseases of the adrenal cortex and those of the adrenal medulla.

TA 83 illustrates pathophysiologic alterations that accompany adrenocortical insufficiency.

Critical Thinking: What are the possible side effects and consequences of long-term steroid therapy?

Critical Thinking: A 62-year-old man has had long-standing adrenal insufficiency and was recently admitted for treatment of pneumococcal pneumonia. His physician has written orders for intravenous fluids, intravenous cortisol, and stat electrolytes. What is the rationale for these orders? Identify three patient-centered goals, and prioritize your nursing interventions.

VIEWSTUDY image #267 shows common characteristics of Cushing's syndrome.

Chapter Outline	Lecture Strategies

Chapter Outline

Pathophysiology/clinical manifestations
    Diagnostic tests
Collaborative management
Nursing management of the patient with Cushing's syndrome
Assessment
Nursing diagnosis
Planning/expected outcomes
Implementation
Evaluation/documentation
Continuity of care
Hyperaldosteronism
Definition/etiology/epidemiology
Pathophysiology

Clinical manifestations
    Diagnostic tests
Collaborative management
Nursing management of the patient with hyperaldosteronism
Assessment
Nursing diagnosis
Planning/expected outcomes
Implementation
Evaluation/documentation
Adrenal medullary disease: pheochromocytoma
Definition
Etiology/epidemiology
Pathophysiology
Clinical manifestations
    Diagnostic tests
Collaborative management
Nursing management of the patient with pheochromocytoma
Assessment
Nursing diagnosis
Planning/expected outcomes

Implementation
Evaluation/documentation
Continuity of care

Lecture Strategies

Critical Thinking: Outline nursing care plans for patients with hypopituitarism, diabetes insipidus, Cushing's syndrome, and Addison's disease.

Critical Thinking: Outline the postoperative goals and nursing priorities for patients undergoing pituitary or adrenal surgery.

Use **TA 84** to discuss pathophysiologic events in hyperaldosteronism.

Ask students to describe signs and symptoms that might be associated with hyperaldosteronism.

Ask students to speculate on the clinical manifestations.

Critical Thinking: Ms. J, a 40-year-old woman, was recently admitted with a diagnosis of possible pheochromocytoma. After eating breakfast she complains of her heart "pounding" in her chest, sweating, and nausea. Identify and prioritize your nursing assessments and interventions.

Critical Thinking: Why is it important to assess coping skills and family functioning of patients with adrenal or pituitary diseases?

Related Skills

1. Using a laboratory setting, ask the students to respond to the following situation by carrying out appropriate nursing actions.
2. May B., 20 years of age, is admitted for evaluation and stabilization following a recent bout of pneumonia. Her diagnosis is Addison's disease. Shortly after admission, she appears confused and complains of abdominal pain and nausea. Her blood pressure is 75/38 (admission blood pressure was 108/62). What will you need to do?

Related Clinical Skills

1. Assign students to patients who are diagnosed with pituitary, hypothalamus, or adrenal disorders. Ensure that students are aware of the emergencies that can arise with these patients and are aware of the appropriate actions to take.
2. Assign the students to a home health nurse. Prepare a postoperative teaching plan for a patient undergoing an adrenalectomy.

CHAPTER 46

Nursing Management of Adults with Thyroid or Parathyroid Disorders

LEARNING OBJECTIVES

1 Correlate the pathophysiology of common thyroid and parathyroid disorders with their typical clinical manifestations.
2 Perform an appropriate nursing assessment for patients with thyroid or parathyroid disorders.
3 Identify nursing goals associated with the commonly encountered nursing diagnoses.
4 Develop strategies for nursing interventions aimed at meeting the defined goals, and discuss the rationale for the use of each strategy.
5 Discuss the nursing implications associated with common medications used to treat thyroid and parathyroid disorders.
6 Develop patient education guides for patients with common disorders of the thyroid or parathyroid glands.
7 Discuss the psychosocial implications of the symptoms associated with thyroid and parathyroid disorders.
8 Identify potential complications of thyroid and parathyroid disorders, and describe appropriate nursing assessment and intervention strategies.

KEY TERMS

Chvostek's sign
exophthalmos
glycosaminoglycans
goiter
mucopolysaccharides
myxedema
nephrocalcinosis
oligomenorrhea
proptosis
tetany
thyrotoxic crisis
thyrotoxicosis
Trousseau's sign

Chapter Outline	Lecture Strategies
Hyperthyroidism	
Graves' disease Definition	Ask students to review the structure, functions, and hormones of the thyroid. **VIEWSTUDY** image #261 illustrates the frontal view of the thyroid gland.
Etiology/epidemiology	**Critical Thinking:** How does Graves' disease cause hypersecretion of thyroid hormone?
Pathophysiology	**Critical Thinking:** What diagnostic tests would be useful in diagnosing Graves' disease?

Chapter Outline	Lecture Strategies
Complications	Ask students to describe the effects and symptoms of hypermetabolism.
Clinical manifestations	
Collaborative management	
Drug therapy	**Critical Thinking:** What patient education is appropriate for patients receiving propylthiouracil?
Treatment of ophthalmopathy	
Sodium ^{131}I	
Surgical intervention	Discuss interactions, side effects, and nursing activities associated with PTU and methimazole.
Nursing management of the patient with Graves' disease	
Assessment	**Critical Thinking:** What components should be included in a nursing history and assessment of Graves' disease?
Nursing diagnosis	
Planning/expected outcomes	
Implementation	
Eye care	
Drug therapy	
Sodium ^{131}I therapy	**Critical Thinking:** What should be included in the care before and after surgery for a patient undergoing thyroidectomy?
Preoperative care	
Postoperative care	**TA 85** shows Chvostek's sign and Trousseau's sign.
Evaluation/documentation	
Continuity of care	
Thyrotoxic crisis	**Critical Thinking:** What are the classic symptoms of thyrotoxicosis?
Thyroiditis	
Hypothyroidism	Ask students to list dietary sources of iodine.
Definition	**Critical Thinking:** What are some early symptoms of hypothyroidism?
Etiology/epidemiology	
Pathophysiology	
Goiter	
Hypometabolism	
Clinical manifestations	
Collaborative management	**Critical Thinking:** What is the goal of hormone replacement therapy in hypothyroidism?
Drug therapy	Ask students to review actions, interactions, side effects, and nursing activities associated with drugs in Table 46-2.
Nursing management of the patient with hypothyroidism	
Assessment	
Nursing diagnosis	
Planning/expected outcomes	
Implementation	Ask students to discuss reasons for the various nursing interventions.
General care	
Drug therapy	**Critical Thinking:** What nursing strategies could be used to increase comfort for a patient with hypothyroidism?
Evaluation/documentation	**Critical Thinking:** How would you evaluate the effectiveness of the care for patients with hypothyroidism?
Continuity of care	

Chapter Outline	Lecture Strategies
Myxedema coma	**Critical Thinking:** Why do patients who develop myxedema coma have such low core body temperatures?
	The symptoms are generally opposite to those in thyroid storm.
	Critical Thinking: What causes a goiter to develop?
Thyroid nodules and cancer	
Hyperparathyroidism	
Definition	Ask students to review location, functions, and secretions of the parathyroid glands.
Etiology/epidemiology	
Pathophysiology	**Critical Thinking:** How does hyperparathyroidism produce symptoms of hypercalcemia?
Clinical manifestations	**Critical Thinking:** What are the common symptoms of hypercalcemia?
Collaborative management	**Critical Thinking:** How is acute hypercalcemia treated?
Surgical management	
Medical management	
Nursing management of the patient with hyper-parathyroidism	
Assessment	Patients with psychiatric symptoms should be evaluated carefully because psychiatric disturbance may result from hyperparathyroidism.
Nursing diagnosis	
Planning/expected outcomes	
Implementation	
Preoperative and postoperative care	
Evaluation/documentation	
Continuity of care	
Hypoparathyroidism	**Critical Thinking:** What patients are at risk for developing hypocalcemia?
Definition	
Clinical manifestations	**Critical Thinking:** What are the classic features of tetany?
Collaborative management	
Nursing management of the patient with hypoparathyroidism	Ask students to recall symptoms of calcium deficiency.
Assessment	
Nursing diagnosis	
Planning/expected outcomes	
Implementation	
Evaluation/documentation	
Continuity of care	**Critical Thinking:** What education should be given to the patient about the ongoing management of hypoparathyroidism?

Related Skills

1. With students in triads, have them practice patient education related to a specific antithyroid drug. The third student will act as an observer and comment on clarity, knowledge, and interaction with the "patient."

Related Clinical Skills

1. Assign students to patients with thyroid or parathyroid problems. Emphasize the need for close monitoring and teaching.
2. Assign students to an elderly patient who has signs and symptoms of calcium deficiency. Develop a teaching plan to correct these symptoms.
3. Assign students to a homebound patient recovering postoperatively from either hyperthyroidism or hyperparathyroidism. Develop a teaching plan about the ongoing pharmacologic management of either disorder.

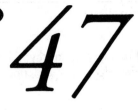

47 Nursing Management of Adults with Diabetes Mellitus

LEARNING OBJECTIVES

1 Define and classify the different types of diabetes mellitus.
2 Distinguish between the pathogenesis associated with insulin- dependent diabetes mellitus and non–insulin-dependent diabetes mellitus.
3 Compare the classifications of diabetes in terms of clinical manifestations.
4 Differentiate among laboratory tests associated with the diagnosis or monitoring of diabetes mellitus.
5 Identify advantages of self-monitoring of blood glucose.
6 List nutrition and exercise goals for diabetes management.
7 Compare and differentiate insulin preparations based on type, source, and concentration.
8 Compare and contrast the various insulin therapy regimens.
9 Describe the action of sulfonylureas.
10 Discuss the impact of diabetes in both young and older adults.
11 Discuss the concept of diabetic control.
12 Explain the basic components of the teaching plan for acute and chronic complications associated with diabetes mellitus.
13 Relate the importance of the concept of self-management in diabetes care.

KEY TERMS

conventional insulin therapy
counterregulatory hormones
diabetes mellitus
diabetic ketoacidosis (DKA)
endocrine
exocrine
euglycemia
glucagon
gluconeogenesis
glycogenolysis
glyconeogenesis
hyperglycemia
hypoglycemia
insulinopenic
intensive conventional therapy (ICT)
islet cell antibodies (ICAs)
islets of Langerhans
lactic acidosis
neuropathy
non–insulin-dependent diabetes mellitus (NIDDM)
paresthesia
polydipsia
polyuria
retinopathy
self-monitoring of blood glucose (SMBG)
sulfonylurea

Chapter Outline	Lecture Strategies

Diabetes mellitus
   Definition
   Classification
      Insulin-dependent diabetes mellitus
      Non–insulin-dependent diabetes mellitus
      Other types of diabetes mellitus
      Impaired glucose tolerance
      Gestational diabetes mellitus	

Chapter Outline	Lecture Strategies

Etiology/epidemiology
   Insulin-dependent diabetes mellitus
      Autoimmune mechanism
      Genetic predisposition
   Non–insulin-dependent diabetes mellitus
      Family history
      Obesity
Pathophysiology
   Insulin secretion
   Insulin receptors and insulin action
Pathogenesis of IDDM and NIDDM
   IDDM
      Glucagon
      Epinephrine
      Growth hormone
      Cortisol
   NIDDM
Clinical manifestations
   Diagnostic tests
      Fasting plasma glucose
      Glycosylated hemoglobin
      Serum fructosamine
      C-peptide
      Urine testing for glucose
      Urine testing for ketones
 	
Self-monitoring of blood glucose
 	
Diet therapy
   Achieving nutritional goals for IDDM
   Achieving nutritional goals for NIDDM
   Nutrition planning
      Calories from carbohydrates
      Calories from fat
      Calories from protein
   Exchange system
   Nutrition education
 	
Exercise therapy
   Exercise planning
   Exercise and IDDM
   Exercise and NIDDM
 	
Drug therapy
   Insulins
      Routes of insulin delivery
      Initiating insulin treatment
	Ask students to differentiate the clinical manifestations and etiology of the two major types of diabetes mellitus.
	
	Critical Thinking: Explain the progression of micro-angiopathy and macroangiopathy in diabetes mellitus in relation to its impact on target organs.
	
	TA 86 is helpful in discussing complications of IDDM and NIDDM.
	
	Describe the use in diagnosing diabetes mellitus of the following: fasting plasma glucose, glycosylated hemoglobin, serum fructosamine, C-peptide, urine testing for glucose, and urine testing for ketones.
	
	Critical Thinking: Discuss the major laboratory tests used to diagnose and monitor diabetes mellitus.
	
	Critical Thinking: What guidelines should be used in recommending SMBG in diabetes management?
	
	Critical Thinking: What are the implications of achieving metabolic control in diabetes mellitus?
	
	Critical Thinking: Compare dietary goals in IDDM versus NIDDM. What is the rationale for each goal?
	
	Ask students to explain how the exchange system works. It is very possible that some students may have had experiences with this system that they can share with the class, if class size and time permit.
	
	Critical Thinking: Describe the exercise guidelines to be provided a patient with IDDM. How do these guidelines differ from those with NIDDM?
	
	Ask, "Why is the choice of insulin therapy a more controversial decision in NIDDM?"

Chapter Outline	Lecture Strategies

Insulin regimens
    Two injections per day
    Three injections per day
    Multidose insulin
    Insulin pumps
  Administration of insulin
  Insulin therapy in NIDDM
Oral hypoglycemic agents
  Metformin
  Acarbose
Combination therapy
	Critical Thinking: What is the rationale for using insulin in patients with NIDDM?
	
	Critical Thinking: How does insulin action differ from that of the oral hypoglycemic agents?
	
	Critical Thinking: Can oral hypoglycemic agents be used in IDDM? Why or why not?

Nursing management of the patient with diabetes
mellitus
 	
  Assessment
  Nursing diagnosis
  Planning/expected outcomes
 	
  Implementation
    Young and middle adulthood
 	
    Older adulthood
 	
  Evaluation/documentation
	VIDEO Volume 7 presents nursing care of the diabetic patient, including coverage of hypoglycemic reaction and foot care.
	
	Critical Thinking: Discuss the psychosocial implications that a diagnosis of diabetes mellitus has for the patient and for the family.
	
	Critical Thinking: Describe the component of the following diabetic teaching plans: survival, in-depth, continuing education.
	
	Ask students to describe how the special considerations of the elderly should influence nursing care plans.
	
	Critical Thinking: What is the role of the nurse in diabetes education? The role of the patient?
	
	Critical Thinking: Identify organizations available to assist the diabetic patient.

Acute complications of diabetes
 	
Diabetic ketoacidosis
  Etiology/epidemiology
  Pathophysiology
  Complications and mortality
  Collaborative management
Nursing management of the patient with diabetic
  ketoacidosis
    Assessment
    Nursing diagnosis
    Planning/expected outcomes
    Implementation
    Evaluation/documentation
Hyperglycemic hyperosmolar nonketotic coma
  Etiology/epidemiology
	
	VIEWSTUDY image #263 illustrates diabetic ketoacidosis.
	
	VIEWSTUDY image #264 demonstrates the pathophysiology of hyperglycemic hyperosmolar nonketosis.
	
	Critical Thinking: Describe the process whereby diabetes mellitus results in hyperglycemia, hyperlipidemia, and hyperaminoacidemia.

Chapter Outline	Lecture Strategies

Nursing management of the patient with hyperglycemic hyperosmolar nonketotic coma
    Assessment
    Nursing diagnosis
    Planning/expected outcomes
    Implementation
    Evaluation/documentation
Hypoglycemia
    Definition
    Etiology
    Clinical manifestations
    Collaborative management
        Somogyi effect
        Dawn phenomenon
 	
        Sick-day management
 	
Nursing care of the patient with diabetic hypoglycemia
    Assessment
    Nursing diagnosis
    Planning/expected outcomes
    Implementation
    Evaluation/documentation
 	
Chronic complications of diabetes: microvascular disease
 	
Diabetic retinopathy
    Pathophysiology
        Nonproliferative retinopathy
        Preproliferative retinopathy
        Proliferative retinopathy
    Collaborative management
Other eye disorders
Nursing management of the patient with diabetic eye disease
    Assessment
    Nursing diagnosis
    Planning/expected outcomes
    Implementation
    Evaluation/documentation
Diabetic nephropathy
    Pathophysiology
Nursing management of the patient with diabetic nephropathy
    Assessment
    Nursing diagnosis
    Planning/expected outcomes
    Implementation
    Evaluation/documentation
Diabetic neuropathy
    Sensorimotor neuropathies
        Diabetic polyneuropathy
	VIEWSTUDY image #262 shows the Somogyi effect.
	
	Ask students to define "Somogyi effect" and "dawn phenomenon."
	
	TA 87 offers a critical thinking guide for discussing hypoglycemia.
	
	Outline preventative measures for hypoglycemia.
	
	Identify the diabetic triopathy of complications: retinopathy, nephropathy, and neuropathy.
	
	Differentiate the manifestations of nonproliferative, preproliferative, and proliferative retinopathy.
	
	Ask students to describe three changes that occur soon after diagnosis of diabetic nephropathy.
	
	Describe distal and contact paresthesias.

Chapter Outline	Lecture Strategies

Autonomic neuropathies
  Gastrointestinal tract
  Genitourinary tract
  Cardiovascular system
  Sudomotor dysfunction
Nursing management of the patient with diabetic neuropathy
  Assessment
  Nursing diagnosis
  Planning/expected outcomes
  Implementation
  Evaluation/documentation

Chronic complications of diabetes: macrovascular disease

Atherosclerosis

Coronary heart disease

Hypertension
Hyperlipidemia
Nursing management of the patient with diabetic atherosclerosis
  Assessment
  Nursing diagnosis
  Planning/expected outcomes
  Implementation
  Evaluation/documentation
Peripheral vascular disease
Diabetic foot
  Etiology
  Pathophysiology
  Clinical manifestations
  Collaborative management
Nursing management of the patient with diabetic foot
  Assessment
  Nursing diagnosis
  Planning/expected outcomes
  Implementation
  Evaluation/documentation
Other peripheral vascular complications
  Skin disorders
  Infections
  Oral complications
Nursing management of the patient with other peripheral vascular complications
  Nursing diagnosis
  Planning/expected outcomes
  Implementation
  Evaluation/documentation
Continuity of care

Lecture Strategies column:

Outline the progressive nature of macrovascular complications associated with atherosclerosis.

Contrast the occurrence of coronary heart disease in the diabetic versus the nondiabetic patient.

Ask students to identify some of the more common sources of breaks in the skin leading to diabetic foot lesions. Use Table 47-8 to discuss warning signs and symptoms.

Related Skills

1. In the laboratory setting, have students practice drawing up and administering different types of insulin. Outline a rotation system for injections. Have students practice using a glucometer.

Related Clinical Skills

1. Assign students to patients newly diagnosed with diabetes. Have them evaluate the patient's knowledge of insulin, meal planning, foot care, and rotation of insulin sites.
2. Have students accompany a home health nurse while he or she is preparing insulin syringes for a homebound elderly patient. Also under the supervision of a home health nurse, have students determine the patient's fasting blood sugar by the use of a glucometer.

CHAPTER 48 Nursing Assessment of the Gastrointestinal System

LEARNING OBJECTIVES

1 Understand the basic structures and functions of the gastrointestinal system.
2 Describe the process by which the body's nutrients are digested and absorbed.
3 Obtain relevant subjective information from the patient who has a gastrointestinal alteration.
4 Using correct technique, examine the patient to obtain appropriate objective information about the gastrointestinal system.
5 Differentiate abnormal from normal subjective and objective findings related to the gastrointestinal system.
6 Describe tests involved in the diagnosis of disorders of the gastrointestinal system.
7 Discuss the patient care that is required for each of the tests involved in the diagnosis of disorders of the gastrointestinal system.

KEY TERMS

Bernstein test
buccal cavity
colon
colonoscopy
endoscopic retrograde cholangiopancreatography
esophagus
esophagogastroduodenoscopy
gallbladder
large intestine
liver
pancreas
percutaneous transhepatic cholangiogram
peristalsis
saliva
small intestine
stomach

Chapter Outline	Lecture Strategies
Anatomy and physiology Structural description	**VIEWSTUDY** image #180 shows the location of organs of the gastrointestinal system. **VIEWSTUDY** image #181 illustrates the parts of the stomach. **VIEWSTUDY** image #182 shows the anatomic location of the large intestine. **VIEWSTUDY** image #183 demonstrates gross structure: liver, gallbladder, pancreas, and the duct system. **VIEWSTUDY** image #184 shows the microscopic structure of a liver lobule. **VIEWSTUDY** image #194 shows a normal esophagus.

Chapter Outline	Lecture Strategies
Mouth	Ask students to describe the functions of saliva.
Esophagus	Ask students to define peristalsis.
	Critical Thinking: What is peristalsis and how does it aid in the digestion and absorption of nutrients?
Stomach Pancreas and liver Small intestine Large intestine Blood supply	Diagrams are useful. Ask students to locate the region of the stomach on themselves.

Chemical digestion and absorption of nutrients
  Carbohydrates
  Proteins
  Fats and fat-soluble vitamins
  Ions
  Water and water-soluble vitamins
	Critical Thinking: Describe the digestive process for each group of essential nutrients. In what GI tract organ does it begin and what are the final products of digestion?

Control of gastrointestinal motility and enzyme
  secretion
  Mouth
  Esophagus
	VIEWSTUDY image #185 shows bilirubin metabolism and conjugation.

Stomach
  Pancreas and gallbladder
  Intestines
  Colon	

Assessment Subjective	**VIEWSTUDY** image #186 depicts the abdominal quadrants.
	Ask students to speculate on areas that should be included in assessment. Much of this information may be obtained during assessment of other systems.

Objective
  General assessment
    Integumentary
    Oral cavity and pharynx
    Cardiovascular
    Respiratory
    Abdomen
	Explain the links between the functions of the gastrointestinal system and the following systems and features: (a) integumentary, (b) oral cavity and pharynx, (c) cardiovascular, (d) respiratory, (e) abdomen, (f) rectum, and (g) genitalia.

	Critical Thinking: Discuss psychologic and sociocultural factors to consider throughout the physical examination of the patient's abdomen.
	Discuss interpretations of the rebound, iliopsoas, obturator, tympany, and fluid wave tests.
Rectum Genitalia	**Critical Thinking:** Design at least three questions to discreetly ask patients about bowel patterns and characteristics of the stools.

Diagnostic and laboratory tests
  Computed tomography of the abdomen
  Ultrasonography
	Critical Thinking: Describe tests that are commonly used in the diagnosis of disorders of the gallbladder.

Chapter Outline	Lecture Strategies

Scintigraphy/nuclear scan
   Patient preparation
Magnetic resonance imaging
   Patient preparation
Diagnostic tests for disorders of the upper
gastrointestinal system
	Ensure that students understand not only the procedures (which may be familiar to some students by now) but also the purposes of scintigraphy and magnetic resonance imaging for gastrointestinal disorders.

Esophageal function studies
      Patient preparation
   Barium swallow
      Patient preparation
	Ask students what they would tell the patient about the test.

Esophagogastroduodenoscopy
      Patient preparation
      Postprocedure care
   Gastric analysis
      Basal gastric secretion rate
      Gastric acid stimulation test
      Patient preparation
   Small bowel biopsy
      Patient preparation
      Procedure
      Postprocedure care
   Blood tests
Diagnostic tests for diseases of the large bowel	

Barium enema
      Patient preparation
   Colonoscopy
      Patient preparation
      Postprocedure care
   Proctosigmoidoscopy
      Patient preparation
   Examinations of the stool
	Critical Thinking: Of what complications must patients who undergo barium studies be warned?

Occult blood test
      Patient preparation
   Stool culture
   Fecal fat
   Fecal urobilinogen
	Compare the usefulness of guaiac and HemoQuant in conducting this evaluation.

Diagnostic tests for diseases of the liver and biliary system	

Liver biopsy
      Patient preparation
      Postprocedure care
	Critical Thinking: Ask the students to explain why the platelet count must be determined before the test.

Laboratory tests for liver function
   Oral cholecystography
      Patient preparation
	Obtain films taken during cholecystography that show a normal gallbladder and one with stones.

Percutaneous transhepatic cholangiogram
      Patient preparation
      Postprocedure care
Diagnostic tests for diseases of the pancreas
   Endoscopic retrograde cholangiopancreatography
      Patient preparation
   Serum amylase and lipase
   Urine amylase	

Related Skills

1. Discuss, demonstrate, and then have students practice abdominal assessment. Select areas of the assessment at random, and have students demonstrate satisfactory performance of this area of the examination. Observe student assessment of bowel sounds.
2. Discuss collection of stool specimens and demonstrate the use of equipment used in the collection of specimens.
3. Arrange for students to visit the radiology department while examinations of the stomach, gallbladder, and liver are being performed.

Related Clinical Skills

1. Assign students to patients who are undergoing diagnostic tests related to disorders of the gastrointestinal system. Have the students prepare a pre- and postprocedure teaching plan for these patients.

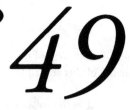

Nursing Management of Adults with Disorders of the Mouth or Esophagus

LEARNING OBJECTIVES

1 Explain the cause, treatment, and prevention of dental problems.
2 Discuss the oral changes and nursing management of the aging patient.
3 Describe the common infections of the oral cavity and treatment.
4 Identify common products for oral hygiene.
5 Explain the etiology of oral cavity carcinoma.
6 Describe nursing interventions for the patient with esophageal disorders.
7 Differentiate between malignant and benign conditions of the esophagus.

KEY TERMS

achalasia
aphthous ulcers
bougienage
candidiasis
dysphagia
erythroplakia
gastroesophageal
    reflux (GERD)
glossectomy
hiatal hernia

leukoplakia
lower esophageal
    sphincter (LES)
odynophagia
periodontal disease
plaque
pyrosis
regurgitation
stomatitis

Chapter Outline	Lecture Strategies

Dental problems

Dental caries
    Definition
    Etiology/epidemiology
    Pathophysiology
    Clinical manifestations

Periodontal disease
    Definition
    Etiology/epidemiology
    Pathophysiology

    Clinical manifestations
Nursing management of the patient with dental
    problems
    Assessment
    Nursing diagnosis
    Planning/expected outcomes

Critical Thinking: Discuss the cause, treatment, and prevention of dental problems.

VIEWSTUDY image #190 shows normal tooth structure.

Critical Thinking: Name the common infections of the oral cavity and medications used to treat them.

VIEWSTUDY image # 191 demonstrates the progression of periodontal disease.

VIEWSTUDY image #192 illustrates periodontitis.

Critical Thinking: What oral changes occur with aging?

Chapter Outline	Lecture Strategies

Implementation
    Oral hygiene
    Nutrition
    Fluoride
    Evaluation/documentation
 	
Disorders of the oral cavity
 	
Vincent's infection
    Definition
    Etiology/epidemiology
    Clinical manifestations
    Collaborative management
Candidiasis
    Definition
    Etiology/epidemiology
    Clinical manifestations
    Collaborative management
Aphthous ulcers
    Etiology/epidemiology
    Clinical manifestations
    Collaborative management
Herpes simplex virus
    Definition
    Etiology/epidemiology
    Clinical manifestations
Nursing management of the patient with oral
    infections
    Assessment
    Implementation
Carcinoma of the oral cavity
    Etiology/epidemiology
 	
    Clinical manifestations
    Collaborative management
        Specific diagnostic measures
        Medical management
        Surgical management
        Complications
Nursing management of the patient with oral cancer
    Assessment
    Nursing diagnosis
    Planning/expected outcomes/implementation
    Evaluation/documentation
    Continuity of care
 	
Esophageal disorders
 	
Gastroesophageal reflux
    Definition/etiology/epidemiology
    Pathophysiology
    Clinical manifestations
    Diagnostic procedures
	Review the classifications, dosages, side effects, and nursing activities associated with the medications.
	
	Emphasize that infections with herpes simplex virus produce systemic symptoms as well as cold sores.
	
	VIEWSTUDY image #193 shows the appearance of the neck after healing from a radical neck dissection.
	
	Break *leukoplakia* down into word components for easier retention.
	
	Ask students to consider how they would react if part of their tongue were removed.
	
	Critical Thinking: Discuss the long-term management and patient education for the person with GERD.

Chapter Outline	Lecture Strategies

Collaborative management
    Medical management
    Complications
    Surgical management
Nursing management of the patient with
  gastroesophageal reflux
  Assessment
  Nursing diagnosis
  Planning/expected outcomes
  Implementation
    Dietary management
    Postural therapy
    Behavior modification

    Drug therapy education
    Postoperative care
  Evaluation/documentation
Hiatal hernia
  Definition
  Etiology/epidemiology
  Clinical manifestations
  Collaborative management
Carcinoma of the esophagus
  Definition
  Etiology/epidemiology
  Pathophysiology
  Clinical manifestations
  Collaborative management
Nursing management of the patient with esophageal
  cancer
  Assessment
  Nursing diagnosis
  Planning/expected outcomes
  Implementation
  Evaluation/documentation
Achalasia
  Definition
  Etiology/epidemiology
  Pathophysiology
  Clinical manifestations
  Collaborative management
Nursing management of the patient with achalasia
Esophageal diverticulum
Esophageal strictures

Diagrams are useful in the visualization of surgeries.

VIEWSTUDY image #198 demonstrates placement of a gastrostomy tube.

VIEWSTUDY image #199 shows a Janeway gastrostomy.

VIEWSTUDY image #200 shows a percutaneous endoscopic gastroscopy.

Patients need instruction in how to take antacids effectively. Have students review dosages, side effects, interactions, and nursing activities associated with antacids.

VIEWSTUDY image #195 demonstrates the Nissen fundoplication for repair of hiatal hernia.

Critical Thinking: What are the differences between malignant and benign conditions of the esophagus?

VIEWSTUDY image #196 illustrates esophageal achalasia.

VIEWSTUDY image #197 shows how pneumatic dilation attempts to treat achalasia.

Critical Thinking: Discuss appropriate nursing interventions for the patient with esophageal disorders.

Related Skills

1. Review and then observe as students practice care of gastrostomy tubes.
2. Review and then observe as students practice mouth care.

Related Clinical Skills

1. Assign students to patients undergoing surgery for disorders of the mouth or esophagus.
2. Assign students to a home health patient with a PEG tube. Have students develop a teaching plan for family members in the care of the PEG tube and enteral feeding.

50 Nursing Management of Adults with Disorders of the Stomach or Duodenum

LEARNING OBJECTIVES

1 Describe the cause of acute and chronic gastritis.
2 Differentiate between chronic gastric and duodenal ulcer disease and acute stress ulcers.
3 Identify subjective data in the assessment of patients with peptic ulcer disease.
4 Compare actions and side effects of the agents used to treat peptic ulcer disease.
5 Describe areas of noncompliance for the patient with peptic ulcer disease.
6 Apply the nursing process to a patient who has peptic ulcer disease.
7 Identify preoperative nursing interventions for the patient undergoing gastric surgery.
8 Identify potential postoperative complications of gastric surgery.
9 Describe nursing interventions for a patient with gastrointestinal tract bleeding.
10 Develop a teaching plan for a patient experiencing the dumping syndrome.
11 Describe the care of the patient after gastric surgery.

KEY TERMS

antrectomy
Billroth I & II procedures
dumping syndrome
duodenal ulcer
gastric ulcer
gastritis
hematochezia

histamine H$_2$ receptor blockers
intrinsic factor
peptic ulcer
pyloroplasty
stress ulcer
vagotomy

Chapter Outline	Lecture Strategies

Acute gastritis
    Definition
    Etiology/epidemiology
    Pathophysiology
    Clinical manifestations
    Collaborative management
Nursing management of the patient with acute gastritis
    Assessment
    Nursing diagnosis
    Planning/expected outcomes
    Implementation
	Critical Thinking: What are the causes of acute and chronic gastritis?
	
	VIEWSTUDY image #201 illustrates the stimuli that are involved in the act of vomiting.
	
	VIEWSTUDY image #203 illustrates disruption of gastric mucosa and pathophysiologic consequences of back-diffusion of acids.

Chapter Outline	Lecture Strategies
	VIEWSTUDY image #204 demonstrates the relationship between mucosal blood flow and disruption of the gastric mucosal barrier.
Chronic gastritis	
Etiology/epidemiology	
Pathophysiology	
Clinical manifestations	
Collaborative management	
Nursing management of the patient with chronic gastritis	
Assessment	
Nursing diagnosis	
Implementation	
Evaluation/documentation	
Peptic ulcer disease	
Definition	**VIEWSTUDY** image #202 shows peptic ulcers.
Epidemiology	Compare and contrast the most common symptoms of peptic ulcer disease.
	Critical Thinking: What are complications that can occur from peptic ulcer disease?
	Critical Thinking: Discuss predisposing factors for gastric ulcer occurrence.
Gastric ulcers	
Etiology	
Pathophysiology	Briefly outline the factors that protect the gastric mucosa. Students should understand the differences in acid production.
Duodenal ulcers	Stress that duodenal ulcers are associated with hypersecretion, and gastric ulcers with lowered gastric mucosal resistance.
Etiology	
Pathophysiology	
Clinical manifestations	**Critical Thinking:** Differentiate between gastric and duodenal ulcer disease and stress ulcers.
	VIEWSTUDY image #205 shows a duodenal ulcer of the posterior wall penetrating into the head of the pancreas, resulting in a walled-off perforation.
Complications	Carefully differentiate between hematemesis and hemoptysis because these may be confused.
Gastrointestinal tract bleeding	**TA 89** shows clinical manifestations of upper GI bleeding.
Hemorrhage	
Perforation	
Penetration	**Critical Thinking:** What are the appropriate nursing interventions for a patient with GI bleeding?
Obstruction	Encourage students to speculate on the clinical manifestations of pyloric obstruction.

Chapter Outline	Lecture Strategies
Collaborative management Pharmacologic therapy	**Critical Thinking:** What are the actions and side effects of major anti-ulcer agents? **Critical Thinking:** Discuss the administration and scheduling of major anti-ulcer agents.
Antacids	Review nursing activities associated with antacids. Discuss the pros and cons of at-home remedies such as baking soda and Tums.

Histamine H_2 receptor blockers
Mucosal healing agents
   Antibiotic therapy
   Diet therapy
   Surgical treatment
      Gastric resection
      Vagotomy
      Pyloroplasty
   Postoperative complications
	Review nursing activities associated with cimetidine and ranitidine.
	
	TA 88 illustrates surgical procedures in peptic ulcer disease.
	
	Critical Thinking: What are the potential postoperative complications of gastric surgery?

Dumping syndrome
      Diarrhea
      Reflux esophagitis
      Nutritional deficits
         Weight loss
         Malabsorption
         Lactose deficiency
	Set up the initial scenario in which food is dumped into the duodenum and jejunum and ask students to speculate on the sequelae.
	
	Review food restrictions of a lactose-free diet.

Vitamin and mineral deficiencies
Nursing management of the patient with peptic ulcer
   disease
   Assessment
   Nursing diagnosis
   Planning/expected outcomes
   Implementation
      Medications
      Diet
      Bleeding/perforation
      Anxiety
   Evaluation/documentation
   Continuity of care
Nursing management of the patient with gastrointestinal bleeding
   Assessment
   Nursing diagnosis
   Planning/expected outcomes
   Implementation
   Evaluation/documentation
Nursing management of the patient who has undergone gastric surgery
   Assessment
	Ask students to speculate as to the cause of the anemias.
	
	Ask students to describe what the nurse might focus on in assessment.
	
	Critical Thinking: List appropriate subjective data in the assessment of patients with peptic ulcer disease.

Chapter Outline	Lecture Strategies

Nursing diagnosis
Planning/expected outcomes
Implementation
Evaluation/documentation
Stress ulcers
   Definition/etiology/epidemiology
   Pathophysiology
   Clinical manifestations/collaborative management
Nursing management of the patient with stress ulcers
Gastric cancer
   Etiology
   Epidemiology
   Pathophysiology
   Clinical manifestations
   Collaborative management
Nursing management of the patient after surgery for
   gastric cancer
   Assessment
   Nursing diagnosis
   Planning/expected outcomes
   Implementation
   Evaluation/documentation
 	
   Continuity of care
	
	Ask students to describe appropriate nursing interventions.
	
	Critical Thinking: Identify nursing interventions for the preoperative patient having gastric surgery.
	
	Critical Thinking: Discuss postoperative care of the patient who has had surgery for gastric cancer.
	
	VIEWSTUDY image #206 shows a total gastrectomy for gastric cancer.

Related Skills

1. Discuss the principles and technique of inserting nasogastric and lavage tubes. Discuss and demonstrate the management of nasogastric suction, irrigations, and lavage.

Related Clinical Skills

1. Assign students to patients who are either awaiting gastric surgery or who are convalescing from gastric surgery, or to patients who are in the initial stages of diagnosis and intervention for peptic ulcer disease. Emphasize the need for thorough assessment and teaching, and provide supervision for procedures as needed.
2. Assign students to a homebound patient who is recovering from gastrectomy. Have students develop a teaching plan focusing on nutritional needs for this patient.

51 Nursing Management of Adults with Intestinal Disorders

LEARNING OBJECTIVES

1 Identify nursing interventions for the patient experiencing constipation and diarrhea.

2 Identify nursing interventions and resources to support the nutritional needs of patients with malabsorption syndromes.

3 Discuss the nursing care related to the prevention and management of intestinal infections.

4 Compare the disease processes of ulcerative colitis and Crohn's disease.

5 Discuss the long-term care requirements of the patient with inflammatory bowel disease.

6 Describe the preoperative and postoperative care for the patient having bowel surgery.

7 Compare the different types of ostomies in terms of their function and care requirements.

8 Identify nursing interventions for irrigation and pouch application for a patient with an ostomy.

9 Discuss peristomal skin problems in terms of causes, prevention, and management.

10 Develop patient education guides for patients with ostomies.

11 Discuss the nursing management for a patient with diverticular disease.

12 Explain the pathophysiology of intestinal obstruction.

13 Identify the nurse's role in screening tests for colorectal cancer.

KEY TERMS

appendicitis
celiac disease
colorectal cancer
colostomy
constipation
Crohn's disease
diarrhea
diverticulitis
diverticulosis
effluent
fistula
Hartmann's pouch
hemorrhoids
hernia
ileoanal anastomosis
ileostomy
Kock's pouch
lactose intolerance
peritonitis
polyps
proctocolectomy
short bowel syndrome
steatorrhea
ulcerative colitis

Chapter Outline	Lecture Strategies
Constipation (inactive colon, colonic stasis)	
Definition	
Etiology/epidemiology	
Pathophysiology	
Clinical manifestations	
Collaborative management	
Diarrhea	
Definition	

Chapter Outline	Lecture Strategies
Etiology/epidemiology	
Pathophysiology	
Clinical manifestations	
Collaborative management	
Nursing management of the patient with constipation or diarrhea	
Assessment	
Nursing diagnosis	
Planning/expected outcomes	
Implementation	
Evaluation/documentation	
Continuity of care	
Malabsorption syndromes	
Lactose intolerance (lactase deficiency)	**Critical Thinking:** Describe the relationship between the intake of lactose and gluten and the development of malabsorption syndromes.
Definition	
Etiology/epidemiology	
Pathophysiology	
Clinical manifestations	Ask students to give examples of foods containing lactose.
Collaborative management	
Adult celiac disease	
Definition	
Etiology/epidemiology	
Pathophysiology	
Clinical manifestations	
Collaborative management	
Nursing management of the patient with malabsorption syndromes	
Assessment	
Nursing diagnosis	
Planning/expected outcomes	
Implementation	**Critical Thinking:** Outline a teaching plan for the patient with a malabsorption syndrome.
Evaluation/documentation	
Continuity of care	
Intestinal infections	**Critical Thinking:** Describe how agent-host factors play a role in the development of an intestinal infection.
Etiology/epidemiology	
Pathophysiology	
Clinical manifestations	
Collaborative management	
Nursing management of the patient with intestinal infections	
Assessment	
Nursing diagnosis	
Planning/expected outcomes	
Implementation	**Critical Thinking:** Identify the nursing interventions for the management of a patient with an intestinal infection.
Evaluation/documentation	
Continuity of care	
Inflammatory bowel syndrome: ulcerative colitis and Crohn's disease	
Definition	Use **TA 90** to discuss similarities and differences in Crohn's disease and ulcerative colitis.
Etiology	
Epidemiology	
Pathophysiology	Emphasize that the underlying process in both diseases is an inflammatory one.

Chapter Outline	Lecture Strategies

Clinical manifestations
    Long-term effects
Collaborative management
    Drug treatment
    Surgical management
	Critical Thinking: Compare and contrast the disease processes of ulcerative colitis and Crohn's disease.
	
	Ask students to delineate on paper differences and similarities in the two diseases from classroom and reading materials.

Nursing management of the patient with inflammatory
    bowel disease
    Assessment
    Nursing diagnosis
    Planning/expected outcomes
    Implementation
    Evaluation/documentation
    Continuity of care
Acute appendicitis
    Definition
    Etiology/epidemiology
    Pathophysiology
    Clinical manifestations
    Collaborative management
Nursing management of the patient with acute
    appendicitis
    Assessment
    Nursing diagnosis
    Planning/expected outcomes
    Implementation
    Evaluation/documentation
    Continuity of care
Diverticular disease
    Definition
    Etiology
	Use a diagram to illustrate the location of the appendix vermiformis.
	
	Appendicitis is commonly known. Students may be able to describe signs and symptoms.
	
	Students will likely be able to define *diverticulitis* once the meaning of *diverticula* is known.

Clinical manifestations Peritonitis	**Critical Thinking:** Explain the problems experienced by the patient with diverticular disease. **VIEWSTUDY** image #214 shows that diverticula are outpouchings of the colon. **VIEWSTUDY** image #215 presents complications of diverticulitis. Ask students to speculate as to the sources of bacteria and chemical irritants.
Collaborative management	Review the actions, side effects, and nursing activities associated with common stool softeners and laxatives.
Surgical treatment	**Critical Thinking:** Describe the postoperative preparation for the patient having bowel surgery. **Critical Thinking:** Identify the primary differences between an ileostomy and a colostomy in terms of function and care requirements.

Chapter Outline	Lecture Strategies

Nursing management of the patient with diverticular disease
    Assessment
    Nursing diagnosis
    Planning/expected outcomes
    Implementation
    Evaluation/documentation
    Continuity of care
	Critical Thinking: Describe how the nurse can prevent and manage peristomal skin problems.
	
	Changes in vision, hearing, and dexterity in the geriatric patient affect the ability to learn self-care quickly.

Abdominal wall hernia
    Definition
    Etiology/pathophysiology/clinical manifestations
    Collaborative management
Nursing management of the patient with abdominal wall hernia
    Assessment
    Nursing diagnosis
    Planning/expected outcomes
    Implementation
    Evaluation/documentation
    Continuity of care
	Demonstrate splinting an incision.

Intestinal obstruction
    Definition
    Etiology/epidemiology
	Ask students which area of the bowel, in terms of lumen, would be most likely to become obstructed.

Pathophysiology
    Clinical manifestations
    Collaborative management
	Outline the mechanisms causing fluid volume deficit.
	
	TA 92 depicts pathophysiologic events in intestinal obstruction.

Nursing management of the patient with intestinal obstruction Assessment	**VIEWSTUDY** image #210 illustrates bowel obstructions. **Critical Thinking:** Relate the assessment findings in intestinal obstruction to the pathophysiologic process. Ask students to describe what they would focus on in an assessment.

Nursing diagnosis
    Planning/expected outcomes
    Implementation
    Evaluation/documentation
    Continuity of care
Polyps
    Definition
    Etiology
    Pathophysiology
    Clinical manifestations
    Collaborative management
	According to Becker's Health Belief Model, the patient would be more likely to take action if he or she believed that (1) he or she was susceptible to malignancy and (2) surgery would help.

Chapter Outline	Lecture Strategies

Nursing management of the patient with familial polyposis and Gardner's syndrome
  Assessment
  Nursing diagnosis
  Planning/expected outcomes
  Implementation
  Evaluation/documentation
  Continuity of care
	Critical Thinking: Describe some of the psychologic effects of bowel diversion surgery.

Ischemic disorders of the colon
  Definition
  Etiology
  Pathophysiology
  Clinical manifestations
  Collaborative management
	Ischemia and infarction may be familiar to students in other areas such as cardiac conditions that have been studied previously. If so, draw upon this knowledge to create various aspects of ischemic bowel disease.

Nursing management of the patient with ischemic disorders of the colon
  Assessment
  Nursing diagnosis
  Planning/expected outcomes
  Implementation
  Evaluation/documentation
  Continuity of care	

Blunt and penetrating trauma
  Definition
  Etiology
  Pathophysiology
  Clinical manifestations
  Collaborative management
	Describe paracentesis and peritoneal lavage in greater detail.

Nursing management of the patient with blunt and penetrating trauma
  Assessment
  Nursing diagnosis
  Planning/expected outcomes
  Implementation
  Evaluation/documentation
  Continuity of care	

Cancer of the colon
  Definition
  Etiology
  Pathophysiology
  Clinical manifestations
  Collaborative management
    Diagnostic testing
    Radiation therapy
    Chemotherapy
    Surgical management
	Critical Thinking: Identify the primary screening examinations for colorectal cancer.
	
	TA 91 illustrates types of colostomies.

Nursing management of the patient with cancer of the colon
  Assessment
  Nursing diagnosis
  Planning/expected outcomes
  Implementation
	VIDEO volume 9 presents nursing care of the patient with colon cancer, including preoperative assessment, stoma placement, surgical care, patient teaching, and postoperative care.
	
	Since nurses may initially find it difficult to confront stomal effluent, discuss ways of coping with this difficulty.

Chapter Outline	Lecture Strategies
Patient teaching Evaluation/documentation Continuity of care	**Critical Thinking:** Develop a teaching plan for the patient with a permanent colostomy. The testing ground for self-care may well be at home, where gaps in knowledge become more apparent. **VIEWSTUDY** image #212 demonstrates loop colostomy. **VIEWSTUDY** image #213 illustrates a cross-sectional view of end stoma.

Hemorrhoids (piles)
  Definition
  Etiology/pathophysiology
  Clinical manifestations
  Collaborative management
	Ask students to describe measures that would ease passage of stools.

Nursing management of the patient with hemorrhoids
  Assessment
  Nursing diagnosis
  Planning/expected outcomes
  Implementation
  Evaluation/documentation
  Continuity of care
Anal fissure and fistula
	Critical Thinking: Describe the nursing care for a patient with hemorrhoids.
	
	VIEWSTUDY image #216 illustrates the anatomic structures of the rectum and anus with external and internal hemorrhoids.
	
	VIEWSTUDY image #217 shows common sites of anorectal abscesses and fistula formation.

Preoperative nursing management of the patient with abdominal surgery
Postoperative nursing management of the patient with abdominal surgery
  Bowel diversion/ileostomy
  Kock's pouch
  Ileoanal reservoir
  Peristomal skin integrity
    Allergic response
    Mechanical trauma
    Chemical irritants
    Infection
  Stoma assessment
  Temporary colostomy
  Permanent colostomy
  Urinary elimination
  Infection
  Sexual dysfunction
  Body image
	Bring a Kock's pouch to class and demonstrate its application.
	
	VIEWSTUDY image #208 demonstrates surgical formation of a continent ileostomy (Kock's pouch).
	
	VIEWSTUDY image #211 demonstrates types of ostomies.

Related Skills

1. Using different types of pouches, discuss and demonstrate care of a colostomy or ileostomy. Have students practice care of a colostomy or ileostomy.
2. Fill pouches one-third full with warm water and have students apply and wear the pouches. Discuss feelings related to wearing the pouch.
3. Set up total parenteral nutrition and discuss uses and care. With students in groups, have students practice site care and line changes, with one student acting as observer.

Related Clinical Skills

1. Assign students to patients undergoing abdominal surgery or to patients who have undergone abdominal surgery. Discuss where to find operative details on the chart that may affect teaching.
2. Arrange for students to accompany a stomal therapist during preoperative and postoperative care.
3. Assign a student to a homebound patient with a newly formed colostomy. Develop a teaching plan for stoma care, nutritional needs, and psychological aspects of living with an ostomy.
4. Contact the American Cancer Society for information concerning a support group for ostomates. Have the student attend a meeting.

52 Nursing Management of Adults with Disorders of the Liver, Biliary Tract, or Exocrine Pancreas

LEARNING OBJECTIVES

1 Relate the pathophysiology and clinical manifestations to the collaborative management of cirrhosis and its complications.
2 Describe the nursing management for a patient with cirrhosis and its complications.
3 Compare the causative factors, routes of infection, incubation period, severity, clinical manifestations, and collaborative management of the various types of hepatitis.
4 Describe the nursing management for a patient with hepatitis.
5 Describe the nursing management for a patient with cancer of the liver.
6 Describe the indications for liver transplantation and care of the patient postoperatively.
7 Differentiate among cholecystitis, cholelithiasis, cholecystectomy, choledocholithiasis, and lithotripsy.
8 Describe the etiology, epidemiology, pathophysiology, clinical manifestations, and collaborative management of patients with cholecystitis and cholelithiasis.
9 Specify the nursing management for patients with disorders of the gallbladder.
10 Describe the etiology, epidemiology, pathophysiology, clinical manifestations, and collaborative management of the patient with pancreatitis.
11 Plan the nursing management for the patient with pancreatitis.
12 Describe the nursing management for the patient with cancer of the pancreas.

KEY TERMS

ascites
cholecystitis
choledocholithiasis
cholelithiasis
cirrhosis
hepatitis
hepatomegaly
jaundice
LeVeen shunt
pancreatitis
paracentesis
portal hypertension
Whipple's procedure

Chapter Outline	Lecture Strategies

Cirrhosis
   Definition
   Etiology/epidemiology
   Pathophysiology
   Clinical manifestations
	Ask students if they associate cirrhosis with any particular factor.
	
	VIEWSTUDY image #220 demonstrates systemic clinical manifestations of liver cirrhosis.
	
	TA 93 details the pathophysiologic events related to liver failure.

Early symptoms
      Hepatic insufficiency
      Skin
      Vitamin synthesis
      Hematopoietic changes
	Ask students why vitamin deficiencies other than A, D, and K may be less evident.

Endocrine/metabolic changes
   Collaborative management
      Complications
         Ascites and edema
            LeVeen shunt
            Paracentesis
         Portal hypertension and esophageal varices
	Ask students to speculate on the type of diet that would be necessary.
	
	VIEWSTUDY image #221 illustrates mechanisms for development of ascites.
	
	Ask students what additional factor(s) will make bleeding difficult to control.

Portal caval shunt
         Hepatic encephalopathy
   Nursing management of the patient with cirrhosis
      Assessment
	TA 94 shows a Sengstaken-Blakemore tube.
	
	Critical Thinking: What is the nursing management of the patient with cirrhosis?

Nursing diagnosis Planning/expected outcomes	**VIEWSTUDY** image #222 shows a LeVeen continuous peritoneovenous shunt. **VIEWSTUDY** image #223 shows portosystemic shunts.

Implementation
      Evaluation/documentation
      Continuity of care
Hepatitis
   Definition
   Etiology/epidemiology
   Pathophysiology
   Clinical manifestations
   Collaborative management
	Critical Thinking: Compare and contrast the causative factors, routes of infection, incubation period, severity, clinical manifestations, and collaborative management of type A, type B, and type non-A, non-B hepatitis.
	
	VIEWSTUDY image #218 depicts clinical and serologic events of a typical patient infected with hepatitis A virus.
	
	VIEWSTUDY image #219 demonstrates clinical and serologic events of a typical patient infected with acute hepatitis B.
	
	Form students into groups of 3 or 4, and ask them to determine priorities in assessment, nursing diagnoses, and planning and expected outcomes to generate appropriate nursing actions. Bring the groups back together to share their thinking.

Chapter Outline	Lecture Strategies
	Ask students to consider whether supplying clean needles to drug addicts to prevent hepatitis and AIDS is useful or not.
Nursing management of the patient with hepatitis	**Critical Thinking:** What is the nursing management of the patient with hepatitis?
Assessment	
Nursing diagnosis	
Planning/expected outcomes	
Implementation	
Evaluation/documentation	
Continuity of care	
Cancer of the liver	
Definition	
Etiology/epidemiology	
Pathophysiology	
Clinical manifestations	
Collaborative management	
Nursing management of the patient with liver cancer	
Assessment	
Nursing diagnosis	
Planning/expected outcomes	
Implementation	
Evaluation/documentation	
Continuity of care	
Liver transplantation	
Definition	
Etiology/epidemiology	
Collaborative management	**Critical Thinking:** Describe the postoperative care for the patient having a liver transplant.
Continuity of care	
Gallstones	**Critical Thinking:** Discuss the differences among cholecystitis, cholelithiasis, cholecystectomy, steatorrhea, and choledocholithiasis.
Definition	Break the terms listed above into word parts to aid in definition.
Etiology/epidemiology	
Pathophysiology	
Clinical manifestations	
Collaborative management	
Nonsurgical stone removal	
Surgical management	Use **TA 95** in explaining the process of endoscopic retrograde cholangiopancreatography.
Nursing management of the patient with gallstones	
Assessment	
Nursing diagnosis	
Planning/expected outcomes	
Implementation	
Preoperative care	
Postoperative care	
Evaluation/documentation	
Continuity of care	
Pancreatitis	**VIEWSTUDY** image #224 illustrates the pathogenic process of acute pancreatitis.
Definition	
Etiology/epidemiology	

Chapter Outline	Lecture Strategies
Pathophysiology	A flow chart of the events is useful.
Clinical manifestations	Ask students to speculate as to why serum and urine amylase levels are increased.
Collaborative management	
Nursing management of the patient with pancreatitis	
Assessment	
Nursing diagnosis	
Planning/expected outcomes	
Implementation	Discuss management of patients in alcohol withdrawal.
Evaluation/documentation	
Continuity of care	
Cancer of the pancreas	
Definition	
Etiology/epidemiology	
Pathophysiology	
Clinical manifestations	
Collaborative management	**VIEWSTUDY** image #225 demonstrates the Whipple procedure, or radical pancreaticoduodenectomy.
Nursing management of the patient with pancreatic cancer	**Critical Thinking:** Compare the nursing management of the patient with pancreatitis to that of the patient with pancreatic cancer.
Assessment	
Nursing diagnosis	
Planning/expected outcomes	
Implementation	
Evaluation/documentation	
Continuity of care	

Related Skills

1. Discuss enteric precautions.
2. Demonstrate and discuss sterile dressings involving a Penrose or Jackson-Pratt drain or a T tube. Have students practice and return a satisfactory demonstration of the dressing.

Related Clinical Skills

1. Assign students to patients who either are undergoing abdominal surgery or have returned from abdominal surgery. When possible, assign students to patients with nasogastric suction or drains.
2. Assign students to a hospice patient with cancer of the liver or pancreas. Develop a teaching plan designed to teach the family and patient about the disease process and pain management.

CHAPTER

53 Nursing Assessment of the Reproductive System

LEARNING OBJECTIVES

1 Know the basic anatomical structure and functions of the male and female reproductive systems.
2 Obtain relevant subjective information from a patient who has a reproductive alteration.
3 Elicit a complete and concise history from a patient who has a reproductive disorder.
4 Accurately examine a patient with a reproductive disorder in an organized manner to obtain appropriate objective data.
5 Record history and physical findings of a patient with a reproductive disorder in a concise, accurate, and logical manner,
6 Differentiate normal from abnormal history and physical findings of a patient with a reproductive disorder.

KEY TERMS

fallopian tubes	penis
follicle stimulating hormone	prostatic specific antigen
hysterosalpingography	scrotum
laparoscopy	semen
luteinizing hormone	sperm
mammography	testes
menstrual cycle	testosterone
ovaries	uterus
	vagina

Chapter Outline	Lecture Strategies

Anatomy and physiology
  Female reproductive system
    Ovaries
	VIEWSTUDY image #272 shows the anatomy of the female reproductive tract.
	
	VIEWSTUDY image #273 shows external female genitalia.
	
	VIEWSTUDY image #270 shows the female breast.
	
	VIEWSTUDY image #271 demonstrates lymphatic drainage of the breast.

Secondary sex organs
  Menstrual cycle and gonadal hormones
    Ovarian cycle
	Critical Thinking: What are the primary and secondary female reproductive organs, and how do the reproductive hormones function to develop and maintain them?

Chapter Outline	Lecture Strategies

Uterine cycle
    Menstruation phase
    Proliferative phase
    Secretory phase
  Secondary sexual characteristics
Male reproductive system
  Testes
	VIEWSTUDY image #275 demonstrates the events of the menstrual cycle.

	VIEWSTUDY image #268 illustrates external and internal male sex organs.
	VIEWSTUDY image #269 demonstrates formation of the ejaculatory ducts.
	VIEWSTUDY image #286 shows areas of the male reproductive system in which problems are likely to develop.
Secondary sex organs Male hormones	**Critical Thinking:** What are the primary and secondary male reproductive organs, and how do the reproductive hormones function to develop and maintain them?

Assessment
  Subjective
  Objective
	Critical Thinking: Design at least three questions to discreetly ask patients about reproductive symptoms.
	
	Critical Thinking: Discuss psychologic and sociocultural factors to consider throughout the physical examination of the patient's reproductive system.

General assessment
  Breast
  Abdominal examination
  Female genitalia
    External genitalia
    Speculum examination
    Bimanual examination
    Rectovaginal examination
  Male genitalia
    Inspection
    Palpation
    Hernia examination
    Rectal examination
Diagnostic and laboratory tests
  Diagnostic tests for conditions of the female
    reproductive system
  Papanicolaou test
    Patient preparation
    Procedure
    Postprocedure care
  Vaginal smear
  Biopsy
    Endometrial biopsy
      Patient preparation
      Procedure
      Postprocedural care
    Cervical biopsy
	Figures 53-5 and 53-6 are useful in illustrating the palpation technique and position of the patient during examination.
	
	TA 96 demonstrates bimanual palpation of the uterus.
	
	TA 97 shows palpation of the prostate gland.

Chapter Outline	Lecture Strategies
Procedure	
Postprocedure care	
Cervical conization	
Breast biopsy	
Patient preparation	
Visual examination	
Colposcopy	
Patient preparation	
Culdoscopy/culdotomy	
Patient preparation	
Postprocedure care	
Laparoscopy	
Patient preparation	
Hysteroscopy	
Patient preparation	
Radiography	
Hysterosalpingography	
Patient preparation	
Postprocedure care	
Acid phosphatase	
Alpha-fetoprotein	
Ultrasonography	
Patient preparation	
Diagnostic tests for diseases of the male reproductive system	
Infusion cavernosgraphy	
Patient preparation	
Nocturnal penile tumescence test	
Semen analysis	
Patient preparation	
Prostatic specific antigen	
Alkaline phosphatase	
Acid phosphatase	
Alpha-fetoprotein	
Ultrasonography	
Patient preparation for ultrasound (transrectal) of the prostate	Explain the process of ultrasonography for the scrotum and for the prostate.
Testicular scintigraphy	Ask students to identify the varying purposes and uses of ultrasonography, testicular scintigraphy, and biopsy of the prostate.
Biopsy of the prostate gland	
Patient preparation	
Postprocedure care	
Diagnostic tests for sexually transmitted diseases	**Critical Thinking:** Describe tests that are used in the detection of chlamydia.

Related Skills

1. Demonstrate and then have students practice external assessments of the female reproductive system. (Pelvic examination may be included in some programs). Discussion of principles and techniques used in assessment may be discussed in the laboratory setting rather than in the classroom.

Related Clinical Skills

1. Assign students to patients who are undergoing diagnostic tests of the reproductive system. Have students prepare the patient, observe the test, and provide aftercare.
2. Assign students to a public health unit. Arrange for them to develop a teaching plan to demonstrate breast self-examination using information from the American Cancer Society.
3. Have students develop a community health fair at a local college or university. Send out samples of questions to students about breast self-examination and testicular self-examination. Instruct students on preventive measures of cancer of the breast and testes.

54 Sexuality and Reproductive Health

LEARNING OBJECTIVES

1 Define sexual health.
2 Discuss sexual development throughout the life span.
3 Describe the human sexual response cycle in men and women.
4 Discuss older adult sexual health issues.
5 Discuss gay and lesbian sexual health issues.
6 Describe the components of a sexual health assessment to maintain a healthy sexuality.
7 Discuss health promotion practices.
8 Contrast various forms of contraception.
9 Differentiate between the major alterations in sexual function that affect healthy sexuality in men and women.

KEY TERMS

anorgasmia
contraception
dyspareunia
erectile dysfunction
homosexuality
hypogonadism
orgasm
Papanicolaou (Pap) smear
premature ejaculation
sexual arousal disorders
sexual desire disorders
sexual health
sexuality
vaginismus

Chapter Outline	Lecture Strategies
Sexuality and sexual health	Ask students to offer their definitions of sexuality. **Critical Thinking:** Discuss the topic of sexual health as it relates to the individual.
Sexual development	**Critical Thinking:** Trace sexual health through each of the developmental phases from young adulthood through older adulthood. Ask students to delineate factors that currently influence their sexual behavior and that of peers. It is essential that partners understand what is *normal* as a means of alleviating some anxiety.

Sexual response cycle
    Preexcitement phase
    Excitement or arousal phase
    Plateau phase
    Orgasm
    Resolution phase
	Critical Thinking: Identify and discuss each phase of the human response cycle.

Chapter Outline	Lecture Strategies
Older adult sexual health issues Physiologic changes in the elderly	**Critical Thinking:** Identify psychologic and social biases that impede older adults in enacting their sexuality.
Gay and lesbian sexual health issues	Ask students to complete a set of sentence starters related to sexual behavior and sexual norms, such as: "Gays are . . . " "Premarital sex is . . . " "What I like best about my sexuality is . . . " Break students into small groups to share the feelings that arise in response to questions.
	Critical Thinking: Discuss reasons that nurses should be sensitive and supportive when assisting gay and lesbian patients with sexual health issues.

Sexual health assessment
    Sexual history
    Physical examination
Health promotion practices
    Breast self-examination
	The patient will be affected by the nurse's level of ease.
	
	Critical Thinking: List and describe preventive health practices related to sexuality and reproductive health.

	VIEWSTUDY image #276 shows breast self-examination and patient instruction.
Mammography Papanicolaou (Pap) Smear Testicular self-examination Contraception	Ask students to explain "mammography's unique contribution to the screening process." Ask students to review the hormonal preparations used in contraception in relation to actions, interactions, side effects, and nursing activities for each.
	Critical Thinking: In counseling patients about contraceptives, list major factors that should be considered. Pay attention to side effects that could be physically dangerous or life-threatening. List chronic health conditions in which specific contraceptives should not be prescribed.
Alterations in sexual function	

Alterations in sexual desire
    Definition
    Etiology/epidemiology
	Critical Thinking: List specific sexual disorders according to when they occur in the sexual cycle. List the major medical interventions for each sexual disorder.

Pathophysiology
    Clinical manifestations
    Collaborative management
	Ask students to define *hypogonadism*.

Nursing management of the patient with sexual desire
    disorder
    Assessment
    Nursing diagnosis
    Planning/expected outcomes
	Critical Thinking: List the basic information necessary to formulate the sexual assessment. Discuss information important to nursing assessment of specific sexual needs.

Chapter Outline	Lecture Strategies
Implementation Evaluation/documentation Continuity of care	**Critical Thinking:** Describe nursing interventions that might make the experience more comfortable and supportive for patients requiring treatment for sexual disorders. Ask, "What kind of special care do patients need while recovering from chronic alcoholism and drug abuse?"

Erectile dysfunction
  Definition
  Etiology/epidemiology
  Pathophysiology
  Clinical manifestations
  Collaborative management
	Explain some of the varied causes of erectile dysfunction.

Nursing management of the patient with erectile
  dysfunction
  Assessment
  Nursing diagnosis
  Planning/expected outcomes
  Implementation
  Evaluation/documentation
	Ask students to design a nursing care plan for the patient with erectile dysfunction.

Female sexual arousal disorder
  Definition
  Etiology/epidemiology
  Pathophysiology
  Clinical manifestations
  Collaborative management	

Nursing management of the patient with female sexual
  arousal disorder
  Assessment
  Nursing diagnosis
  Planning/expected outcomes
  Implementation
  Evaluation/documentation
  Continuity of care
	Describe the varying aspects of counseling for the patient with a disorder of female sexual arousal.

Dyspareunia and vaginismus
  Definition
  Etiology/epidemiology
  Pathophysiology
  Clinical manifestations
  Collaborative management
	Explain the difference between dyspareunia and vaginismus.

Nursing management of the patient experiencing
  discomfort related to sexual activity
  Assessment
  Nursing diagnosis
  Planning/expected outcomes
  Implementation
  Evaluation/documentation
  Continuity of care
	Guide students in drawing up a nursing management scheme for the patient experiencing discomfort in relation to sexual activity.

Female orgasmic disorder
  Definition
  Etiology/epidemiology
  Pathophysiology
  Clinical manifestations
  Collaborative management
	Compare and contrast nursing management for patients experiencing inhibited male or female orgasms.

Chapter Outline	Lecture Strategies

Nursing management of the patient experiencing
  inhibited female orgasm
  Assessment
  Nursing diagnosis
  Planning/expected outcomes
  Implementation
  Evaluation/documentation
  Continuity of care
Male orgasmic disorder
  Definition
  Etiology/epidemiology
  Pathophysiology
  Clinical manifestations
  Collaborative management
Nursing management of the patient with inhibited
  male orgasm
  Assessment
  Nursing diagnosis
  Planning/expected outcomes
  Implementation
  Evaluation/documentation
  Continuity of care
Premature ejaculation
  Definition
  Etiology/epidemiology
  Clinical manifestations
  Collaborative management
Nursing management of the patient with premature
  ejaculation
  Assessment
  Nursing diagnosis
  Planning/expected outcomes
  Implementation
  Evaluation/documentation

Ask students to detail four aspects which must be covered in the nursing history of the patient with premature ejaculation.

Related Skills

1. Demonstrate (as appropriate) and discuss the correct use of a cervical cap, diaphragm, foams, creams, and suppositories.
2. Role-play the collection of a sexual history. Discuss approaches to interviews involving sexual histories.

Related Clinical Skills

1. Place students in rape crisis centers or in emergency departments that deal frequently with rape victims. Ask them to particularly observe approaches to these patients.
2. Assign students to a public health unit screening for sexually transmitted diseases. Interview clients who are being screened for STDs.

55 Nursing Management of Women with Reproductive System Disorders

LEARNING OBJECTIVES

1 List common disorders of the female reproductive tract.
2 Identify risk factors for gynecologic disorders.
3 List common nursing diagnoses for patients with gynecologic disorders.
4 Develop a care plan for a patient undergoing gynecologic surgery.
5 Identify a treatment plan and follow-up care for patients with a specific benign gynecologic disorder.
6 Identify the two most common benign breast disorders.
7 List the risk factors for breast cancer.
8 Identify the current therapies for breast cancer.
9 List the nursing interventions for patients with metastatic breast cancer.

KEY TERMS

cervical intraepithelial neoplasia (CIN)
climacteric
dysfunctional uterine bleeding (DUB)
dysmenorrhea
endometriosis
fibroadenoma
fibrocystic disorder
hypermenorrhea
leiomyomas
leukorrhea
metrorrhagia
pelvic inflammatory disease (PID)
premenstrual syndrome (PMS)
toxic shock syndrome (TSS)
vulvovaginitis

Chapter Outline	Lecture Strategies
Disorders of the female genital tract	
Vulvovaginitis	Ask students to define the term *vulvovaginitis* by breaking it into its word parts.
Definition	
Etiology	
Epidemiology	**Critical Thinking:** How is the vagina normally protected from infection?
Clinical manifestations	
Collaborative management	
Nursing management of the patient with vulvovaginitis	**Critical Thinking:** What are four risk factors for developing vulvovaginal infections?
Assessment	
Nursing diagnosis	
Planning/expected outcomes	
Implementation	
Continuity of care	
Pelvic inflammatory disease	
Definition	
Etiology/epidemiology	
Pathophysiology	Ask students to speculate as to how PID would be diagnosed.

Chapter Outline	Lecture Strategies
Clinical manifestations Collaborative management	**VIEWSTUDY** image #280 demonstrates common routes of spread of pelvic inflammatory disease. **Critical Thinking:** What is the most serious consequence of pelvic inflammatory disease?
Nursing management of the patient with pelvic inflammatory disease Assessment Nursing diagnosis Planning/expected outcomes Implementation Evaluation/documentation	Ask students to speculate on the reasons for semi-Fowler positioning.
Continuity of care Toxic shock syndrome Definition Etiology/epidemiology Pathophysiology Clinical manifestations	The dilemma that is posed in many health care situations is that what is desirable for the caregiver may not be desirable for the patient. **Critical Thinking:** What laboratory values are elevated in toxic shock syndrome?
Collaborative management Nursing management of the patient with toxic shock syndrome Assessment Nursing diagnosis Planning/expected outcomes Implementation Evaluation/documentation Continuity of care Abnormal uterine bleeding Definition Etiology Clinical manifestations	Discuss what is meant by beta-lactamase-resistant penicillins. **Critical Thinking:** What patient teaching is appropriate for the patient with toxic shock syndrome? Present the various terms, and ask students to attempt definitions from knowledge of word parts. **Critical Thinking:** What is dysfunctional uterine bleeding?
Collaborative management Nursing management of the patient with abnormal uterine bleeding Assessment Nursing diagnosis Planning/expected outcomes Implementation Evaluation/documentation Continuity of care Premenstrual syndrome Definition	Review the action, interaction, side effects, and nursing activities associated with MPA. Until recently, PMS was poorly understood and seldom acknowledged.
Etiology Pathophysiology Clinical manifestations Collaborative management	**Critical Thinking:** What are some theories about the cause of premenstrual syndrome?

Chapter Outline	Lecture Strategies
Nursing management of the patient with premenstrual syndrome	
Assessment	
Nursing diagnosis	
Planning/expected outcomes	**Critical Thinking:** What dietary modifications can be used to decrease the symptoms of premenstrual syndrome?
Implementation	
Evaluation/documentation	
Dysmenorrhea	
Definition	
Etiology	**Critical Thinking:** What is the greatest single cause of absenteeism among women?
Pathophysiology	
Clinical manifestations	
Collaborative management	**VIEWSTUDY** image #278 depicts treatment strategies for premenstrual syndrome.
Nursing management of the patient with dysmenorrhea	
Menopause and climacteric	
Definition	
Etiology	Ask students what they associate with menopause.
Pathophysiology	**Critical Thinking:** List several physiologic changes that occur in women as a result of menopause.
Clinical manifestations	
Collaborative management	Review the side effects, interactions, and nursing activities associated with estrogen preparations.
Nursing management of the patient during climacteric	
Assessment	
Nursing diagnosis	
Planning/expected outcomes	**Critical Thinking:** What patient teaching is appropriate for the woman going through the "change of life"?
Implementation	
Evaluation/documentation	
Continuity of care	
Endometriosis	
Definition	**VIEWSTUDY** image #281 shows common sites of endometriosis.
Etiology/epidemiology	
Clinical manifestations	Women who experience the symptoms are often labeled as neurotic.
Collaborative management	
Nursing management of the patient with endometriosis	
Assessment	
Nursing diagnosis	**Critical Thinking:** Suggest a common nursing diagnosis for the woman with endometriosis.
Planning/expected outcomes	
Implementation	
Leiomyoma	
Definition	
Etiology/epidemiology	
Pathophysiology	
Clinical manifestations	Ask students to speculate as to what symptoms would arise from the pressure.
Collaborative management	**TA 98** shows an abdominal hysterectomy.
Hysterectomy	**Critical Thinking:** What dietary modifications are important in the patient with leiomyomas?

Chapter Outline	Lecture Strategies
Nursing management of the patient with leiomyoma	
Assessment	
Nursing diagnosis	
Planning/expected outcomes	**Critical Thinking:** What should be included in the postoperative care for a patient undergoing hysterectomy?
Implementation	
Evaluation/documentation	
Continuity of care	
Cervical polyps	
Definition/etiology	
Pathophysiology	
Clinical manifestations	
Collaborative management	
Nursing management of the patient with cervical polyps	
Endometrial polyps	
Definition/etiology	
Pathophysiology	
Clinical manifestations/collaborative management	**Critical Thinking:** What is the most common method for obtaining endometrial cells for study?
Dilatation and curettage	
Nursing management of the patient undergoing dilatation and curettage	
Uterine displacements	**VIEWSTUDY** image #284 shows uterine prolapse.
Definition/etiology	
Pathophysiology/clinical manifestations	
Collaborative management	
Uterine prolapse	A diagram of the reproductive tract is useful in visualizing the prolapse.
Etiology/pathophysiology	
Clinical manifestations	Describe a pessary to the students.
Collaborative management	A diagram is useful in visualizing the rectocele.
Cystocele	
Rectocele	The anteroposterior colporrhaphy may be known as an A&P repair.
Nursing management of the patient with uterine displacement	
Vaginal fistulas	
Definition/pathophysiology	**VIEWSTUDY** image #285 illustrates common fistulas involving the vagina.
Clinical manifestations	Ask students what characteristics they might expect of vaginal drainage.
Collaborative management	
Nursing management of the patient with a vaginal fistula	
Cancer of cervix	
Etiology/pathophysiology	
Clinical manifestations	
Collaborative management	**Critical Thinking:** How is cervical cancer treated?
Chemotherapy	
Recurrent disease	

Chapter Outline	Lecture Strategies

Nursing management of the patient with cancer of the cervix
  Assessment
  Nursing diagnosis
  Planning/expected outcomes
  Implementation
  Evaluation/documentation
  Continuity of care	

Nursing management of the patient undergoing internal irradiation
  Assessment
  Nursing diagnosis
  Planning/expected outcomes
  Implementation
  Evaluation/documentation
  Continuity of care
	Elicit and discuss the reactions of students to caring for patients undergoing irradiation.

Cancer of endometrium
  Etiology
  Pathophysiology
  Clinical manifestations
  Collaborative management
    Hormonal therapy
    Chemotherapy
	Critical Thinking: What patients are at risk for developing endometrial cancer?

Cancer of the ovary
  Etiology
  Pathophysiology
  Clinical manifestations
  Collaborative management
    Chemotherapy
    Second-look surgery
    Radiation therapy	

Nursing management of the patient with ovarian cancer
  Assessment
  Nursing diagnosis
  Planning/expected outcomes
  Implementation
  Evaluation/documentation
  Continuity of care
	Critical Thinking: What patient teaching is appropriate for a patient receiving internal irradiation?

Cancer of the vulva
  Etiology
  Pathophysiology
  Clinical manifestations
  Collaborative management
    Stage 0
    Stage I
    Stage II and III
    Stage IV
    Radiation therapy	

Nursing management of the patient with cancer of vulva
  Assessment
  Nursing diagnosis	

Chapter Outline	Lecture Strategies
Planning/expected outcomes Implementation Evaluation/documentation Continuity of care	**Critical Thinking:** What nursing strategies could be used to increase comfort in a patient with a vulvectomy?
Breast disorders	

Benign breast disorders
  Definition
  Etiology/epidemiology
  Pathophysiology
  Clinical manifestations
Fibrocystic disorder
  Definition
  Clinical manifestations
  Collaborative management
    Dietary measures
    Hormones
    Other methods
Fibroadenoma
  Definition
  Clinical manifestations
Mammary duct ectasia
  Definition
  Clinical manifestations
Nursing management of the patient with benign breast
  disorders
  Assessment
  Nursing diagnosis
  Planning/expected outcomes
  Implementation
  Evaluation/documentation
  Continuity of care
	Critical Thinking: What are the two most common benign breast disorders?
	
	Critical Thinking: What diagnostic tools are used to differentiate between breast cancer and benign breast disorders?

Cancer of the breast
  Etiology/epidemiology
  Pathophysiology
  Clinical manifestations
    Diagnostic studies
	Critical Thinking: What are five risk factors for breast cancer?
	
	The psychological implications of scheduling a mastectomy to immediately follow a biopsy have made this practice less common.

Collaborative management	**Critical Thinking:** What are the three therapeutic modalities for breast cancer? Use diagrams to help students visualize surgery.
Surgery Staging Nursing management of the patient undergoing breast cancer surgery	**VIDEO** Volume 6 presents nursing care of the breast cancer patient, including coverage of screening, pre- and postoperative care, and rehabilitation. **Critical Thinking:** What nursing measures are used for a patient who is newly diagnosed with breast cancer?

Chapter Outline	Lecture Strategies
	Critical Thinking: How might the surgery for breast cancer alter self concept?
Radiation therapy Nursing management of the patient undergoing radiotherapy Chemotherapy Reconstruction	**TA 99** shows a modified radical mastectomy. **Critical Thinking:** What are the nursing interventions for postmastectomy patients?
Recurrent breast cancer metastasis	**Critical Thinking:** What are the most common sites of breast cancer metastasis? What are two nursing measures to be taken for each site?
Nursing management of the patient with metastatic breast cancer	Invite representatives from Reach to Recovery to discuss their experiences and their group.

Related Skills

1. Discuss and teach breast self-examination..
2. Using a model, demonstrate the setup and procedure for giving a vaginal douche. Review perineal care with and without a catheter. Have students return a satisfactory demonstration of one or both skills.
3. Have students practice postmastectomy exercises in the laboratory setting.

Related Clinical Skills

1. Assign students to patients undergoing surgery for gynecological problems. Emphasize the need for teaching and support.
2. Assign students to a homebound patient with a new mastectomy. Develop a teaching plan for exercises and care of the mastectomy site.
3. Allow a student to go with a Reach for Recovery volunteer from the American Cancer Society to visit a patient who has breast cancer and is contemplating mastectomy.

56 Nursing Management of Men with Reproductive System Disorders

LEARNING OBJECTIVES

1 Identify the principal pathophysiologic process associated with benign prostatic hypertrophy.
2 List four common clinical manifestations of benign prostatic hypertrophy.
3 Describe the purpose of the voiding diary in patients with benign prostatic hypertrophy.
4 Identify three complications of hormonal therapy for prostatic cancer.
5 List three nursing strategies for preventing disruption of the urethrovesical anastomosis after radical prostatectomy.
6 Describe an exercise regimen for the patient with stress urinary incontinence after radical prostatectomy.
7 State the most common initial symptom of testicular cancer.
8 Outline the elements of a teaching plan for the patient learning to inject a vasodilator for erectile dysfunction.

KEY TERMS

benign prostatic hypertrophy (BPH)
double voiding
erectile dysfunction
nocturia
obstructive uropathy
penile prosthesis
radical prostatectomy
trabeculation
transurethral resection
urge incontinence

Chapter Outline	Lecture Strategies

Benign prostatic hypertrophy
  Definition
  Etiology/epidemiology
	Use a diagram to illustrate the anatomical location of BPH.
	
	VIEWSTUDY image #287 shows benign prostatic hyperplasia.

Pathophysiology Endocrine control and prostatic hyperplasia	Review dihydrotestosterone and endogenous estradiol and their functioning.

Bladder outlet obstruction
Clinical manifestations
Collaborative management
  Medical interventions
  Surgical interventions
	Critical Thinking: How does BPH alter urinary elimination patterns? What complications are associated with urinary obstruction?
	
	Critical Thinking: What is the goal of transurethral resection? What is the nursing care of a three-way Foley catheter after surgery?

Chapter Outline	Lecture Strategies
Nursing management of the patient with benign prostatic hypertrophy Assessment Nursing diagnosis Planning/expected outcomes	**TA 100** illustrates transurethral resection of the prostate. Use diagrams to illustrate the other surgeries. **VIEWSTUDY** image #288 demonstrates four types of prostatectomy.
Implementation	**Critical Thinking:** What can the nurse do to help the patient alleviate and cope with symptoms of altered urinary elimination? **Critical Thinking:** How can the nurse assess for bleeding after surgery? How is TUR syndrome manifested? Ask students to speculate about why double voiding and avoidance of large fluid intake at meals will help manage urinary symptoms.
Postoperative care	Review the setup for a continuous bladder irrigation.
Medical therapy Evaluation/documentation	Review the actions, uses, side effects, interactions, and nursing activities associated with antiandrogens.
Continuity of care	**Critical Thinking:** What kinds of instruction should the nurse give the patient before discharge regarding stress urinary incontinence? recurrence of bladder obstruction?
Cancer of the prostate Definition Etiology/epidemiology Pathophysiology Clinical manifestations Collaborative management Radiotherapy Hormonal therapy Surgical interventions Nursing management of the patient with cancer of the prostate Assessment Nursing diagnosis Planning/expected outcomes Implementation Choosing no therapy Radiotherapy Hormonal therapy	**Critical Thinking:** Describe a nursing strategy for assessing pain in the patient with prostatic cancer and bony metastasis. **Critical Thinking:** What symptoms are common after radiotherapy, and how may the nurse minimize them? Discuss feelings and perceptions of the students related to teaching of sexual matters with older men.

Chapter Outline	Lecture Strategies
Radical prostatectomy	**Critical Thinking:** What are the two major long-term effects of radical prostatectomy, and what are the related nursing interventions?
Evaluation/documentation Continuity of care	**Critical Thinking:** What are the four major aspects of nursing care during long-term rehabilitation of a patient with prostatic cancer? Describe the major interventions for each.

Testicular cancer
   Definition
   Etiology/epidemiology
   Pathophysiology
     Germ cell tumors
     Non-germ cell tumors
     Metastatic testicular tumors
   Clinical manifestations
   Collaborative management
     Surgical management
     Radiotherapy and chemotherapy
     Advanced disease
	Critical Thinking: What are the symptoms of testicular tumors? How can the nurse teach patients to detect possible warning signs of cancer?
	
	Critical Thinking: Outline the nursing care of the patient after radiotherapy and chemotherapy and after surgery.

Nursing management of the patient with testicular
   cancer
   Assessment
   Nursing diagnosis
   Planning/expected outcomes
   Implementation
     Surgery
     Radiotherapy and chemotherapy
   Evaluation/documentation
   Continuity of care
Erectile dysfunction
   Definition
   Etiology/epidemiology
   Pathophysiology
     Hormonal disorders
     Vascular disorders
     Neurologic disorders
     Other medical disorders
     Surgical and traumatic disorders
     Drugs
     Psychogenic dysfunction
   Clinical manifestations
   Collaborative management
     Hormonal therapy
     Therapy for vascular disorders
     Mechanical devices
     Prosthetic therapy
     Psychologic therapy
	Ask students to list conditions that affect erectile function.
	
	A diagram is useful in visualization.

Chapter Outline	Lecture Strategies

Nursing management of the patient with erectile dysfunction
   Assessment
   Nursing diagnosis
   Planning/expected outcomes
   Implementation
      Hormonal therapy
      Vascular therapy
      Mechanical devices
      Penile prosthesis care
   Evaluation/documentation
   Continuity of care
	Critical Thinking: What factors are involved in erectile dysfunction? How can the nurse assess the effect of dysfunction on the patient and his partner? Describe the nursing care of the patient with a penile prosthesis. What must the nurse teach the patient to ensure continual care?

Related Skills

1. Explain and demonstrate irrigation of the three-way Foley catheter in a patient with a TUR.

Related Clinical Skills

1. Assign students to patients who are undergoing prostatectomies or orchiectomies. Ensure that care takes into account patient teaching and the patient's sexuality.

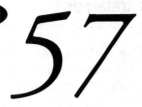

57 Nursing Management of Adults with Sexually Transmitted Diseases

LEARNING OBJECTIVES

1 Discuss the epidemiology of sexually transmitted diseases.
2 Identify the signs and symptoms of common sexually transmitted diseases.
3 Describe medical treatment of specific sexually transmitted diseases.
4 Plan nursing care for adults with sexually transmitted diseases.
5 Develop teaching plans for patients with sexually transmitted diseases.

KEY TERMS

bacterial vaginosis
candidiasis
chancroid
donovanosis
genital warts
gonorrhea
herpes genitalis
lymphogranuloma venereum
molluscum contagiosum
sexually transmitted diseases (STDs)
syphilis
trichomoniasis

Chapter Outline	Lecture Strategies

Sexually transmitted diseases
  Definition
  Etiology/epidemiology
	The concern with AIDS may have overshadowed the concern with other more traditionally defined STDs.
	
	Prepare a short true/false pre-quiz on STD prevention.

Nursing management of the patient with a sexually transmitted disease Assessment	**Critical Thinking:** Describe the psychologic reaction to an STD diagnosis and the nursing interventions required. **Critical Thinking:** What should be included in a teaching plan for a patient with a sexually transmitted disease? **Critical Thinking:** Outline the major nursing interventions for a patient with a sexually transmitted disease.

Herpes genitalis
  Definition
  Etiology/epidemiology
  Pathophysiology
  Clinical manifestations
  Collaborative management
	Critical Thinking: Explain what tests you would expect to see used to diagnose syphilis, herpes, and gonorrhea.

Chapter Outline	Lecture Strategies

Nursing management of the patient with herpes genitalis
    Assessment
    Nursing diagnosis
    Planning/expected outcomes
    Implementation
    Evaluation/documentation
    Continuity of care
	Critical Thinking: Describe the important patient care needs that should be addressed in a care plan for a patient diagnosed with herpes.

Syphilis
    Definition
    Etiology/epidemiology
    Pathophysiology
    Clinical manifestations
    Collaborative management
	Discuss common myths on how syphilis can be transmitted.
	
	Syphilis may produce mental retardation in the fetus. Summarize the stages.

Nursing management of the patient with syphilis
    Assessment
    Nursing diagnosis
    Planning/expected outcomes
    Implementation
    Evaluation/documentation
    Continuity of care	

Gonorrhea
    Definition
    Etiology/epidemiology
    Pathophysiology
    Clinical manifestations
    Collaborative management
	Ask, "Who is most susceptible to gonorrhea?"
	
	Ask students to suggest symptoms of gonorrhea.
	
	Review the side effects, interactions, and nursing activities associated with drugs taken for gonorrhea.

Nursing management of the patient with gonorrhea
    Assessment
    Nursing diagnosis
    Planning/expected outcomes
    Implementation
    Evaluation/documentation
    Continuity of care	

Chancroid
    Definition
    Etiology/epidemiology
    Pathophysiology
    Clinical manifestations
    Collaborative management	

Nursing management of the patient with chancroid
    Assessment
    Nursing diagnosis
    Planning/expected outcomes
    Implementation
    Evaluation/documentation
    Continuity of care
	In addition to routine nursing implications for patients with STDs, stress the need for patients diagnosed with chancroid to wash the genital area more frequently with soap and water to reduce the risk of contracting STDs in the future.

Chlamydia
    Definition
    Etiology/epidemiology
    Pathophysiology	

Chapter Outline	Lecture Strategies
Clinical manifestations	
Collaborative management	
Nursing management of the patient with chlamydia	
Assessment	
Nursing diagnosis	
Planning/expected outcomes	
Implementation	
Evaluation/documentation	
Continuity of care	
Genital warts	
Definition	
Etiology/epidemiology	
Pathophysiology	
Clinical manifestations	
Collaborative management	Refer students to Table 57-6 in discussing the collaborative management of genital warts.
Nursing management of the patient with genital warts	
Assessment	
Nursing diagnosis	
Planning/expected outcomes	
Implementation	
Evaluation/documentation	
Continuity of care	
Lymphogranuloma venereum	
Definition	
Etiology/epidemiology	
Pathophysiology	
Clinical manifestations	
Collaborative management	Review actions, interactions, side effects, and nursing activities associated with tetracycline.
Nursing management of the patient with lympho-	
granuloma venereum	
Assessment	
Nursing diagnosis	
Planning/expected outcomes	
Implementation	
Evaluation/documentation	
Continuity of care	
Donovanosis	Point out that donovanosis is rare in the United States.
Definition	
Etiology/epidemiology	
Pathophysiology	
Clinical manifestations	
Collaborative management	
Nursing management of the patient with donovanosis	
Assessment	
Trichomoniasis	
Definition	
Etiology/epidemiology	
Pathophysiology	
Clinical manifestations	
Collaborative management	

Chapter Outline	Lecture Strategies
Nursing management of the patient with trichomoniasis 　Assessment 　Nursing diagnosis 　Planning/expected outcomes 　Implementation 　Evaluation/documentation 　Continuity of care	Patients should be warned that taking metronidazole for trichomoniasis may turn urine dark orange or brown. If students are becoming saturated with the various names, etiologies, and clinical manifestations, place a few of the diseases on the overhead or board, and ask them to quickly write as much as they can remember of the diseases.
Bacterial vaginosis 　Definition 　Etiology/epidemiology 　Pathophysiology 　Clinical manifestations 　Collaborative management Nursing management of the patient with bacterial vaginosis 　Assessment 　Nursing diagnosis 　Planning/expected outcomes 　Implementation 　Evaluation/documentation 　Continuity of care Vaginal candidiasis 　Definition 　Etiology/epidemiology 　Pathophysiology 　Clinical manifestations 　Collaborative management Nursing management of the patient with vaginal candidiasis 　Assessment 　Nursing diagnosis 　Planning/expected outcomes 　Implementation 　Evaluation/documentation 　Continuity of care Molluscum contagiosum 　Definition 　Etiology/epidemiology 　Pathophysiology 　Clinical management 　Collaborative management Nursing management of the patient with molluscum contagiosum 　Assessment 　Nursing diagnosis 　Planning/expected outcomes 　Implementation 　Evaluation/documentation 　Continuity of care	**Critical Thinking:** Compare the signs and symptoms of vaginosis with the signs and symptoms of pelvic inflammatory disease. Molluscum contagiosum is not necessarily transmitted by sexual contact.

Related Skills

1. Divide group into triads. With one student as an observer, ask the remaining pair to role-play an AIDS patient who is experiencing a great deal of anger over diagnosis and the limitations of the medical system and a nurse who is caring for the patient. Switch roles in 20 minutes and again in 20 minutes. Observers are to provide feedback to the caregiver as to the effectiveness of interventions and approaches. The triads are to discuss feelings and reactions to being faced with anger. Debrief by bringing the total group back and reviewing general responses and interventions.
2. Review standard precautions.
3. Demonstrate the collection of specimens from rectal, vaginal, and skin lesions for culture and sensitivity.

Related Clinical Skills

1. Assign students to patients who are being treated for STDs. Encourage students to focus on psychological care, barrier technique, and patient teaching.
2. Assign students to a public health clinic that screens for STDs. Have the students interview patients who come to the clinic for testing. Have the students develop a teaching plan that focuses on prevention.
3. Hold a health fair at a local university or college and have students answer questions about STDs. Develop literature on the do's and don'ts of safe sex.

CHAPTER

58 Nursing Assessment of the Integumentary System

LEARNING OBJECTIVES

1 Know the structure of the skin and its main functions.
2 Elicit a complete and concise history from a patient with an integumentary disorder.
3 Accurately examine a patient with an integumentary disorder in an organized manner to obtain appropriate objective data.
4 Record the history and physical findings of a patient with an integumentary disorder in a concise, accurate, and logical manner.
5 Differentiate normal from abnormal history and physical findings of a patient with an integumentary disorder.
6 Describe diagnostic procedures that are involved in the diagnosis and detection of skin disorders.
7 Discuss patient preparation and care related to the procedures for diagnosing skin disorders.

KEY TERMS

biopsy
ceruminous glands
core temperature
dermis
epidermis
immunofluorescence
intradermal skin test

melanin
patch test
primary lesions
sebaceous glands
secondary lesions
sudoriferous glands
Wood's light

Chapter Outline	Lecture Strategies
Anatomy and physiology Structural description	Ask students to recall details of the anatomy and physiology of the skin.
Epidermis Dermis	The upward migration of old cells is an important process in some pathological processes. **Critical Thinking:** How do the epidermis and dermis differ in structure? **VIEWSTUDY** image #65 shows a microscopic view of skin in longitudinal section.
Hair, nails, and glands Functions of skin Protection from dehydration and mechanical injury	Ask students to speculate about the function of the accessory structures.

Chapter Outline	Lecture Strategies
Temperature control	**Critical Thinking:** How does the skin help regulate body temperature?
Other functions	Ask students to describe other functions of the skin.
Assessment Subjective	**Critical Thinking:** Design at least three questions to discreetly ask patients about skin breakdown in the perineal area.
Objective General assessment Skin Hair Nails	**Critical Thinking:** Discuss psychologic and ethnic factors to consider throughout the physical examination of the patient's integument. **Critical Thinking:** Discuss special considerations in regard to skin integrity in older adults.
Diagnostic and laboratory tests Biopsy Patient preparation Scrapings Culture Wood's light Cytology Immunofluorescence Skin tests for allergies Patch test Intradermal skin test	**Critical Thinking:** Describe the care and preparation of a patient who is undergoing skin biopsy. **Critical Thinking:** Describe the procedure for an intradermal skin test.

Related Skills

1. Demonstrate assessment of the integument, and then have students practice the assessment in pairs.

Related Clinical Skills

1. Assign students to patients who are undergoing skin biopsy. Have them prepare the patients and stay with them during the procedure.
2. Assign students to patients with specific skin alterations, either as a result of a skin disorder or as a result of another skin condition. For all patients that are assigned, have the students focus on and document specific observations related to the skin.
3. Assign students to a homebound patient. Have them focus on and document skin integrity in these older adults.

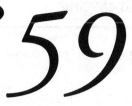

Nursing Management of Adults with Skin Disorders

LEARNING OBJECTIVES

1 Describe the general treatment modalities for skin disorders.
2 Help the patient and family cope with the psychologic trauma of dermatologic disorders.
3 Discuss nursing care for the patient with pruritus.
4 Use the nursing process to provide care for patients with inflammatory, infectious, autoimmune, or neoplastic skin disorders.
5 Discuss patient education needs in secretory disorders.
6 Discuss the pathophysiology and treatment of psoriasis.
7 Contrast extrinsic and intrinsic risk factors related to the development of pressure ulcers.
8 Develop a plan of care for the patient with a risk of developing pressure ulcers.
9 Compare the types of neoplastic skin disorders.
10 Identify special considerations for the elderly patient, the African-American patient, and the patient with HIV.

KEY TERMS

basal cell carcinoma
carbuncles
cellulitis
debridement
dermatitis
eczema
exfoliative dermatitis
folliculitis
furuncles

herpes zoster
maceration
malignant melanoma
pemphigus vulgaris
pressure ulcer
pruritus
psoriasis
scleroderma
topical medications

Chapter Outline	Lecture Strategies
Common interventions for skin disorders	**Critical Thinking:** Describe the nurse's responsibility for the general aspects of dermatologic care (i.e., dressings, phototherapy, photoprotection).
Topical medications	Ask students to speculate as to why inflamed skin would absorb topical medication more readily.

Corticosteroids
Therapeutic baths
Dressings
   Open dressings
   Occlusive dressings
	Ask students to give reasons for the hypothermia that is experienced when wet dressings are applied.

Chapter Outline	Lecture Strategies

Common skin disorders

Pruritus
Nursing management of the patient with pruritus
    Assessment
    Nursing diagnosis
    Planning/expected outcomes
    Implementation
    Evaluation/documentation

Critical Thinking: Pruritus is a common aspect of skin disorders. Develop a plan of care for the patient with acute pruritus; with chronic pruritis.

Inflammatory skin disorders

Dermatitis
Nursing management of the patient with dermatitis
    Assessment
    Nursing diagnosis
    Planning/expected outcomes
    Implementation
Exfoliative dermatitis
Nursing management of the patient with exfoliative
    dermatitis
    Assessment
    Nursing diagnosis
    Planning/expected outcomes
    Implementation
Eczema
Nursing management of the patient with eczema
    Assessment
    Nursing diagnosis
    Planning/expected outcomes
    Implementation
    Evaluation/documentation
    Continuity of care
Psoriasis
    Definition
    Etiology
    Clinical manifestations/pathophysiology

Compare and contrast pustular psoriasis and exfoliative psoriasis.

    Collaborative management

Discuss the proper application of tar and retinoid preparations.

Nursing management of the patient with psoriasis

Critical Thinking: Your patient has been diagnosed with psoriaisis. Plan a teaching strategy for the patient who will be discharged in 3 days.

Infectious skin disorders

Folliculitis, furuncles, and carbuncles
Nursing management of the patient with folliculitis,
    furuncles, and carbuncles
Cellulitis

Point out that furuncles can be very painful.

Chapter Outline	Lecture Strategies
Nursing management of the patient with cellulitis	
Herpes zoster	
Definition/etiology	
Clinical manifestations	Review the actions, side effects, interactions, and nursing activities associated with acyclovir.
Collaborative management	
Nursing management of the patient with herpes zoster	
Fungal infections	
Parasitic skin disorders	Review the proper application of Kwell. The eggs of head lice can be detected as small silvery attachments on the hair shaft that cannot easily be removed.
Pediculosis	
Scabies	
Nursing management of the patient with parasitic skin disorders	
Autoimmune disorders	
Pemphigus vulgaris	
Nursing management of the patient with pemphigus vulgaris	
Assessment	
Nursing diagnosis	
Planning/expected outcomes	Ask students what might signal infection in this patient.
Implementation	
	Critical Thinking: Describe how infection can be contained in patients with pemphigus; with scabies.
Evaluation/documentation	
Continuity of care	
Toxic epidermal necrolysis	
Nursing management of the patient with toxic epidermal necrolysis	
Scleroderma	
Clinical manifestations/pathophysiology	
Nursing management of the patient with scleroderma	
Dermatomyositis	
Nursing management of the patient with dermatomyositis	
Pressure-related conditions	
Pressure ulcers	
Definition	**Critical Thinking:** List and describe the intrinsic and extrinsic factors related to pressure ulcers. How could the risk factors be modified?
Etiology	
Pathophysiology	
	VIEWSTUDY image #67 demonstrates staging of pressure sores.
	VIEWSTUDY image #68 shows a stage IV pressure ulcer.
	Ask students to identify the most common sites for ulcer development.

Chapter Outline	Lecture Strategies
Nursing management of the patient with pressure ulcers	**Critical Thinking:** Discuss your feelings about caring for patients with open, draining skin lesions. How could you help the patient improve his or her self-concept?
	Ask students to speculate on risk factors for development of pressure sores.

Assessment
Nursing diagnosis
Planning/expected outcomes
Implementation
  Prevention
  Wound management
    Wound cleansing
    Debridement
    Wound dressings
    Surgery
Evaluation/documentation
Continuity of care
	Review the actions, side effects, and nursing activities associated with debriding agents.

	Critical Thinking: Your patient is a 30-year-old quadriplegic who has undergone surgical repair of a pressure ulcer. Develop a teaching plan for him to prevent recurrence and allow the flap to heal.
Skin cancer	**Critical Thinking:** Describe the skin cancers and their appearance.
	VIEWSTUDY image #66 demonstrates the ABCDs of melanoma.

Basal cell carcinoma
Squamous cell carcinoma
Malignant melanoma
  Definition/etiology
  Clinical manifestations
  Collaborative management
Nursing management of the patient with malignant melanoma
Assessment
Nursing diagnosis
Planning/expected outcomes
Implementation
Evaluation/documentation
Continuity of care
Special patient populations
  The geriatric patient
    Changes associated with aging
    Skin growths in the elderly
  The African-American patient
    Common conditions
  The patient with HIV
	Critical Thinking: Your patient is a 35-year-old mother who is to have a wide excision of a melanoma on her leg. Plan her care, using nursing and interpersonal processes.
	
	Ask students to differentiate the following: Seborrheic keratoses, senile lentigenes, acrochordon, and cherry angiomas.
	
	Ask students to define some of the following: *Voight's lines, atopic dermatitis, Fox-Fordyce disease, hot-comb alopecia, traction alopecia, pomade acne, acne keloidalis nuchae, dermatosis papulosis nigra, pseudofolliculitis,* and *sickle-cell leg ulcers.*

Related Skills

1. Review and demonstrate occlusive dressings, wet-to-dry dressings, and open, wet dressings. Have students practice and return a satisfactory demonstration of one of the dressings, chosen at random.

Related Clinical Skills

1. Assign students to patients undergoing therapy for skin disorders. Observe students for their responses to lesions, and discuss how the student might deal with a sight that is repugnant.
2. Assign students to follow an enterostomal therapy nurse while he or she performs wound care.
3. Assign students to a homebound patient who requires dressing changes on a wound

60 Nursing Management of Adults with Burns

LEARNING OBJECTIVES

1 Differentiate superficial partial-thickness, deep partial-thickness, and full-thickness injury in relation to the level and severity of injury.
2 Define *eschar* and describe its effects on the healing of burn wounds.
3 Describe the physiologic alterations in selected body systems caused by thermal, electrical, or chemical burns.
4 Using the nursing process, outline the care of the patient with a minor burn injury who is undergoing outpatient treatment.
5 Discuss the care of the patient in the emergent, acute, and rehabilitation phases of a moderate to severe burn.
6 Discuss the needs and contributions of the family or significant others in the care and successful recovery of the burn patient.
7 Discuss the nurse's role in fluid resuscitation of the burn patient.
8 Outline the nursing care requirements related to the psychosocial needs of the burn patient.
9 Describe the nursing responsibilities related to surgical and nonsurgical wound care, including debridement, excision, and graft care.

KEY TERMS

autograft
biologic dressings
chemical burn
deep partial-thickness burn
electrical burn
eschar
escharotomy
fascial excision

fasciotomy
full-thickness burn
homograft
meshed graft
partial-thickness burn
sheet graft
tangential excision
xenograft

Chapter Outline	Lecture Strategies
Burn injury	**TA 101** illustrates the layers of skin involved in burn injury.
Etiology	**VIEWSTUDY** image #69 shows types of burn injury.
Pathophysiology Integumentary system	**Critical Thinking:** What layers of the skin are altered in a full-thickness burn? A partial-thickness burn? Describe each of these burns; include color, blister formation, and severity. **VIEWSTUDY** image #71 shows a cross-section of skin, indicating the degree of burn and structures of skin involved.

Chapter Outline	Lecture Strategies
	VIEWSTUDY image #72 demonstrates how, at the time of major burn injury, the capillaries increase in permeability.
	Critical Thinking: What does eschar look like? Why is it important to remove it from the burn wound?
	VIEWSTUDY image #74 shows escharotomy of the chest and abdomen.
Cardiovascular system Pulmonary system Renal system	Provide students with the basic disruption and encourage them to generate the sequelae. For example, if RBCs cannot leave the vascular system, what will be the effect on circulation?
Gastrointestinal system	Ensure that the students are familiar with the symptoms of paralytic ileus and gastroduodenal stress ulcer.
Additional system derangements Electrical burns Chemical burns Infection Healing	Ask students to speculate as to the physiological basis for some of these changes. (For example, "What is the physiological basis for an increase in glucose levels?")
	VIEWSTUDY image #70 shows electrical injury.
	Discuss the events involved in the healing of deeper wounds.
	Ask students to review the functions of the epidermis.
Collaborative management	Ask students to speculate as to goals that they would see as being appropriate for the burned patient.
Prehospital care	**VIEWSTUDY** image #73 illustrates the effects of burn shock during the first 24 hours.
Emergency department care	Although relief of pain may seem a more immediate need to the patient and family, it is important to explain that other treatments have greater priority in the very initial stages of treatment.
Inhalation injury	**VIEWSTUDY** image #75 shows a patient with massive upper airway edema.
Burn assessment	Present students with problems involving calculations of burn area.
Fluid resuscitation	**TA 102** shows how to calculate fluid needs in burn patients.
Wound treatment	Review the side effects and application of silver sulfadiazine and mafenide acetate.
Gastrointestinal system Musculoskeletal system	**VIEWSTUDY** image #78 shows a patient being treated with mafenide (Sulfamylon).

Chapter Outline	Lecture Strategies
Pain control Nonsurgical treatment Surgical treatment	
	VIEWSTUDY image #77 demonstrates operative debridement of full-thickness burns.
Types of excision Grafts	Slides are particularly useful in illustrating the types of excisions and grafts.
	VIEWSTUDY image #79 illustrates a surgeon harvesting skin from a patient's thigh.
	VIEWSTUDY image #80 shows a patient with cultured epithelial autograft.
	Critical Thinking: What is the difference between a split-thickness and mesh skin graft? Describe the nursing care requirements of each.
Biologic and synthetic skin substitutes Electrical burns Chemical burns Tar burns Nursing management of the patient with burns	Stress that these dressings are only temporary.
	VIDEO volume 5 presents nursing care of the burn patient, including etiology/epidemiology, assessment, diagnoses, and interventions.
	Critical Thinking: What are some important factors in the successful rehabilitation of the burn patient? What factors are most detrimental to the burn patient?
Assessment Nursing diagnosis Planning/expected outcomes	**Critical Thinking:** Name three areas that require assessment by the nurse when treating the severely burned patient, and explain what information can be gathered from the assessment.
Implementation Emergent phase Acute phase Infection control Comfort and pain management	Ask students to speculate on nursing care activities in this period. **Critical Thinking:** Write two sample nursing interventions related to the nursing diagnosis "Pain related to the burn injury."
Splinting and positioning	**VIEWSTUDY** image #81 shows contracture of axilla. **Critical Thinking:** Write one long-term goal and one short-term goal appropriate to the nursing diagnosis in the previous question.
Fluid resuscitation	Ask students to speculate as to what they would evaluate in assessing the adequacy of fluid resuscitation. **Critical Thinking:** Using the Brooke formula, calculate the fluid requirements of a patient with 75% third-degree burns who weighed 230 pounds on admission.

Chapter Outline	Lecture Strategies

Nutrition
Gastrointestinal management
Wound care
    Sheet grafts
    Mesh grafts
    Donor site
Outpatient care of minor burn wounds
Evaluation/documentation
	Critical Thinking: What are the basic nursing activities in outpatient burn care? What areas are to be covered in the outpatient teaching plan?

Continuity of care	Obtain slides showing pressure garments and ask a member of the rehabilitative team to discuss measurement and care of the garment.
Psychologic adaptation	**Critical Thinking:** What nursing interventions could be implemented for the family of a burn patient? What kind of information would be valuable for the nurse to gather about the family?
Rehabilitation Reintegration	**Critical Thinking:** Describe the environmental considerations necessary for the burn patient, and discuss the rationale for each.

Related Skills

1. Set up an area of the laboratory as protective isolation. Using this set-up as a demonstration and practice area, review the principles and practices of isolation. Have students practice and demonstrate satisfactory application of an isolation gown and sterile gloves.
2. Invite an occupational therapist to discuss the principles of hand splinting and the use of pressure garments.
3. Demonstrate and then observe the students practicing therapeutic positioning.

Related Clinical Skills

1. Assign students to patients with burns. More advanced students may be assigned to patients who are in the acute phase of burn care, whereas beginning students may be assigned to patients in the rehabilitative stages of care.
2. Assign students to patients who return home after rehabilitation from burns. Develop a teaching plan that focuses on restoring ADLs at home, coping with changes and dressing changes if needed.

61

Nursing Management of Adults Undergoing Cosmetic or Reconstructive Surgery

LEARNING OBJECTIVES

1 Explain the intended outcomes of cosmetic and reconstructive surgery.
2 Discuss the effects of plastic surgery on body image.
3 Describe the preoperative teaching and evaluation measures for the cosmetic or reconstructive surgery patient.
4 Identify postoperative nursing care for the cosmetic and reconstructive surgical patient.
5 Describe the changes in physical appearance that occur with the various types of cosmetic and reconstructive surgery.
6 Discuss the nursing interventions to detect and prevent common postoperative complications of cosmetic and reconstructive surgery.
7 State the goals and interventions for major nursing diagnoses after cosmetic and reconstructive surgery.
8 Describe home care instructions for the cosmetic and reconstructive surgical patient.

KEY TERMS

abdominoplasty
augmentation mammoplasty
breast reconstruction
blepharoplasty
blow-out fracture
flaps
malocclusion
mentoplasty
rhinoplasty
rhytidectomy
skin graft
suction assisted lipectomy (SAL)

Chapter Outline	Lecture Strategies
General nursing management	**Critical Thinking:** What are the intended outcomes of cosmetic and reconstructive surgery?
	Critical Thinking: What determines a successful surgical result?
	Critical Thinking: List factors that determine the surgical setting for a plastic surgical procedure.
	Critical Thinking: Why do patients elect to have cosmetic surgery?

Chapter Outline	Lecture Strategies
Preoperative nursing management	**Critical Thinking:** What are the preoperative teaching interventions for the cosmetic and reconstructive surgical patient?
	Critical Thinking: Identify the necessary factors to evaluate the psychosocial status of the plastic surgery patient.
	Critical Thinking: List five major nursing diagnoses that are most appropriate for patients who will undergo cosmetic and reconstructive surgery. Discuss the goals and nursing interventions for each diagnosis.
Postoperative nursing management	Patients who are unprepared for the realities of their postoperative experience may be very distraught by the failure to immediately achieve the desired effect.
	Critical Thinking: List five major nursing diagnoses that are most appropriate for patients in the immediate postoperative period of cosmetic and reconstructive surgery. Discuss the goals and nursing interventions for each diagnosis.
Cosmetic surgery	**Critical Thinking:** What effect does plastic surgery have on body image?

Blepharoplasty
  Definition
  Etiology
  Clinical manifestations
  Collaborative management
	A diagram is useful in visualizing this surgery.

Nursing management of the patient undergoing
  blepharoplasty
  Assessment
  Nursing diagnosis
  Planning/expected outcomes
	Critical Thinking: What are the expected changes in physical appearance that occur with the various types of cosmetic and reconstructive surgery?

	Critical Thinking: List nursing interventions to detect and prevent common complications of cosmetic and reconstructive surgery.

Implementation
  Evaluation/documentation
  Continuity of care
Rhinoplasty
  Definition
  Etiology
  Clinical manifestations
  Collaborative management
	Ask students to describe measures that will reduce swelling around the eyes.

Nursing management of the patient undergoing
  rhinoplasty
  Assessment
  Nursing diagnosis
  Planning/expected outcomes
  Implementation
  Evaluation/documentation
	Ask students to describe interventions that would be useful in achieving these nursing goals.

Chapter Outline	Lecture Strategies
Continuity of care	**Critical Thinking:** Describe home care instructio for the various cosmetic and reconstructive surgical pr cedures. Some patients are very disturbed by the bruising ar swelling around the eyes.
Mentoplasty	Ask students to describe the purpose and process mentoplasty.

Rhytidectomy
  Definition
  Etiology
  Clinical manifestations
  Collaborative management
Nursing management of the patient undergoing
  rhytidectomy
  Assessment
  Nursing diagnosis
  Planning/expected outcomes
  Implementation
	The lay term for this procedure is face lift.
	
	Patients may be very anxious to remove the dressin and then may be very disappointed by what they see.

Evaluation/documentation
  Continuity of care
Brow/forehead lift
Chemical face peel
  Definition
  Etiology
  Clinical manifestations
  Collaborative management
    Phenol peel
    Trichloroacetic acid peel
	Students should be able to suggest factors for evaluati of a rhytidectomy.
	
	Describe the procedure for a TCA peel.

Nursing management of the patient undergoing a
  chemical face peel
  Assessment
  Nursing diagnosis
  Planning/expected outcomes
  Implementation
  Evaluation/documentation
  Continuity of care
	Students will be able to identify areas of evaluation.

Dermabrasion
  Definition
  Etiology
  Clinical manifestations
  Collaborative management
Nursing management of the patient undergoing
  dermabrasion
  Assessment
  Nursing diagnosis
  Planning/expected outcomes
  Implementation
  Evaluation/documentation
  Continuity of care
	Ask students to define the term after consideration the word parts.
	
	Ask students to suggest why the family's reaction to alterations in appearance are evaluated after each visi

Chapter Outline	Lecture Strategies
Collagen injection	
Definition	
Etiology	
Clinical manifestations	
Collaborative management	
Nursing management of the patient undergoing collagen injections	
Assessment	
Nursing diagnosis	
Planning/expected outcomes	
Implementation	
Evaluation/documentation	If possible, obtain preoperative and postoperative photographs to show the physical results of collagen injection and to discuss their use in documentation.
Continuity of care	
Abdominoplasty	
Definition	It is important to emphasize that this surgery is not a substitute for weight control.
Etiology	
Clinical manifestations	
Collaborative management	**Critical Thinking:** What must the nurse observe for in postoperative abdominoplasty where more than three pounds of fat have been removed?
Nursing management of the patient undergoing abdominoplasty	
Assessment	
Nursing diagnosis	
Planning/expected outcomes	Ask students to speculate as to why the stooped position would be helpful.
Implementation	
	Demonstrate the correct method of evaluating abdominal tissue for intact skin integrity after abdominoplasty.
Evaluation/documentation	
Continuity of care	A diagram is useful in visualizing the procedure.
Suction-assisted lipectomy	
Definition	
Etiology	
Collaborative management	
Nursing management of the patient undergoing suction-assisted lipectomy	
Assessment	
Nursing diagnosis	
Planning/expected outcomes	
Implementation	
Evaluation/documentation	Review how to evaluate adequate fluid volume.
Continuity of care	
Augmentation mammoplasty	By examining the words and word parts, students will be able to reach a definition quite readily.
Definition	
Etiology	
Clinical manifestations	
Collaborative management	
Nursing management of the patient undergoing augmentation mammoplasty	
Assessment	
Nursing diagnosis	
Planning/expected outcomes	
Implementation	
Evaluation/documentation	
Continuity of care	

Chapter Outline	Lecture Strategies

Reconstructive surgery
 	
Skin grafts
Flaps
Nursing management of the patient with flaps and grafts
Tissue expansion
 	
Replantation
Breast reconstruction
   Definition
   Etiology
   Clinical manifestations
   Collaborative management
Nursing management of the patient undergoing breast
   reconstruction
   Assessment
   Nursing diagnosis
   Planning/expected outcomes
   Implementation
   Evaluation/documentation
   Continuity of care
Reduction mammoplasty
Maxillofacial trauma
   Facial fractures
   Nasal fractures
   Mandibular fractures
   Maxillary fractures
   Zygomatic fractures
   Orbital floor fractures
Nursing management of the patient with facial fractures
   Assessment
   Nursing diagnosis
   Planning/expected outcomes
   Implementation
   Evaluation/documentation
   Continuity of care
	Ask students to identify the advantages and indications for tissue expansion.
	
	Ask, "When is replantation indicated? What affects its degree of success?"

Related Skills

1. Demonstrate use of a Water-Pik in mouth care.
2. Discuss and demonstrate suture line care for a patient who has undergone cosmetic or reconstructive surgery.

Related Clinical Skills

1. Assign students to patients who have undergone cosmetic or reconstructive surgery. Emphasize the need to be supportive of the decisions of these patients and the need to communicate realistic postoperative expectations.
2. Assign a student to follow a postoperative patient to the home setting. Develop a teaching plan for a patient who has undergone a reconstructive surgical procedure. Interview family members about changes that the patient has undergone and how these changes will affect the family system.

Answers to Case

Study Worksheets and

Critical Thinking Guides

Answers to Case Study Worksheets

Case Study 1
The Patient with Chronic Obstructive Pulmonary Disease, Having an Episode of Acute Respiratory Distress

1. The nurse should include questions about the onset, character and duration of dyspnea; whether a precipitating event such as an infection had been identified; and what measures or medications Mrs. Antonio had tried. The patient should be assessed for presence of adventitious breath sounds; asymmetry of chest wall excursions; alteration in level of consciousness or mentation due to hypercapnia; fever or indications of malnutrition; cigarette smoking; and sleep and activity patterns.

2. Reexpansion of the right lung: decreased dyspnea, breath sounds, symmetrical expansion of chest, character and amount of chest tube drainage, chest x-rays . . .
Improvement of respiratory failure: mental and emotional status, skin color, arterial blood gases, pulse oximetry . . .

3. Intravenous aminophylline is given to promote bronchodilation. Inhaled beta agonists are given for bronchodilation and to improve clearance of secretions. Corticosteroids seem to speed recovery and decrease time on mechanical ventilation. Low-dose subcutaneous heparin is given to avoid pulmonary emboli. Stress ulcer prophylaxis is often given to ventilator patients because of the high incidence of GI bleeding. Specially formulated gavage tube feedings are given to prevent further cachexia and to avoid hypophosphatemia or high glucose loads. Crystalloid intravenous fluids are used to maintain adequate hydration.

4. The nurse checks the ventilator settings including mode, FIO_2 respiratory rate, tidal volume, peak inspiratory pressure and alarm status.

5. The nurse checks the patient's ability to tolerate gavage tube feedings: residual amounts, bowel sounds, and consistency of bowel movements. The effectiveness of the formulation can be monitored by daily weights and integrity of skin and mucus membranes. Safety measures that should be used include elevating the head of bed, checking for tube placement before adding formula, and adding food coloring to formula for ease of identification.

6. Key points in limiting exacerbations of Mrs. Antonio's pulmonary disease include exercising to increase functional ability; planning activities to avoid exhaustion; using home oxygen to avoid oxygen desaturation; learning dyspnea-introducing techniques (diaphragmatic breathing, pursed-lip breathing, and relaxation therapy); observing sputum and reporting changes; and maintaining adequate dietary intake.

Case Study 2
The Patient with Tuberculosis

1. People at greatest risk for developing tuberculosis include those who live in overcrowded conditions such as slums and shelters for the homeless and who are intravenous drug users or alcoholics or are malnourished. Persons in crowded, impoverished working conditions exposed to high-risk populations from developing countries are at high risk for exposure to drug-resistant organisms, leading to failure of treatment.

2. The lesions of tuberculosis may be seen on chest x-ray film as small nondescript densities (early), as cavitation with tissue destruction (advanced), or as scarring and calcification (posttreatment). Chest x-rays cannot be used to determine if the tuberculosis is active or inactive. Pulmonary function tests help to identify only if scarring is causing restrictive lung disease. Microscopic examination of sputum and culture of the tuberculosis organism is required for definitive diagnosis.

3. Effectiveness of therapy depends greatly on the client's willingness and ability to take medications on a regular basis for as long as 6 to 9 months. His previous experience when treated for tuberculosis should be discussed to identify compliance problems. It is important to identify the patient's close personal contacts. Information about the patient's living conditions; number of persons sleeping in a room; the ventilation, frequency and proximity; and age and health status of close personal contacts will be helpful in advising him about home care. Key to his compliance is his understanding and acceptance of responsibility for his own role in the treatment plan. Members living in the home may be high risk for tuberculosis. They will need to be evaluated and possibly placed on prophylactic therapy.

Case Study 3
The Patient with Primary Hypertension

1. Mr. George's age, sex, personality, lifestyle habits (heavy alcohol use and little physical activity) and weight place him in the moderate to high risk categories.

2. The complications of untreated primary hypertension include strokes, premature cardiovascular disease, accelerated atherosclerosis, retinal damage, left ventricular hypertrophy, and renal damage.

3. Modifying Mr. George's lifestyle will be a big challenge for him and for the nurse. First, the nurse assesses Mr. George's knowledge and understanding of the disease and how he thinks it will affect his lifestyle and his self-concept. This could help give clues as to what might motivate him. Nurses can enhance compliance through reminders, contracts, self-monitoring records, tailoring interviews to the client's needs, reinforcement, use of support systems, and making home visits. Getting Mr. George actively involved in making constructive plans is an essential requirement on the road to controlling his blood pressure.

Case Study 4
The Patient with Parkinson's Disease

1. Parkinson's disease can affect cognitive function and emotional stability and is progressive in its effects on motor function. Therefore, assessment should include a thorough review of the patient's knowledge of the illness and medication regimen; motor assessment individualized to the person; and patient and family coping in the areas of communication, decision making, and concerns about safety.

2. In making her decision the daughter should consider the mother's response to therapy; trends in the mother's self-care deficit; the reliability of the home care worker; the daughter's ability to continue commuting on weekends to care for her mother; and the balance between the mother's desire to stay in familiar surroundings and the daughter's peace of mind concerning long distance supervision of care.

3. While being weaned from medications, Mrs. Norris may need help with meals, bathing, dressing, toileting and oral hygiene. She will be less active unless nursing interventions are planned to have her sit up and do range of motion exercises. She should be evaluated daily for her ability to swallow, and foods that are easy to chew may need to be ordered.

Case Study 5
The Patient with a Cerebrovascular Accident

1. The admission assessment of Mrs. King should include evaluation of motor function and strength of extremities; testing of sensory perception involving face, arms, and legs; observation of level of consciousness, orientation and ability to follow directions; and ability to understand and express thoughts verbally.

2. Right hemisphere dysfunction involves problems with sensory- perception, visual-spatial processing, awareness of body space, impulsive actions, carrying out self-care actions, and left-sided motor deficit.

3. Some resources that may be tapped to help Mr. King include a home health agency to provide workers to assist with activities of daily living, physical therapists to prescribe an exercise program, and nurses to monitor Mrs. King's health status. Meals on Wheels services can usually provide one hot meal a day, and many communities have volunteer pools that do errands and grocery shopping.

4. The location of Mrs. King's CVA will cause a visual-spatial processing deficit. This problem, when accompanied by a diminished visual field, will make it very likely she will injure herself repeatedly, due to an inability to judge spatial distances. Examples would be constant bumping into furniture or being involved in an automobile accident due to inability to judge distances.

Case Study 6
The Patient with Lumbar Intervertebral Disk Disease

1. Assessment of Mark's motor strength and sensory function is important to establish a baseline. He should be asked if he has experienced any problems with urinary retention or constipation, either in the past or since his recent pain. With Mark's lifestyle it is a possibility that this problem is due to repeated small traumas. He may have been tolerating minor problems for a while. It is also important to explore the psychological impact of this problem on Mark. How willing is he to comply with a regimen that emphasizes rest and immobility? Will his student obligations interfere with his role as a patient? The nurse should also assess his knowledge and use of body mechanics.

2. Mark has probably learned the expected action and side effects of his prescribed medications. His nurse should review these and then ask him to discuss his plan for coping with the effects of the medications during school hours. Unless Mark can verbalize a strategy that contains adequate safeguards, the nurse should warn him of the jeopardy to his health, his anticipated career, and those with whom he comes in contact.

3. The nurse can suggest proper body mechanics, a firm mattress or bed board, a back support or corset, stress reduction and relaxation techniques, cold or hot showers or packs, and abdominal and back strengthening exercises. Mark could also be encouraged to ask his physician to recommend a structured exercise program with physical therapy.

Case Study 7
The Patient with Right Above-the-Knee Amputation

1. A teaching plan needs to be developed to instruct the patient on home safety, such as arranging pathways and furniture to promote support in ambulation, and preventing accidents from bumping or falling and injuring the operative or other side.

2. Instruct on cleansing and gently drying the stump and in massaging and exposing it to air for 20 minutes, as well as on reapplying the dressing or bandage, with proper wrapping. Instruct on avoiding use of powders or lotions on the stump; application of a stump sock daily after cleansing and drying the stump; and padding pressure areas on the skin and stump.

3. Nursing diagnoses that would be applicable to a patient with an amputation include body image disturbance, ineffective individual coping, and impaired social interaction.

Case Study 8
The Patient with a Total Hip Replacement

1. Preoperative instruction for Mr. Petry is very important. Do not assume that he will remember the routine from his previous surgery. Instructions include the activity and the limitations that are required postoperatively. Activity may include the use of a continuous passive motion machine. Abduction is managed with an abduction pillow. He should be instructed about site care, dressing changes, suction devices, exercises, pain relief measures and symptoms of dislocation.

2. In the immediate postoperative period Mr. Petry's vital signs are checked for early signs of hypovolemia. Blood loss from drainage collection devices or on dressing is monitored. Peripheral pulses and neurovascular status are monitored due to the potential for neurovascular impairment and venous stasis. Mr. Petry's nutritional status, hydration, skin intactness, and wound healing or presence of infection are also important. Mr. Petry needs to know the "Dos and Don'ts" of safeguarding his hip: Do keep legs apart while sitting or lying; use a pillow between legs as a reminder; sit on a high, firm chair; use caution when getting in and out of a bath tub; walk with assistive devices; use an elevated toilet seat; notify physician if the operative site shows signs of infection. Do not sit in low, soft chairs; do not cross legs, turn hip or knee inward, or bend past 90 degrees to put on shoes or socks.

3. The nurse assesses for the signs of dislocation: shortening of the affected leg, sudden pain, and inability to move the extremity.

4. Blood loss is monitored and measured or estimated. If the patient is using anticoagulant therapy, he should be checked for bleeding from nose and gums and in urine and stool. Drainage in excess of 150 ml per hour or 500 ml in the first 24 hours is reported to the physician.

Case Study 9
The Patient with Osteoarthritis

1. Instruct the patient to elevate the leg to reduce swelling. Use cold packs for 10 to 15 minutes four times a day. Instruct on administration of analgesics, as ordered by the physician.

2. Instruct the patient to coordinate medication for pain with activities and to avoid overwork or activities that cause stress to joints. Instruct to avoid stressful situations; damp, moist environments; or extremes in environmental temperatures. Instruct to avoid prolonged activities, including walking, standing, and sitting, as well as sudden movements. Instruct in prescribed limitations of joints, 1-hour rest periods throughout the day to rest affected parts, and scheduling of activities to avoid fatigue and joint injury.

3. Instruct the patient to provide safe environment to reduce injury from falls, including removal of small rugs, use of night lights and handrails, use of cane or walker, wearing good-fitting sturdy shoes, and clearing all pathways.

Case Study 10
The Patient with Hypothyroidism

1. Lack of thyroid hormone decreases metabolic rate and can cause every form of lipid metabolism disorder. These are linked to hypertension and coronary artery disease. Since Mrs. Quinones has been self-medicating without physician supervision for 25 years, it is very likely that her once-adequate dose has been inadequate for many years.

2. Mrs. Quinones is a candidate for myxedema coma complication because she is 80 years old, has received inadequate health care follow-up for many years, and has just suffered from a condition leading to a period of severe decrease in cardiac output and hypoxia.

3. The classic changes seen in hypothyroidism include dry, coarse, yellowish skin; puffy face and hands; thickened and brittle nails; and thin and fragile hair. Behavior symptoms may indicate she is depressed, withdrawn, or apathetic.

4. At her age, Mrs Quinones is likely to be forgetful about taking her medications. She may need help in identifying a system for taking her thyroid supplement at the same time each day and on an empty stomach. She may find that a 7-day pill box kept by her toothbrush would help. She should identify someone who can check her pulse twice a week and should verbalize her intention to adhere to a schedule for physician follow-up.

Case Study 11
The Patient with Insulin-Dependent Diabetes Mellitus

1. Diabetic ketoacidosis develops as a result of severe insulin deficiency and excess levels of the counterregulatory hormones. DKA is the occurrence of ketoacidosis secondary to diabetes mellitus. Ketoacidosis is the result of insufficient cellular glucose utilization, intense lipolysis, and accelerated hepatic ketogenesis. As a result of insulin deficiency, plasma glucose, fatty acid, ketone, and hydrogen ion levels increase. This elevated glucose level results in water moving from the intracellular to the extracellular compartment, resulting in polydipsia and polyuria.

2. Infusion pumps are used to administer IV solution to protect the patient from an excess fluid overload, which could result in respiratory difficulties.

3. Provide emotional support. Reinforce teaching about the importance of receiving insulin even if food intake has been reduced.

4. Refer the mother to the ADA office for general literature. Encourage her to attend an ADA support group for patients and families with diabetes.

Case Study 12
The Patient with Decubitus Ulcer

1. This type of wound would heal by secondary intention, in which granulation tissue fills in the wound. Measure the length, width, and depth of the wound at each visit. Take pictures to continue to evaluate wound care. Assess for signs and symptoms of infection (such as drainage with purulent smell), increased body temperature, and redness extending around the wound.

2. Using aseptic technique and standard precautions, clean the inside of the wound with normal saline. Apply gauze soaked in normal saline to pack the inside of the wound, and cover with large abdominal pads (wet-to-dry technique). Using paper tape, tape the ABD pads in place. Check with the physician or enterostomal therapist for more specific wound-care orders.

3. Instruct caregivers on proper body alignment and positioning in bed to prevent skin tears from shearing skin. Evaluate the patient's need for equipment, such as supplies to decrease pressure, alternating pressure mattress, and heel and elbow protectors. Instruct on turning every 2 hours; instruct on the importance of proper nutrition for wound healing.

Case Study 13
The Patient with Liver Failure

1. The role of the nurse when caring for a patient with a Sengstaken-Blakemore tube is threefold: maintain and monitor the therapeutic effects of the tube; ensure the patient's safety; and provide for patient comfort. The nurse should label each of the tube's lumina with its designation and the amount of air pressure that is appropriate. If gastric lavage is ordered, the nurse should ensure that isotonic solutions are used. If iced saline is ordered, the nurse must guard against a piece of ice entering the tube. To ensure client's safety: the head of his bed is elevated 30 to 45 degrees; a foam rubber block (nasal cuff) is used to protect the nose from pressure; balloons are deflated periodically; tube placement is checked periodically. To promote the client's comfort, oral care is provided regularly each shift; back rubs and repositioning can reduce fatigue while bed rest is required.

2. Once hemorrhage had occurred, Mr. Trisch was at risk for developing hypovolemic shock and any of its complications. The hemorrhage could have been preceded by occult bleeding into the intestinal tract. This often contributes to development of hepatic encephalopathy, as the failing liver is unable to detoxify the metabolites of protein.

3. Measures to prevent or control complications would include: oxygen administration; hemoglobin, hematocrit, sodium and potassium samples to guide replacement therapy; type and crossmatch for fresh blood products; cathartics and enemas to remove blood from the intestinal tract; and neomycin to destroy colonic bacteria.

4. The protein helps facilitate cellular regeneration, but Mr. Trisch's wife needs to monitor him for changes in mental status that could indicate impending hepatic encephalopathy.

5. The nurse could set up consultations with a psychologist or social worker and support groups for the family of an alcoholic.

Case Study 14
The Patient with Prostate Cancer

1. Ask about pain regularly. Assess pain systematically. Believe the patient and the family about their reports of pain and what relieves it. Choose pain control options appropriate for the patient, family, and setting. Deliver interventions in a timely, logical, coordinated fashion. Empower patients and their families. Enable patients to control their course to the greatest extent possible.

2. Assess how the patient addressed his spiritual needs prior to the cancer. If he has not been to church regularly but would like to reestablish contact, notify a priest with whom he is most comfortable to give spiritual guidance. Make sure that all sacraments that are part of his religion are honored and received when necessary (Sacrament to the Sick, Last Rites). Encourage the family to participate whenever possible during these rituals.

3. Instruct the family members on the phases of dying. Administer pharmacologic comfort measures for temperature elevation. Continue administering pain medication to assist with respiratory discomfort during the dying phases. Stay with the family if death appears to be imminent. Continue providing emotional support to the family members and the patient. Call the priest to be with them if necessary.

Answers to Critical Thinking Guides

The Patient with Essential Hypertension

A Nursing assessment
- three B/P readings: 170/110, 166/106, 182/118
- stress
- type A personality
- diet high in fat, sugar, Na, and calories
- 25 lbs. overweight, concentrated in abdominal area
- smokes 2 packs of cigarettes per day

B Nursing interventions
- instruct patient on what HTN is, risk factors, causes, treatment, long-term complications, lifestyle, medications, relationships of treatment to control of complications
- assist patient in obtaining home B/P monitoring equipment and instruction in its use
- assess cost of new medications and patient's financial resources to buy medication

C Nursing interventions
- provide sample meal plans and food guides
- instruct patient and spouse on relationship of calories, Na, and fat intake to control of B/P and complications
- help patient set realistic goal of 1 to 2 lb. per week weight loss
- explain importance of reading food labels and limiting fast food

D Patient outcomes
- patient will select foods within Na, fat, and caloric limits
- patient will achieve and maintain desired body weight

E Nursing interventions
- assist patient to identify support systems
- allow patient uninterrupted time to verbalize concerns about diagnosis and treatment
- assist patient in identifying personal strengths to build a positive self-image
- instruct in stress management techniques, exercise, assertiveness training, meditation, and relaxation training
- refer to counseling or support groups for smoking cessation and weight management

The Patient with End-Stage Renal Disease

A Nursing assessment
- B/P 192/110, P108, R22
- orthopnea
- grayish pallor
- pulmonary rales
- 3+ edema of ankles
- JVD
- palpable liver (2-3 finger breadths)
- hematuria
- flank pain

B Diagnostic tests
- urinalysis
- CBC
- blood chemistries
- chest x-ray
- CT scan of abdomen
- IVP
- Renal scan

C Nursing interventions
Assess for adequate diuresis:
- urine output increased
- vital signs: B/P, pulse decrease
- neck veins flat
- decreased edema, weight loss
- breath sounds clear

Assess for inadequate diuresis:
- poor urinary output
- B/P, pulse, respiration remain elevated
- neck veins distended
- increasing edema, weight gain
- continued pulmonary rales

Prepare for emergency dialysis

D Nursing interventions
- administer ion-exchange resin
- follow-up blood work
- monitor patient for adverse reaction
- if K^+ remains elevated, prepare for emergency dialysis
- monitor cardiac rhythm

E Nursing interventions
- patient education, assess compliance
- assess alternate ingestion modes of Na, K^+ fluids, such as OTC medications

The Patient with Parkinson's Disease

A Physical assessment
   - ST memory loss
   - shuffling gait
   - resting tremors
   - sexual dysfunction
   - bradykinesia
   - rigidity
   - anxiety and depression
   - alteration in elimination

B Nursing interventions: patient education
   - signs and symptoms of infection
   - increase fluid intake
   - acidic urine
   - schedule catheter change
   - sterile system

C Nursing interventions
   - bowel training
   - patient education: fluid and dietary requirements
   - maintain or enhance activity level

The Patient with a Cerebrovascular Accident

A Nursing assessment
   - vital signs: B/P 194/108, P112, R8, axillary temp 99.8
   - right facial drooping, drooling
   - responds only to painful stimuli
   - nail beds cyanotic
   - right arm and leg flaccid
   - + Babinski's reflex
   - PO_2, 60; CO_2, 34
   - seizure

B Nursing interventions
   - mobilize secretions using chest percussion
   - suction as necessary
   - administer bronchodilators, if ordered
   - assess ability to cough
   - assess respiratory status: depth of respiration, air exchange, congestion
   - monitor ABGs
   - administer O_2 as ordered

C Nursing interventions
   - prepare for possible nasotracheal intubation, artificial airway
   - stand-by ventilator, respiratory therapy
   - monitor effectiveness of mechanical ventilation by respiration assessment and ABGs

D Nursing interventions
   Assess neurologic vital signs, change in mental status, cranial nerve function, muscular tone and strength, reflexes
   Assess hx. of seizures: frequency, duration, and severity
   Seizure care:
   - lay patient flat
   - protect from injury
   - maintain airway
   - administer anticonvulsants, as ordered

The Patient with Glaucoma

A Nursing assessment
   - loss of peripheral vision
   - increased IOP
   - diabetes
   - positive maternal history
   - other medications
   - last eye exam
   - vision changes
   - self care

B Diagnostic tests
   - tonometer
   - visual field testing

C Implement emergency measures to decrease intraocular pressure
   - miotics (Pilocarpine)
   - carbonic anhydrase inhibitors (Glamox)

D Assess for visual impairment needs
   - assess for degree of loss of vision
   - assess self-care deficits
   - assess problems with activities of daily living
   - assess for ability to administer eye drops
   - assess for social isolation and support systems

E Environmental assessment
   - assess home for scatter rugs, grab bars, mobility aids, room lighting, or any hazards

F Patient teaching
   - use of eye drops
   - turn head from side to side
   - familiarization with surroundings
   - side rails at night

The Patient with a Total Hip Replacement

A Nursing interventions
- assess for basis, location, duration, and intensity of pain
- administer prescribed medications and observe for side effects
- teach use of PCA, if prescribed
- promote diversional activities
- use relaxation therapy and other measures to promote comfort
- encourage position changes
- assess for complications, such as dislocation of hip prosthesis, shortening of affected leg, sudden pain, inability to move the extremity, or infection
- if on CPM, assess for pressure areas to groin, knee, and under straps, or positive Homan's sign

B Nursing interventions
- promote balance of rest with activity
- alternate rest periods in morning and evening
- evaluate ability to perform self-care activities
- coordinate with patient assessment and use of health care team services, such as occupational therapy and physical therapy
- encourage range of motion and stretching exercises, physical therapy, as ordered
- identify and encourage use of assistive devices
- teach measures to prevent dislocation of joint prosthesis

C Patient outcomes
- patient is able to progress to highest level of mobility possible within physical restrictions
- patient demonstrates an increased ability to engage in self-care behaviors and activities of daily living
- functional ROM of operated joint

D Patient outcomes
- no evidence of infection, such as fever, increased pain, or purulent drainage

E Patient outcomes
- patient will be able to care for self with maximum degree of independence available

F Nursing interventions
- notify physician if site becomes reddened, drainage occurs, or if painful ambulation occurs, as it might mean loosening of prosthesis
- evaluate weight bearing of affected extremity and use of any assistive ambulatory device
- instruct in exercise and activity
- assess home for environmental modifications, such as elevated toilet seat, bath/shower seat, extension devices
- return visit to physician
- diet therapy to prevent constipation
- use of high, hard back chairs, trapeze, or elevated toilet seat, as appropriate

The Patient with Hypothyroidism

A Nursing assessment
- fatigue
- dry skin/hair
- intolerance to cold
- difficulty with mental functioning
- constipation

B Patient teaching
- regular schedule for levothyroxine
- takes drug on empty stomach
- checks and records pulse regularly
- reports heart rate of 100 and above to doctor
- reports signs of CHF, such as weight gain

C Patient outcomes
- patient will accept altered body function and appearance
- patient will be able to make lifestyle changes

D Nursing interventions
- encourage patient to verbalize feelings regarding changes in body and fears
- assess self-esteem at intervals (weekly)
- provide education for patient and family
- assess role and relationships within the family
- assess support systems
- praise patient's positive attributes, such as intelligence, personality, etc.

The Patient with Diabetes Mellitus

A History
- diabetes type I
- repetitive trauma to foot
- jogger
- insulin-dependent diabetes
- diabetic retinopathy

B Assessment
- ulcer 3 cm with yellow and black tissue
- 1800-calorie diet
- check pedal, popliteal, and femoral pulses
- check for trophic changes in nails, infection
- check for sensory and motor deficits (pain, temperature, deep tendon reflexes)

C Nursing interventions
- culture wound if ordered
- apply antibacterial solutions if ordered
- cover ulcer with gauze
- should be in non–weight-bearing situations
- change dressing daily using aseptic techniques

D Nursing interventions: foot care patient education
Inspection
- assess feet daily
- see a foot doctor if corns, calluses, swelling or infection is present

Bathing and socks
- bathe feet daily in warm water
- use a mild soap, dry well
- soften skin with creams or lotions
- wear cotton socks
- never wear garters or hose with elastic tops

Toenail care
- cut or file nails to follow natural curve of toe
- see foot doctor for ingrown toenails
- trim toenails after bathing

Shoes
- check for fit; if necessary have special shoes made
- check for stones in shoes
- check shoe for ridges, wrinkles, or seams

Circulation
- quit smoking
- exercise with a brisk, daily walk
- avoid extremes of heat and cold

The Patient with Breast Cancer and Bone Metastasis

A Nursing assessment
  • risk factors: history, menopause at age 52, nulliparous, age 62, Jewish
  • 0 BSE, 0 mammograms
  • Pain: incisional, bone
  • concern over appearance

B Diagnostic studies
  • preop mammogram
  • premastectomy biopsies
  • bone scan
  • CT scan

C Nursing interventions
  • good hand washing with all patient contact
  • administer antibiotics, if ordered
  • monitor WBC count for elevation
  • assess patient for signs and symptoms of infection: fever, purulent wound drainage, malaise, or diaphoresis
  • on discharge from hospital, instruct patient on signs and symptoms of infection, wound site care, and care of wound drains

D Nursing interventions
  • physical therapy to decrease lymphedema or pneumomassage appliance to promote lymphatic drainage
  • instruct patient to avoid procedures such as B/P readings, injections, IVs, blood drawing
  • instruct patient to guard against injury from burns or needle pricks

E Patient outcome
  • patient is able to accept physical changes and integrate these into a positive body image and make lifestyle adjustments

F Nursing interventions
  • encourage patient to verbalize feelings about physical changes
  • encourage patient to look at affected area, verbalize how body has changed and visit with family and friends
  • assist patient to achieve maximum independence with ADLs
  • refer patient to Reach for Recovery program or counseling

G Nursing interventions
  • assess pain location, intensity, and duration by asking patient to describe pain
  • administer medication prescribed for pain relief, as ordered
  • assess pain relief and duration of relief
  • nursing measures to promote comfort: relaxation, repositioning, and heat or cold applications
  • instruct patient to protect from risk for fracture
  • protect bony prominences when moving, transferring
  • monitor serum calcium, assess mental state, encourage fluid intake

Test Bank

Test Bank Format

This Test Bank contains questions covering content related to adult health nursing. Divided into 61 chapters, the Test Bank is composed of independent questions, with correct answers with rationales and item codes for each question.

The questions duplicate those found in the computerized format of the Test Bank. These questions are provided in print form to allow faculty who are not using the computerized version to construct tests, as well as to provide a printed version of the questions for faculty using the computerized version.

The Questions

All questions are written in a multiple-choice format that corresponds to questions used on the National Council Licensure Examination for RNs (NCLEX-RN). There are three incorrect options and one correct answer for each question.

Each question is coded by the step of the nursing process, the clinical area, the client need, the category of concern (the specific topic), and the focus of concern.

1. **Nursing process:** Questions are written for each step of the nursing process. These codes can be used to select questions testing nursing process applications.

   Assessment - The student gathers subjective and objective information about the patient, identifies signs and symptoms, or completes a database.

   Analysis - The student interprets data in order to identify the patient's actual or potential health care needs and to formulate nursing diagnoses.

   Planning - The student establishes priorities for care, develops short-term and long-term goals, and collaborates with other health care personnel.

   Implementation - The student chooses appropriate nursing interventions, provides a rationale for nursing actions, helps the patient and significant others meet health care goals, or instructs the patient and family about self-care or health care practices.

   Evaluation - The student determines effectiveness of nursing actions, compares actual with intended patient care outcomes, or suggests alternative care plans.

2. **Clinical area:** Questions are coded for the clinical areas of *Medicine/Surgery, Childbearing and Women's Health, Pediatrics*, and *Mental Health*; these codes can be used to select questions testing students' knowledge of clinical concepts. As ***ADULT HEALTH NURSING*** is a textbook focusing on key medical-surgical nursing concepts, most questions in this Test Bank are coded Medicine/Surgery.

3. **Client need:** Questions are coded for the client needs listed below. These questions can be used to test students' knowledge of patients' health care needs that must be addressed by the nurse.

   • Support and promotion of **physiologic and anatomic equilibrium**

   • An **environment** that is safe and conducive to effective therapeutic care

- **Education** and other forms of health promotion to prevent, minimize, or correct actual or potential health problems

- Support and promotion of **psychosocial and emotional equilibrium**

4. **Focus of care:** Questions are coded for each focus of care listed below. These questions can be used to test students' knowledge of nursing actions which span the various steps in the nursing process, clinical areas, client needs, and categories of concern.

   Acute Care
   Community-Based Care
   Older Adult Care
   Health Maintenance/Promotion
   Long-Term Care

5. **Category of concern:** Questions are written to cover the categories of concern listed below, which are specific content areas within the broad clinical areas from which the material has been drawn. These codes allow the selection of questions targeted at specific content areas covered in *ADULT HEALTH NURSING*.

   Medicine/Surgery
   Blood and immunity
   Cardiovascular
   Drug-related responses
   Emotional needs related to health problems
   Endocrine
   Fluid and electrolyte
   Gastrointestinal
   Growth and development
   Integumentary
   Neuromuscular
   Reproductive and genitourinary
   Respiratory
   Skeletal

CHAPTER 1   Infection

Analysis
Medicine/Surgery
Physiologic and Anatomic Equilibrium
Community Health
Blood and Immunity

1. **A community health nurse is reviewing data on the number of communicable diseases reported among her clients. The process by which infection is produced is:**
   1. Causative agent, susceptibility of host, carrier
   2. Susceptibility of host, pathogen, portal of entry
   3. Carrier, pathogen, portal of entry, susceptibility of host
   4. Pathogen, dose, portal of entry, susceptibility of host

RATIONALE

(4) Client safety depends on the nurses' ability to understand the progression of events in the infective process.
   1. The causative agent or pathogen must first be present in sufficient quantity and gain entrance into the host.
   2. The susceptibility of the host is significant once the pathogen has gained entry.
   3. Many pathogens do not require a carrier.

Analysis
Medicine/Surgery
Physiologic and Anatomic Equilibrium
Acute Care
Blood and Immunity

2. **On the second postoperative day, the nurse notices that the client's incision is infected. This infection is called:**
   1. Latent
   2. Secondary
   3. Nosocomial
   4. Opportunistic

RATIONALE

(3) Infections in hospitalized individuals who do not have an infection before admission are called nosocomial. Clients are at increased risk for this type of infection when barriers such as the skin are disrupted.
   1. Latent infections follow the same course as acute primary infections; however, the organism remains in the body.
   2. Secondary infections develop from a second organism after a primary infection has resolved.

   4. Opportunistic infections occur because of the failure of one or more components of the immune system.

Analysis
Medicine/Surgery
Physiologic and Anatomic Equilibrium
Acute Care
Blood and Immunity

3. **Surgical unit nurses assess their clients carefully for signs of infection. The most common hospital-acquired infection is:**
   1. Wound
   2. Respiratory
   3. Pneumonia
   4. Urinary tract

RATIONALE

(4) The most commonly acquired infections are those of the urinary tract that develop in clients with indwelling catheters.
   1. Wound infections occur with traumatic injuries and improper aseptic technique.
   2. Respiratory infections are increased in clients with respiratory diseases.
   3. Pneumonia is one type of respiratory infection

Assessment
Medicine/Surgery
Physiologic and Anatomic Equilibrium
Acute Care
Blood and Immunity

4. **The nurse assessing the client for valuable signs of the prodromal stage of an infection will observe for:**
   1. Pain
   2. Flushing
   3. Diaphoresis
   4. Low-grade fever

RATIONALE

(4) Low-grade fever is a clinical manifestation of the immune system's battle to control the organism.
   1. Pain is not a common prodromal sign.
   2. Flushing is not related to this infective stage.
   3. Diaphoresis is not observed.

Analysis
Medicine/Surgery
Physiologic and Anatomic Equilibrium
Acute Care
Blood and Immunity

5. **A nurse is caring for a client with a drug-resistant infection. These infections are transmitted primarily by:**
   1. Contaminated linen
   2. Colonized clients and health care workers
   3. Improperly cleaned respiratory equipment
   4. Contaminated ventilation vents and medication

RATIONALE

(2) Nosocomial infections caused by drug-resistant microorganisms are primarily transmitted by colonized clients and health care workers.

1. Linen is disinfected, which usually destroys all microorganisms.
3. Respiratory equipment that is not properly cleaned can cause nosocomial infections, but is not the primary source.
4. Contaminated vents and medication are secondary sources of drug-resistant infections.

Assessment
Medicine/Surgery
Physiologic and Anatomic Equilibrium
Acute Care
Blood and Immunity

6. A clinic nurse is assessing a client with a possible infection as a result of a cut on the arm. A key assessment finding that indicates infection is:
1. Hyperthermia
2. Leukocytosis
3. Phagocytosis
4. Decreased sedimentation rate

RATIONALE

(1) Fever is usually considered the key assessment parameter in clients who have an adequate number of leukocytes.

2. Leukocytosis is an increased number of white blood cells identified by obtaining a blood sample.
3. Phagocytosis refers to the process of organism ingestion by granulocytes and monocytes.
4. The sedimentation rate is increased by infection and inflammation.

Analysis
Medicine/Surgery
Physiologic and Anatomic Equilibrium
Acute Care
Blood and Immunity

7. The nurse is asked to retrieve a client's differential count from the computer. The client is suspected of having an infection. The significance of this test is:
1. It indicates stability of red blood cells.
2. It classifies the white blood cells present.
3. It is indicative of the seriousness of infection.
4. It tells where in the body the infection is located.

RATIONALE

(3) In clients who are not immunosuppressed, the increase in leukocytes is directly proportional to the severity of the infection and the client's response to therapy.

1. This is not a function of the differential count.
2. The differential count indicates the percentage of each of the five different types of leukocytes.
4. Elevation of certain types of leukocytes are related to certain types of infections, but the exact location is not identified by this test.

Analysis
Medicine/Surgery
Physiologic and Anatomic Equilibrium
Acute Care
Blood/Immunity

8. A client's differential count indicates a "shift to the left." This means:
1. Increased blood volume
2. Increased immature neutrophils
3. Decreased immature neutrophils
4. Decreased plasma concentration

RATIONALE

(2) The shift to the left shows a release of immature neutrophils from the bone marrow, indicating infection.

1. The differential count does not relate to blood volume.
3. The immature neutrophils are increased.
4. The plasma concentration is not measured by this segment of the test.

Planning
Medicine/Surgery
Physiologic and Anatomic
    Equilibrium
Acute Care
Blood and Immunity

9. The nursing director of a surgical unit informs the staff of an increased number of nosocomial infections on the unit, and a plan to eliminate them. The most effective method of decreasing pathogen transmission is:
1. Handwashing
2. Antibiotics
3. Isolation
4. Disinfection

RATIONALE

(1) Handwashing by all persons who come in contact with a client will reduce the spread of infection.

2. Antibiotics are needed after the infection has spread.
3. Isolation techniques are not needed in every case.
4. Disinfection of equipment is important, although some organisms do not survive outside the body.

Implementation
Medicine/Surgery
Physiologic and Anatomic Equilibrium
Acute Care
Blood and Immunity

10. **Health care workers are frequently exposed to blood-borne pathogens. The infection control nurse advises everyone to:**
   1. Be immunized
   2. Wear uniforms
   3. Bandage cuts
   4. Use standard precautions

RATIONALE

(4) Standard precautions are applied to the care of all clients, since it is difficult to know which clients are carriers of blood-borne pathogens.
   1. Immunization is not available against all pathogens.
   2. Clothing alone will not protect against pathogens. Gloves and masks may be needed.
   3. Covering cuts or abrasions is important, but pathogens can enter through other routes.

Implementation
Medicine/Surgery
Physiologic and Anatomic Equilibrium
Acute Care
Blood and Immunity

11. **A client with measles is placed in isolation by the nurse. The type of isolation will be:**
   1. Strict
   2. Enteric
   3. Contact
   4. Respiratory

RATIONALE

(4) Measles requires respiratory restrictions. Clients with infectious diseases should be placed in a private room with their own bathroom.
   1. Strict is not a category of isolation precautions.
   2. Enteric is a type of contact isolation used when pathogens are transmitted by the gastrointestinal route.
   3. Contact isolation is used when microorganisms are transmitted by direct or indirect contact.

Implementation
Medicine/Surgery
Physiologic and Anatomic Equilibrium
Acute Care
Blood and Immunity

12. **The physician suspects an infectious process and orders a culture and antibiotics. In order to carry out the orders effectively, the nurse will:**
   1. Initiate the antibiotics before the cultures are taken
   2. Start the antibiotics after the cultures are obtained
   3. Delay the administration of the antibiotics until the results of the culture are known
   4. Recognize that the results of the culture and sensitivity don't affect the selection of antibiotics

RATIONALE

(2) Antibiotics are started after the cultures are obtained to avoid a false reading.
   1. Beginning the antibiotics first may destroy some microorganisms.
   3. Broad-spectrum antibiotics are started immediately and changed if needed when the culture results are known.
   4. The culture and sensitivity results are crucial. The pathogen must be identified as well as the drugs that destroy it.

CHAPTER 2 Fluids, Electrolytes, and Acid-Base Balance

Analysis
Medicine/Surgery
Physiologic and Anatomic Equilibrium
Acute Care
Fluid and Electrolyte

1. **In an emergency situation when fluid replacement is needed, isotonic solutions such as 5% dextrose in water or 0.9% sodium chloride solution are used. They cause:**
   1. Cell swelling
   2. Cell replication
   3. Minimal fluid movement
   4. Increased cell shrinkage

RATIONALE

(3) Isotonic solutions are similar in composition to cellular fluid. They cause little movement of fluid from the cell into the bloodstream or vice versa.
   1. Cell enlargement is caused by the administration of hypotonic solution.
   2. Cell replication is not affected by intravenous solutions such as these.
   4. Cell shrinkage is caused by hypertonic solutions, which draw fluid from the cells.

Evaluation
Medicine/Surgery
Physiologic and Anatomic Equilibrium
Acute Care
Fluid and Electrolyte

2. **A client has received a large amount of hypertonic glucose, and the nurse observes that the urinary output has decreased. This is a result of the release of the antidiuretic hormone, which causes:**

1. Decreased urine concentration
2. Increased serum hypertonicity
3. Increased water resorption by the renal tubules
4. Decreased water resorption by the renal tubules

RATIONALE

(3) Antidiuretic hormone (ADH) is the water-conservation hormone. Increased production of ADH results in increased resorption of water by the kidney through osmosis.
1. The urine becomes more concentrated.
2. The increased water resorption lowers the serum tonicity.
4. Water resorption is increased.

Analysis
Medicine/Surgery
Physiologic and Anatomic
Equilibrium
Acute Care
Fluid and Electrolyte

3. In reviewing an article in a nursing journal on regulation of fluid and electrolyte balance, the nurse reads about volume receptors in the walls of the right and left atria. The nurse knows that these:
1. Shrink, signal the brain, decrease intravascular volume.
2. Shrink, signal the brain, increase intravascular volume.
3. Stretch, send signals to the brain resulting in increased urinary output.
4. Stretch, send signals to the brain, resulting in decreased urinary output.

RATIONALE

(3) Excessive intravascular volume causes stretching of these receptors, which sends a message to the brain signaling the kidney to increase the filtration rate and urinary output.
1. The receptors do not shrink.
2. The intravascular volume is decreased by the stretching of these receptors.
4. The urinary output is increased.

Evaluation
Medicine/Surgery
Physiologic and Anatomic
Equilibrium
Acute Care
Fluid and Electrolyte

4. The nurse has administered fluids to a client who is dehydrated. Effectiveness of the treatment can be evaluated by the presence of:
1. Dry skin
2. Pulse rate of 80
3. Distended neck veins
4. Decreased blood pressure

RATIONALE

(2) Dehydrated clients usually have tachycardia because of decreased intravascular volume. It returns to normal as the client is rehydrated.
1. Dry skin indicates dehydration.
3. Distended neck veins indicate fluid volume overload.
4. Decreased blood pressure indicates dehydration.

Evaluation
Medicine/Surgery
Physiologic and Anatomic Equilibrium
Acute Care
Fluid and Electrolyte

5. The nurse's most accurate evaluation of fluid volume loss in a client with fluid excess is by:
1. Daily weight
2. Checking the skin turgor with calipers
3. Measuring urinary output by using an indwelling urinary catheter
4. Measuring output including perspiration, vomiting and colostomy drainage

RATIONALE

(1) Weight is the most accurate indicator of fluid gain or loss.
2. Skin turgor is affected by many things, including age.
3. Measuring urinary output is one way to determine fluid status, but it can be misleading if the client has renal disease.
4. Measuring output alone will not provide an accurate evaluation of fluid loss.

Evaluation
Medicine/Surgery
Physiologic and Anatomic Equilibrium
Acute Care
Fluid and Electrolyte

6. The medical intensive care unit nurse who is caring for a client who has third-space loss of body fluid from ascites notices that the daily weights have not changed, but that the client continues to have a low blood pressure and a fast heart rate. This could be the result of:
1. Intravascular volume deficit
2. Intravascular volume excess
3. Extracellular volume deficit
4. Intravenous fluid overload

RATIONALE

(1) Ascites is a buildup of fluid in the abdominal cavity. Even though the client is retaining fluid in one area, fluid replacement and careful monitoring is needed to maintain the intravascular fluid volume.

2. The client has a intravascular volume loss.
3. Ascites causes extracellular volume excess.
4. Excess intravenous fluid administration results in increased blood pressure.

> Assessment
> Medicine/Surgery
> Physiologic and Anatomic Equilibrium
> Acute Care
> Fluid and Electrolyte

7. **The medical unit nurse is assessing a client for signs of hypocalcemia, which include:**
   1. Hypotension, headache
   2. Depression, flabby muscles
   3. Diarrhea, bradycardia, weight loss
   4. Muscle cramps, tingling of fingers, tetany

RATIONALE

(4) Decreased serum calcium causes spontaneous discharge of sensory and motor fibers in peripheral nerves, resulting in tetany.
   1. These are generalized signs not specific to hypocalcemia.
   2. Flabby muscles are a result of hypercalcemia.
   3. These are symptoms that can result from several electrolyte imbalances.

> Planning
> Medicine/Surgery
> Physiologic and Anatomic Equilibrium
> Long-term care
> Fluid and electrolyte

8. **The discharge planning nurse is preparing a client for intravenous therapy in the home. The care plan will include:**
   1. Pharmacist scheduling
   2. Caregiver education
   3. Laboratory testing
   4. Coordination of physician visits

RATIONALE

(2) Many clients receive intravenous therapy at home. Education of the caregiver should begin before discharge and should include several teaching sessions.
   1. Pharmacists are not usually involved in this treatment.
   3. Laboratory testing is usually scheduled by the caregiver.
   4. The discharge planner may be responsible for scheduling physician visits, but this is not the priority.

> Assessment
> Medicine/Surgery
> Physiologic and Anatomic Equilibrium
> Acute Care
> Fluid and Electrolyte

9. **The nurse on a renal unit who is administering intravenous fluids to a client with renal disease knows that this client is at risk for vascular overload. The nurse assesses frequently for:**
   1. Renal overload
   2. Renal shutdown
   3. Pulmonary edema
   4. Dependant edema

RATIONALE

(3) With renal disease, excess fluid results in retention of sodium and water, resulting in symptoms of congestive heart failure including pulmonary edema.
   1. Clients with renal disease usually already have some degree of renal overload.
   2. Many clients have renal shutdown that requires treatment.
   4. Clients with renal disease frequently have varying degrees of edema.

> Assessment
> Medicine/Surgery
> Physiologic and Anatomic Equilibrium
> Acute Care
> Fluid and Electrolyte

10. **A client is receiving Ringer's lactate solution to replace fluid losses. The nurse is monitoring for signs of fluid overload, which may include:**
    1. Crackles
    2. Confusion
    3. Increased urinary output
    4. Decreasing abdominal girth

RATIONALE

(1) Signs of too rapid fluid replacement are crackles, shortness of breath and edema.
    2. Confusion is a sign of electrolyte imbalance.
    3. Increased urinary output indicates increased renal filtration.
    4. Decreasing abdominal girth is a sign of fluid loss from the abdominal cavity.

> Implementation
> Medicine/Surgery
> Physiologic and Anatomic Equilibrium
> Acute Care
> Fluid and Electrolyte

11. **An emergency room nurse is asked to administer an intravenous infusion of hypertonic dextrose and insulin to a client who has hyperkalemia. This treatment causes:**
    1. Potassium levels to increase
    2. Potassium to enter the renal tubule
    3. A permanent shift of potassium
    4. Potassium to enter the intracellular compartment

RATIONALE

(4) The potassium enters the intracellular compartment and decreases the serum potassium level.

1. Potassium levels are lowered
2. Potassium enters the cell, not the renal tubule.
3. The effects of this treatment are temporary. The infusion should not be stopped suddenly.

> Analysis
> Medicine/Surgery
> Physiologic and Anatomic Equilibrium
> Acute Care
> Fluid and Electrolyte

12. A telemetry unit nurse is monitoring a client with hypokalemia. Electrocardiogram changes that might be present include:
    1. Peaked T waves
    2. Flattened T waves
    3. Elevated ST segment
    4. Absent U waves

RATIONALE

(2) Flattened T waves are associated with hypokalemia.

1. Peaked T waves are associated with hyperkalemia.
3. The ST segments are depressed in clients with hypokalemia.
4. U waves are usually present in cases of hypokalemia.

> Planning
> Medicine/Surgery
> Physiologic and Anatomic Equilibrium
> Long-term Care
> Fluid and Electrolyte

13. A home health nurse is developing a care plan for a client who is receiving digitalis and a diuretic. The client will be monitored for:
    1. Renal failure
    2. Digitalis toxicity
    3. Metabolic acidosis
    4. Bowel obstruction

RATIONALE

(2) There is an increased chance of digitalis toxicity because of low potassium levels.

1. Renal failure may not be a direct result of digitalis and diuretic use.
3. Potassium loss can lead to metabolic alkalosis.
4. Digitalis and diuretic use do not cause bowel obstruction.

> Analysis
> Medicine/Surgery
> Physiologic and Anatomic Equilibrium
> Acute Care
> Fluid and Electrolyte

14. The nurse is analyzing the laboratory results of a client and notices a high calcium level. One of the primary causes of hypercalcemia is:
    1. Hypomagnesemia
    2. Hyperparathyroidism and malignancy
    3. Hypoparathyroidism and renal disease
    4. Increased ingestion of calcium-rich foods

RATIONALE

(2) The parathyroid gland stimulates calcium release. Multiple myeloma, vitamin D overdose, and prolonged immobilization may also contribute to this disorder.

1. Hypomagnesemia is associated with hypocalcemia.
3. Lower parathyroid levels relate to hypocalcemia.
4. Increased calcium intake usually has minimal effect on the serum calcium level.

> Analysis
> Medicine/Surgery
> Physiologic and Anatomic Equilibrium
> Acute Care
> Fluid and Electrolyte

15. A nurse reviewing an arterial blood gas report notices a value that indicates alkalosis. It is:
    1. Serum pH above 7.45
    2. Urine pH less than 6.0
    3. PCO_2 greater than 40 mm Hg
    4. Bicarbonate less than 27 mEq/L

RATIONALE

(1) A serum pH greater than 7.45 is the primary indicator of alkalosis.

2. Urine pH is not evaluated to determine serum pH.
3. PCO_2 greater than 40 mm Hg indicates acidosis.
4. A bicarbonate level of 22 to 26 mEq/L is normal.

> Implementation
> Medicine/Surgery
> Physiologic and Anatomic Equilibrium
> Acute Care
> Fluid and Electrolyte

16. A client is anxious and is hyperventilating. In order to prevent respiratory alkalosis the nurse will:
    1. Administer oxygen
    2. Instruct the client to pant
    3. Have the client breathe deeply and slowly
    4. Have the client breathe into a paper bag

RATIONALE

(4) Rebreathing carbon dioxide will increase the level of carbon dioxide in the blood and prevent respiratory alkalosis.

1. Anxious clients usually do not allow the placement of a mask or nasal prongs.

2. Panting will worsen the respiratory alkalosis.
3. A client who is hyperventilating usually needs further interventions in order to breath slowly.

CHAPTER 3 Pain

Implementation
Medicine/Surgery
Education
Health Maintenance
Neuromuscular

1. **In keeping with the World Health Organization's statement, "Every client has a right to adequate pain control," a nurse educator instructs staff to:**
   1. Rely on observable signs of pain
   2. Always consider clients as potential malingerers
   3. Assume that they are the authority on pain
   4. Believe that clients may have pain without observable signs

RATIONALE

(4) Nurses have incorrectly been informed that clients in pain have observable signs and symptoms. This is true only for clients with sudden, severe pain.
   1. Clients may have pain but not look as if they do.
   2. It is rare for a client to pretend to have pain (be a malingerer).
   3. The client is the only authority on pain, not the health professional.

Planning
Medicine/Surgery
Physiologic and Anatomic Equilibrium
Health Maintenance
Drug-related Responses

2. **The oncology unit nurse plans the timing and dosing of pain medication considering the risk of addiction to be:**
   1. Rare
   2. High
   3. Variable
   4. Gender based

RATIONALE

(1) Data in the literature suggest that the risk of addiction is rare among clients receiving opioids for pain.
   2. The risk is low.
   3. Many factors affect addiction, but the risk is low.
   4. The available data indicate that the danger of addiction to pain medication is vastly overrated.

Planning
Medicine/Surgery
Psychosocial Equilibrium
Acute Care
Drug-related Response

3. **The nurse may justify the use of a placebo to determine whether a client really had pain:**

1. At any time
2. When ordered
3. At no time
4. When the client cannot speak

RATIONALE

(3) There is no reason to justify using a placebo to determine whether a client really has pain.
   1. Placebos are not the objective test for pain.
   2. Nurses may refuse to administer placebos.
   4. Placebo use is inappropriate in this case.

Implementation
Medicine/Surgery
Psychosocial Equilibrium
Health Maintenance
Emotional Needs

4. **A major goal of nursing is to establish trust and rapport with the client. To the client with pain the nurse may say:**
   1. "I've given your medication as ordered."
   2. "Your pain can't be that severe, you are very quiet."
   3. "I believe you are in pain and I will help you to relieve it."
   4. "Your family will be here shortly and that will help your pain."

RATIONALE

(3) This statement lowers the client's anxiety level. Anxiety is the most important factor affecting a person's ability to tolerate and cope with pain.
   1. Therapies other than medication effectively relieve pain.
   2. Clients in pain often do not display physical signs.
   4. Clients can be distracted by family visits or other events, but the reduction in the pain level is short lived.

Planning
Medicine/Surgery
Physiologic and Anatomic Equilibrium
Acute Care
Emotional Needs

5. **In developing a care plan for a client, a nurse on an orthopedic unit will use the recommended clinical approach for pain management identified by the letters:**
   1. A, B, C, D, E
   2. P, Q, R, S, T
   3. H, E, L, P, S
   4. P, A, I, N, O

RATIONALE

(1) Ask, assess, believe, choose, deliver, empower, enable are the key words identifying the correct steps to follow in the treatment of pain.

2. These letters identify cardiac wave forms visible on the electrocardiogram.
3. These letters have no significance.
4. These letters have no significance.

Assessment
Medicine/Surgery
Psychosocial Equilibrium
Health Maintenance
Emotional Needs

6. **The nurse in a pain clinic knows that many factors affect a person's perception of pain, one of which is:**
1. Occupation
2. Religion
3. Socioeconomic status
4. Proximity to other persons in pain

RATIONALE

(2) Factors that affect a person's perception of pain include culture, religion, age, gender, past experience, and emotional factors such as anxiety.
1. Occupation has no specific effect on pain perception.
3. Persons have varying responses to pain regardless of their economic level.
4. Reaction to pain is an individual response. Clients in the same room have different responses to painful stimuli.

Analysis
Medicine/Surgery
Physiologic and Anatomic Equilibrium
Long-term Care
Neuromuscular

7. **A nurse in a pain clinic provides clients with chronic back pain information on the transmission of pain. The teaching plan identifies nociceptors as:**
1. Pain conduction fibers
2. Central nervous system fibers
3. Receptors that respond to injury
4. Chemical substances that initiate pain impulses

RATIONALE

(3) Nociceptors are specialized endings on neurons that respond to injury or painful stimuli.
1. Peripheral nerve fibers conduct the pain impulse to the central nervous system.
2. Impulses from the peripheral nerve fibers travel to the substantia gelatinosa in the dorsal horn of the spinal cord.
4. Chemical substances such as histamine and prostaglandins are released after nociceptor stimulation.

Implementation
Medicine/Surgery
Physiologic and Anatomic Equilibrium
Acute Care
Neuromuscular

8. **The nurse on a surgical unit uses massage as one intervention to relieve pain. The massage will:**
1. Distract the client
2. Decrease anxiety
3. Relieve pain by stimulating nerve fibers
4. Stimulate production of pain-inhibiting chemicals

RATIONALE

(3) Cutaneous stimulation relieves pain by stimulating large nerve fibers to close the gate to pain transmission.
1. Distraction includes talking and visualization.
2. Massage does decrease anxiety, but it also relieves pain.
4. This is not the mechanism of action of this therapy.

Analysis
Medicine/Surgery
Physiologic and Anatomic Equilibrium
Acute Care
Drug-related Response

9. **The nurse has received a physician's order for meperidine for postoperative pain. Expected effects of this drug include:**
1. Hypnotic effects
2. Increased tolerance to pain
3. Decreased perception of pain
4. Absence of any sensation of pain

RATIONALE

(3) Meperidine and other narcotic analgesics act at the central nervous system level to block pain perception.
1. Opioids do not produce hypnosis.
2. The pain tolerance level is not specifically affected.
4. Anesthetic agents block nerve impulses; meperidine does not.

Implementation
Medicine/Surgery
Physiologic and Anatomic Equilibrium
Acute Care
Drug-related Response

10. **Morphine is being given for the control of cancer pain. The nurse anticipates that the physician will order:**
1. Oral solution regularly
2. Sustained-release tablets infrequently
3. Frequent small doses intramuscularly
4. Occasional large doses intramuscularly

RATIONALE

(1) Cancer pain experts recommend concentrated oral morphine solution around the clock.
2. Sustained-release tablets regularly around the clock are recommended.

3. Intramuscular injections are painful and the absorption is erratic.
4. This dosing schedule is not recommended.

Evaluation
Medicine/Surgery
Physiologic and Anatomic Equilibrium
Acute Care
Neuromuscular

11. **To adequately evaluate the effectiveness of therapies for pain control, the nurse should:**
1. Be casual and informal
2. Not bother if the client is quiet
3. Use a pain assessment tool
4. Rely on the client's feedback

RATIONALE

(3) A systematic approach to collecting information about pain enables the nurse to better evaluate and plan interventions for pain relief.
1. It is necessary to use some type of formal tool that gives nurses a common language for evaluating pain relief.
2. Clients may be in pain even when they are quiet.
4. Clients often do not discuss their pain levels or ask for additional therapies.

Planning
Medicine/Surgery
Physiologic and Anatomic Equilibrium
Acute Care
Drug-related Response

12. **When planning medication therapy for a client with severe pain from a compression fracture of the vertebrae, the nurse will:**
1. Give opioids
2. Give nonopioid analgesics
3. Deliver both opioids and nonopioids
4. Use alternate therapies without medication

RATIONALE

(3) Opioids work at the level of the central nervous system, while nonopioids work at the level of the periphery. If the two types of drugs are combined, the pain can be attacked at two different levels.
1. Opioids alone are less effective than when combined.
2. Nonopioid analgesics are the first step in the analgesic ladder and potentiate the effect of opioids in the treatment of severe pain.
4. Alternate therapies should be used in combination with medication.

Evaluation
Medicine/Surgery
Physiologic and Anatomic Equilibrium
Acute Care
Drug-related Response

13. **The nurse returns to the bedside 30 minutes after administering nonopioid analgesic to a client with arthritis. The pain level has diminished significantly. Nonopioid analgesics are potent antiinflammatory agents that:**
1. Produce amnesia
2. Increase pain tolerance
3. Inhibit the synthesis of prostaglandins
4. Increase the synthesis of prostaglandins

RATIONALE

(3) Prostaglandins are fatty-acid substances that cause pain, edema, and inflammation when released into the body.
1. Amnesia is a loss of memory, an effect not produced by these drugs.
2. The pain tolerance level is not directly altered.
4. The prostaglandin synthesis is decreased.

Planning
Medicine/Surgery
Physiologic and Anatomic Equilibrium
Long-term Care
Drug-related Response

14. **In counseling a client about the analgesic effects of nonopioids, the nurse ensures that the "ceiling effect" is understood. The implications to the client will be:**
1. Not to exceed the recommended dosage
2. Take twice the recommended dose as needed
3. The drug is not effective if used alone
4. Once a certain dosage level is reached, side effects are minimal

RATIONALE

(1) There is a ceiling to the analgesic effect of the nonopioids beyond which no additional analgesic effect is produced but the side effects are increased.
2. Double dosing is not beneficial and may be harmful.
3. Nonopioids are effective when taken without other medication.
4. Increased dosing results in increased side effects.

Assessment
Medicine/Surgery
Physiologic and Anatomic Equilibrium
Long-term Care
Drug-related Responses

15. **On a return visit to the pain clinic, a client complains of tinnitus. The nurse questions the client about the use of:**
1. Aspirin
2. Meperidine
3. Morphine
4. Acetaminophen

RATIONALE

(1) In high doses, aspirin causes tinnitus.
2. Meperidine does not cause this symptom.
3. This is not a symptom associated with morphine.
4. Acetaminophen in high doses causes liver failure.

Evaluation
Medicine/Surgery
Physiologic and Anatomic Equilibrium
Older Adult Care
Drug-related Response

16. An elderly client who exercises routinely is given a nonsteroidal drug for inflammation of the hip. The client returns to the clinic in a week stating that the medication is not working. The nurse explains that:
    1. The dosage is the highest possible
    2. The effectiveness increases over time
    3. Maximum effectiveness should have been achieved
    4. The drug will be changed immediately

RATIONALE

(2) The antiinflammatory drug may take 3 to 4 weeks to achieve the optimal analgesic effect in clients with serious inflammatory problems.
    1. The elderly are always started on the lowest possible dosage.
    3. Maximum effect increases with time.
    4. One drug should be given an adequate trial with maximum doses before switching to another.

Planning
Medicine/Surgery
Education
Long-term
Drug-related Response

17. An oncology nurse is preparing a client for discharge home. The intravenous medications have been changed to oral. The dosage will be:
    1. Doubled
    2. Lowered
    3. Unchanged
    4. Increased

RATIONALE

(4) The most important point to remember about opioids is that their oral and parenteral doses are not interchangeable. Oral doses are usually higher.
    1. The equianalgesic chart indicates that oral doses are usually increased but not always doubled.
    2. The doses are lowered if the change is from oral to intravenous.
    3. There is a change of dosage when the medication is administered by different routes.

Evaluation
Medicine/Surgery
Education
Long-term Care
Drug-related Responses

18. A client with cancer who has recently started taking opioids is complaining of nausea and vomiting. The nurse advises:
    1. Take an antiemetic; the problem should resolve in 1 week.
    2. Take an antiemetic; this is a common problem with opioids
    3. Discontinue the medication. This is probably an allergic response.
    4. Doubling the dose of opioid and taking an antiemetic.

RATIONALE

(1) Antiemetics are usually effective, and the side effects of opioids are time limited and easily managed.
    2. The side effect of nausea or vomiting varies from client to client.
    3. Nausea and vomiting are often mistaken for allergic reactions.
    4. The opioid dose should not be doubled.

Assessment
Medicine/Surgery
Physiologic and Anatomic Equilibrium
Long-term Care
Drug-related Responses

19. A client with cancer has been receiving opioids for pain. The medication effects had been lasting for 4 hours but now last 3. The nurse identifies:
    1. Substance abuse
    2. Drug tolerance
    3. Psychologic addiction
    4. Physical dependance

RATIONALE

(2) Tolerance is a physiologic characteristic where increasingly larger doses of opioid are needed to provide the same effect.
    1. Abuse of medication is rare among cancer clients.
    3. Psychologic addiction occurs when the client needs the drug even when there is no longer a physical requirement for it.
    4. Physical dependance or addiction is rare in cancer clients.

Implementation
Medicine/Surgery
Physiologic and Anatomic Equilibrium
Acute Care
Drug-related Response

20. For the most effective postoperative pain relief, meperidine should be given:

1. When requested
2. Before painful activities
3. Before family visits
4. When the pain is severe

RATIONALE

(2) It is more effective to prevent pain than to reduce the intensity. Analgesics work best when given regularly.
1. Clients often do not self-report pain.
3. This may be unnecessary and result is social isolation.
4. Less medication is required if given before the pain level becomes intense.

> Analysis
> Medicine/ Surgery
> Physiologic and Anatomic Equilibrium
> Acute Care
> Drug-related Response

21. The nurse discusses using a patient-controlled analgesic (PCA) pump with a client's surgeon. The order is written and an expected outcome of using the pump is:
1. Increased risk of overdose
2. Increased use of the narcotic
3. Decreased tolerance to the narcotic
4. Increased patient control of drug administration

RATIONALE

(4) The best way to treat pain is to prevent it. Patient-controlled analgesia is ideal because it allows the client more control of drug administration.
1. The pump has a lock-out mechanism to prevent overdose.
2. PCA use usually results in less narcotic administration.
3. Tolerance is not directly related to pump usage.

> Assessment
> Medicine/Surgery
> Physiologic and Anatomic Equilibrium
> Acute Care
> Drug-related Response

22. A client is receiving opioids through an epidural catheter. The client must be monitored carefully for:
1. Pain control
2. Slowed breathing
3. Allergic reaction
4. Hallucinations

RATIONALE

(2) Close monitoring with frequent vital signs, apnea monitoring, and naloxone availability are all necessary for this client. Respiratory depression can occur up to 24 hours after medication administration.

1. The level of pain relief should be monitored also, but is not the priority.
2. Allergic reaction can occur but usually is an immediate occurrence.
4. This is not a usual side effect from this therapy.

> Evaluation
> Medicine/Surgery
> Physiologic and Anatomic Equilibrium
> Acute Care
> Drug-related Response

23. Naloxone is needed to reverse the respiratory depressant effect of an opioid. The nurse should continue to monitor the client because:
1. Hyperthermia may develop
2. The heart rate may increase
3. Naloxone causes increased sedation
4. The effect of the opioid lasts longer than the naloxone

RATIONALE

(4) The effect of naloxone is short lived and respiratory depression can recur.
1. This is not a usual side effect.
2. This may be a desired effect.
3. Naloxone reverses the effect of the opioid.

> Planning
> Medicine/Surgery
> Education
> Health Maintenance
> Neuromuscular

24. In teaching a class on noninvasive pain relief techniques to new employees, the nurse instructs them to:
1. Perform therapies without a physician's order
2. Practice the technique before needing to use it
3. Use the techniques only in combination with medication
4. Begin the therapy when the pain level becomes intense

RATIONALE

(2) It is best to practice the noninvasive therapy with the client before the time that it is needed.
1. A physician's order should be obtained if there is any doubt about the safety of the method or its legality.
3. These therapies can be effective when used alone.
4. For best results, start the therapy before the pain begins or shortly thereafter.

> Analysis
> Medicine/Surgery
> Education
> Long-term Care
> Neuromuscular

25. A home health nurse has a client with chronic pain. Recent acupuncture treatments appear to have decreased the pain intensity. When asked, the nurse explains that it works by:
   1. Endorphin blockage
   2. Endorphin release
   3. Distraction and imagery
   4. Relaxation and heat

RATIONALE

(2) It is postulated that acupuncture causes the release of endorphins and stimulates large nerve fibers to close the gate to pain impulses.
   1. Endorphin levels are increased.
   3. These techniques may be used in combination with acupuncture.
   4. Heat is not generated.

> Implementation
> Medicine/Surgery
> Psychosocial
> Long-term Care
> Older-adult Care

26. A nurse in a long-term care facility has a client who has complained of pain infrequently for several days. The nurse assesses the client and:
   1. Fears overmedicating the client
   2. Considers this a ploy to gain attention
   3. States a belief in the presence of the pain
   4. Accepts that pain is a normal part of aging

RATIONALE

(3) Assessing the pain systematically and believing the client are part of the recommended clinical approach to pain treatment.
   1. Studies show that elderly clients often receive fewer analgesics than do other clients.
   2. The elderly often fail to report pain and even deny its existence.
   4. Despite what many people think, pain is not and should not be a normal part of aging.

CHAPTER 4   Neoplasia

> Analysis
> Medicine/Surgery
> Physiologic and Anatomic
>   Equilibrium
> Long-term Care
> Blood and Immunity

1. A radiation safety inspector was recently diagnosed with cancer. The type of cancer associated with this occupation is:
   1. Leukemia
   2. Sarcoma
   3. Adenocarcinoma
   4. Wilms' tumor

RATIONALE

(1) High dose ionizing radiation is associated with leukemias because the hematopoietic system is very radiosensitive.
   2. Sarcoma is not associated with radiation exposure.
   3. Adenocarcinoma is not common with this occupational risk.
   4. Wilms' tumor is a cancer of the kidney found in children.

> Evaluation
> Medicine/Surgery
> Physiologic and Anatomic Equilibrium
> Long-term Care
> Blood and Immunity

2. A client with an adenocarcinoma of the colon returns to the clinic after therapy to have blood drawn for a carcinoembryonic antigen level. The nurse explains that this test will:
   1. Estimate chemotherapy level
   2. Monitor responses to treatment
   3. Identify normal cell damage
   4. Locate areas of metastasis in the body

RATIONALE

(2) CEA is one type of oncofetal antigen that is released by colon cancer cells. It cannot be used solely to diagnose cancer but is used to monitor a client's response to treatment. A rise in CEA may indicate a recurrence or spread of the cancer.
   1. The antigen may give some indication of the effect of the chemotherapy but not the level.
   3. This test does not indicate damage that normal cells may have received as a result of therapy.
   4. Specific metastatic locations are not identified by this test.

> Implementation
> Medicine/Surgery
> Education
> Community-based Care
> Reproductive

3. Education is the key to successful screening and detection. The nurse has presented a class on the American Cancer Society's recommendations for early detection. In the instruction the nurse specifies that women should have a mammogram:
   1. Biannually
   2. Quarterly
   3. Monthly
   4. Annually

RATIONALE

(4) Mammography should be done once a year for women over 50.

1. Twice a year is excessive unless there is active breast disease.
2. Four times a year is inappropriate.
3. Monthly mammography is inappropriate and potentially harmful.

Evaluation
Medicine/Surgery
Physiologic and Anatomic Equilibrium
Acute Care
Reproduction

4. **A client has had a breast biopsy after the placement of a needle to identify the tumor site. The client is at risk for:**
   1. Pain
   2. Nausea
   3. Edema
   4. Bleeding

RATIONALE

(4) Bleeding and infection are potential hazards of any biopsy procedure.
1. Pain is an easily managed problem after this procedure.
2. Nausea is rare in this situation.
3. Edema is usually minimal because of the application of a pressure dressing.

Implementation
Medicine/Surgery
Psychosocial
Long-term Care
Emotional Needs

5. **The husband of a young woman who is receiving treatment for recurrent breast cancer starts to cry when the nurse asks how the client is doing. Intervention might include:**
   1. Acknowledging his grief
   2. Completing nursing care quickly
   3. Quietly leaving the room to ensure privacy
   4. Focusing attention onto the client

RATIONALE

(1) Loss of function or body part results in a grieving process. Both the client and the family must be informed that this grieving is a normal event and be supported as they go through it.
2. Oncology clients and their families need emotional support.
3. This would further isolate the client and family member.
4. The client's significant others need care and support also.

Implementation
Medicine/Surgery
Physiologic and Anatomic Equilibrium
Acute Care
Reproduction

6. **A client is receiving internal radiation therapy for uterine cancer. She calls the nurse into the room because one of the radioactive seeds has fallen on the floor. The nurse should:**
   1. Ask the client to retrieve it
   2. Call the radiation safety officer
   3. Use tongs to place it into a lead lined container
   4. Block off the room until the physician arrives

RATIONALE

(3) A lead-lined container should be in the room of any client who is receiving radiation therapy from an encapsulated source. The nurse should use long forceps to handle the radioactive seed.
1. Radioactive material should never be touched with bare hands.
2. The radioactive material should be contained as soon as possible.
4. The physician may not be immediately available. An unenclosed radioactive source in a client's room is a hazard and should be contained immediately.

Implementation
Medicine/Surgery
Physiologic and Anatomic Equilibrium
Education
Integumentary

7. **A client is receiving radiation therapy and has port markings in place. The nurse's advice on skin care is:**
   1. Apply lotion to keep skin soft
   2. Keep the area as dry as possible
   3. Use an astringent after washing the site
   4. Use rubbing alcohol to strengthen the skin

RATIONALE

(2) The skin in the area of the port markings should be kept as dry as possible and if necessary, gently rinsed with water.
1. Lotions should not be used.
3. Astringents may dry the skin
4. Alcohol can also damage the skin.

Implementation
Medicine/Surgery
Education
Acute Care
Emotional Needs

8. **A client is receiving radiation therapy and is afraid to play with the grandchildren because of fear of being "radioactive." The nurse responds:**
   1. "You are not radioactive."
   2. "Only your urine and body secretions are radioactive."
   3. "Only your blood is radioactive, but it will not contaminate anyone."
   4. "You are radioactive while receiving treatment but not afterward."

RATIONALE

(1) Clients receiving external radiation are not radioactive at any time.

2. Urine and body secretions may become radioactive when a client has received internal radiation.
3. External radiation does not contaminate a client's blood.
4. The client is not radioactive at any time.

Implementation
Medicine/Surgery
Physiologic and Anatomic Equilibrium
Acute Care
Gastrointestinal

9. **A client who is receiving radiation therapy has been experiencing nausea, vomiting, and diarrhea. The most appropriate nursing intervention is:**
   1. Maintain accurate intake and output records
   2. Offer dry toast and crackers after treatment
   3. Administer an antiemetic 1 hour before treatment
   4. Encourage the intake of carbonated fluids 30 minutes before the radiation therapy

RATIONALE

(3) The antiemetic will prevent or minimize nausea and vomiting if administered before the radiation treatment.

1. The best therapy is aimed at stopping the vomiting and diarrhea, although recording intake and output is important.
2. The symptoms should be treated prophylactically
4. Carbonated fluids may worsen the symptoms.

Planning
Medicine/Surgery
Physiologic and Anatomic
   Equilibrium
Long-term Care
Integumentary

10. **A young woman with breast cancer is receiving chemotherapy known to cause alopecia. The plan of care will encourage:**
    1. Hair brushing
    2. Purchase of a wig
    3. The client to have a permanent
    4. Scalp rubs with hydrogen peroxide

RATIONALE

(2) Clients can purchase wigs before hair loss to match the color and texture of their own hair before hair loss occurs.

1. This may increase hair loss.
3. Chemicals which curl hair are harsh and contraindicated.
4. Hydrogen peroxide use is not appropriate.

Planning
Medicine/Surgery
Education
Long-term Care
Gastrointestinal

11. **An elderly client who has recently started chemotherapy for cancer tells the nurse that she has noticed painful, bleeding ulcerations in her mouth. The plan of care will include:**
    1. Gargle with an antiseptic solution
    2. A liquid diet until the ulcers heal
    3. Brushing the teeth with a soft-bristled toothbrush
    4. Rinsing with a salt and baking soda solution

RATIONALE

(4) These solutions provide comfort and promote healing for mouth ulcerations.

1. Antiseptic solutions often contain alcohol, which can cause stinging.
2. This may interfere with adequate nutrition.
3. Brushing with a toothbrush may cause bleeding.

Planning
Medicine/Surgery
Physiologic and Anatomic Equilibrium
Acute Care
Blood and Immunity

12. **A client is scheduled to receive the biologic response modifier interleukin-2. The plan of care will include:**
    1. Exercise
    2. Regular diet
    3. Vigorous skin care
    4. Rest and liquids as tolerated

RATIONALE

(4) The interleukins are a group of cytokines that function as communicators between lymphocytes. They are not directly toxic to cancer cells; they stimulate or enhance the immune system. They can cause severe toxicity, including flu-like syndrome.

1. These drugs cause fatigue.
2. Nausea and vomiting is a frequent side effect.
3. Skin rash and erythema often occur.

Planning
Medicine/Surgery
Psychosocial
Long-term Care
Emotional Needs

13. **A home health nurse caring for a client with advanced cancer hears frequent references to dying and an afterlife. The plan of care will include:**
    1. Referral to a member of the clergy
    2. Physical care only
    3. Allowing the client to discuss spirituality
    4. Exploration of these statements in depth

(3) Spiritual care needs of the cancer client are often of less priority than physical care needs. Every nurse can at least listen to the client's discussion of spiritual issues.

1. Some clients may wish to speak to a member of the clergy whereas others will not.
2. The care plan should include psychosocial as well as physical and spiritual aspects.
4. This may be beyond the capabilities of many nurses and clients.

> Analysis
> Medicine/Surgery
> Education
> Long-term Care
> Emotional Needs

14. **A school teacher recently diagnosed with a malignant growth requests an explanation of the term. The nurse explains that:**
    1. The rate of growth is slow
    2. The tumor is encapsulated
    3. Cells are well differentiated
    4. This cancer invades other tissue

RATIONALE

(4) Malignant growths are characterized by their ability to invade surrounding tissue, presence of undifferentiated cells, and their rapid growth and metastatic capabilities.

1. The rate of growth is rapid.
2. The tumor invades adjacent tissue.
3. There is some lack of differentiation in all malignancies.

CHAPTER 5 Shock

> Analysis
> Medicine/Surgery
> Physiologic and Anatomic Equilibrium
> Acute Care
> Cardiovascular

1. **The intensive care unit nurse admitting a client with shock chooses a nursing diagnosis that is appropriate for all forms of shock. It is:**
   1. Social isolation
   2. Altered tissue perfusion
   3. Fluid volume deficit
   4. Decreased cardiac output

RATIONALE

(2) All forms of shock create a decrease in tissue perfusion with altered cellular function.

1. Many clients in shock have strong social support.
3. Fluid volume deficit is common in hypovolemic shock.

4. Decreased cardiac output occurs with cardiogenic shock.

> Assessment
> Medicine/Surgery
> Physiologic and Anatomic Equilibrium
> Acute Care
> Respiratory

2. **A farmer is brought to the emergency room with symptoms of anaphylactic shock. As part of the assessment the nurse inquires about:**
   1. Insect bites
   2. Dietary changes
   3. Hours spent outdoors
   4. Fiber content of clothing

RATIONALE

(1) Anaphylactic shock follows a severe allergic reaction in which the client is exposed to an antigen such as drugs, contrast media, blood products or insect stings to which he or she has been previously sensitized.

2. This results in gastrointestinal symptoms.
3. Prolonged sun exposure may result in heat stroke.
4. Certain fabrics may cause contact dermatitis.

> Assessment
> Medicine/Surgery
> Physiologic and Anatomic Equilibrium
> Acute Care
> Cardiovascular

3. **The nurse admits to the intensive care unit from the emergency room an attorney who has suffered an acute myocardial infarction. The blood pressure is 80/50 mm Hg. This type of shock is:**
   1. Septic
   2. Vasogenic
   3. Cardiogenic
   4. Hypovolemic

RATIONALE

(3) Death of heart muscle, termed myocardial infarction, can place the client at risk to develop cardiogenic shock.

1. Sepsis results from a bacterial infection.
2. Vasogenic shock is triggered by central nervous system changes.
4. Hypovolemic shock occurs from fluid loss.

> Evaluation
> Medicine/Surgery
> Physiologic and Anatomic Equilibrium
> Acute Care
> Cardiovascular

4. **In evaluating the effectiveness of interventions for any client in shock, the nurse would check the:**
   1. Temperature
   2. Lactic acid level

3. Hemoglobin and hematocrit
4. Sensation in the lower extremities

RATIONALE

(2) All forms of shock decrease tissue perfusion, which alters cellular metabolism. The lactic acid level correlates with anaerobic metabolism.

1. Shock clients may be normo-, hypo-, or hyperthermic.
3. This laboratory value is altered in hypovolemic shock.
4. Neurogenic shock may cause this symptom.

Assessment
Medicine/Surgery
Physiologic and Anatomic Equilibrium
Acute Care
Neuromuscular

5. **Neurologic assessment of a client with progressive shock would reveal:**
   1. Incoherence
   2. Unresponsiveness
   3. Seizure activity
   4. Restlessness and agitation

RATIONALE

(2) In the progressive stage of shock, there is an inadequate oxygenation of the brain and the level of consciousness deteriorates; the client is no longer responsive to verbal and painful stimuli.

1. This may be seen in the initial stage.
3. This may occur with neurogenic shock.
4. These are early signs of shock.

Analysis
Medicine/Surgery
Physiologic and Anatomic Equilibrium
Acute Care
Cardiovascular

6. **Dobutamine is administered to a client with traumatic internal bleeding to:**
   1. Prevent atelectasis
   2. Correct metabolic acidosis
   3. Dilate arteries to vital organs
   4. Increase force of myocardial contraction

RATIONALE

(3) Inotropic agents are specific drugs used to increase the force of myocardial contraction in the shock client. Dopamine is also frequently used.

1. This drug has no effect on the alveoli.
2. This is a secondary effect as tissue perfusion is increased.
3. Vasodilation does not occur.

Planning
Medicine/Surgery
Physiologic and Anatomic Equilibrium

Acute Care
Cardiovascular

7. **In planning the care of a client who is demonstrating signs of shock after spinal anesthesia, the nurse would anticipate:**
   1. Providing a cooling mattress
   2. Administering warmed intravenous fluids
   3. Elevating the head of the bed 15 degrees
   4. Placing the client in the Trendelenburg position

RATIONALE

(3) Proper head positioning allows for adequate sympathetic outflow. Spinal shock occurs from the blockage of sympathetic innervation to the peripheral vessels resulting in vasodilation.

1. Hyperthermia is not related to this shock state.
2. This is not appropriate.
3. Having the head dependent may worsen the condition.

Analysis
Medicine/Surgery
Physiologic and Anatomic Equilibrium
Acute Care
Cardiovascular

8. **A client recovering from a massive myocardial infarction has a Swan-Ganz catheter in place. The pulmonary artery wedge pressure is 8 mm Hg. This value is:**
   1. Low
   2. High
   3. Normal
   4. Critically low

RATIONALE

(3) A Swan-Ganz catheter is floated into the pulmonary artery, where pressure measurements can be taken on the right and left side of the heart and the pulmonary circulation. Pulmonary artery wedge pressure indirectly measures left ventricular pressure.

1. The lower limit of normal for this value is 6 mm hg.
2. The upper limit of normal for this value is 12 mm hg.
4. Values below 6 are low.

CHAPTER 6 The Critically Ill Adult with Multiple Organ Dysfunction Syndrome

Analysis
Medicine/Surgery
Physiologic and Anatomic Equilibrium
Acute Care
Cardiovascular

1. **A critical care unit nurse is caring for a critically ill client. A pending diagnosis is that of multiple**

organ dysfunction syndrome (MODS). This is confirmed with the identification of:
1. Widespread infection
2. Presence of drug resistant bacteria
3. Dysfunction of two or more organ systems
4. Presence of disease of unknown cause

RATIONALE

(3) MODS is a nonspecific complication of critical illness or injury involving progressive, sequential dysfunction of two or more organ systems.
1. MODS is not always caused by infection.
2. This is not a criterion for this diagnosis.
4. This is not a criterion for this disease.

> Analysis
> Medicine/Surgery
> Physiologic and Anatomic Equilibrium
> Acute Care
> Blood and Immunity

2. **The nurse is assigned to care for a client who has an inflammatory response clinically identical to sepsis, except that there is no infection present. This condition is called:**
1. Arthritis
2. Anaphylactic shock
3. Multisystem organ failure
4. Systemic inflammatory response syndrome (SIRS)

RATIONALE

(4) An inflammatory response identical to sepsis without the presence of infection can occur as a result of trauma, burns, pancreatitis or ischemia.
1. This is inflammation of the joint spaces.
2. This causes a reaction in the respiratory tract and skin.
3. SIRS is the process through which triggers are released that begin to effect multiple organs.

> Planning
> Medicine/Surgery
> Physiologic and Anatomic Equilibrium
> Acute Care
> Cardiovascular

3. **The nurse is asked to obtain equipment needed to monitor the cardiac output of a client. This will include:**
1. Swan-Ganz catheter
2. Arterial catheter
3. Ventriculostomy catheter
4. Sequential compression device

RATIONALE

(1) This is a pulmonary artery catheter that can be used to monitor fluid status and cardiac function.
2. This is used to monitor pressure in a peripheral artery.
3. This is used to measure intracranial pressure.

4. This is used to exert pressure on the lower extremities to prevent venous stasis.

> Analysis
> Medicine/Surgery
> Physiologic and Anatomic Equilibrium
> Acute Care
> Cardiovascular

4. **The nurse is caring for a client who has cardiac failure. The first line intervention in severe cardiovascular disorders is:**
1. Drug therapy
2. Permanent pacemaker
3. Hemodynamic monitoring
4. Cardiopulmonary resuscitation

RATIONALE

(1) Inotropic medications are used to increase the strength of cardiac contractions and to increase cardiac output.
2. These may be used if there is a problem with heart rate or electrical conduction in the heart.
3. This is used to evaluate the effectiveness of drug therapy.
4. This is a therapy that is used when all others have failed.

> Evaluation
> Medicine/Surgery
> Physiologic and Anatomic Equilibrium
> Acute Care
> Blood and immunity

5. **The medical intensive care unit nurse is evaluating the results of laboratory work on a client with systemic inflammatory response syndrome. The expected findings include:**
1. Heart rate of 80
2. Respiratory rate of 14
3. Body temperature of 38° C
4. WBC count of 14,000/mm^3

RATIONALE

(4) A WBC count greater than 12,000/mm^3 or less than 4000/mm^3, or with more than 10% immature neutrophils is characteristic of the disease.
1. Heart rates greater than 90 are expected.
2. Tachypnea with a rate greater than 20 breaths/minute or hyperventilation with a PCO_2 less than 32 mm Hg is expected.
3. The temperature range is expected to be greater than 38° C or less than 36° C.

> Planning
> Medicine/Surgery
> Physiologic and Anatomic Equilibrium
> Acute Care
> Gastrointestinal

6. **A client with multisystem organ failure has an oral endotracheal tube. The plan to provide nutritional support that maintains gut integrity will include:**
   1. Enteral feeding
   2. Fluid restriction
   3. Intravenous fluid
   4. Total parenteral nutrition

   RATIONALE

   (1) Enteral feedings are encouraged because they prevent the mucosal lining from becoming atrophied.
   2. These clients need fluid replacement.
   3. This therapy alone contributes to gut atrophy.
   4. This supplies nutrients but does not stop the atrophy of the gut.

   > Analysis
   > Medicine/Surgery
   > Psychosocial
   > Acute Care
   > Blood and Immunity

7. **A client is moved from the general medical-surgical unit to the intensive care unit. This transfer will increase the risk of infection and other complications by:**
   1. Intact skin
   2. Presence of invasive devices
   3. Potential overload of nutritional support
   4. Administration of low doses of antibiotics

   RATIONALE

   (2) Critical care units can can increase the risk of complications from the use of invasive lines.
   1. Intact skin is an effective defense against infection.
   3. This is a relatively unlikely complication.
   4. Low doses of antibiotics rarely cause problems.

   > Evaluation
   > Medicine/Surgery
   > Psychosocial
   > Acute Care
   > Cardiovascular

8. **A care plan for a client who is critically ill will include the major goal of:**
   1. Adequate circulating volume
   2. Decreasing oxygen delivery
   3. Maximizing oxygen demand
   4. Meeting psychologic requirements

   RATIONALE

   (1) The primary goals for the critically ill client focus on minimizing infections and inflammatory stimuli and maintaining adequate preload and circulating volume.
   2. Oxygen delivery and consumption should be enhanced.

   3. Oxygen demand should be minimized and metabolic requirements should be met.
   4. These are addressed after critical physical needs are met.

   > Assessment
   > Medicine/Surgery
   > Psychosocial
   > Acute Care
   > Cardiovascular

9. **A client is septic and has a cardiac output of 10 L/min. Myocardial depression occurs early in septic shock and multisystem organ failure, so the increase in contractility cannot be the cause of the increased cardiac output. The other factor contributing to the elevated cardiac output is:**
   1. Hyperdynamic state increases preload
   2. Sympathetic stimulation increases preload
   3. Autonomic stimulation increases preload
   4. Parasympathetic stimulation increases preload

   RATIONALE

   (2) This increases venous return and preload; along with tachycardia, the increased preload increases cardiac output.
   1. This state is the source of the problem.
   3. The sympathetic nervous system is one branch of the autonomic nervous system.
   4. This decreases preload.

   > Assessment
   > Medicine/Surgery
   > Physiologic and Anatomic Equilibrium
   > Acute Care
   > Cardiovascular

10. **The nurse notices that a client has generalized peripheral edema, yet his pulmonary capillary wedge pressure and urine output are low. He is not volume overloaded. The source of edema is:**
    1. Vasoconstriction
    2. Selective vasodilation
    3. Decreased capillary permeability
    4. Increased capillary permeability

    RATIONALE

    (4) The endothelial lining of the vascular system becomes damaged and capillaries become permeable. Fluid leaks into the tissue and yields generalized peripheral edema.
    1. Vasoconstriction alone does not cause this.
    2. Vasodilation is not the source of the problem.
    3. The permeability is increased.

    > Planning
    > Medicine/Surgery
    > Physiologic and Anatomic Equilibrium
    > Acute Care
    > Respiratory

11. A client develops nosocomial pneumonia 6 days after admission to the intensive care unit. This is related to the stress ulcer prophylaxis of antacids and H2 blockers. The connection between this therapy and the pneumonia is:
    1. Overgrowth of bacteria in the nose
    2. Overgrowth of bacteria in the stomach
    3. Overgrowth of bacteria in the mouth
    4. Colonization of bacteria in the endotracheal tube

RATIONALE

(2) Prophylaxis of antacids and H2 blockers has been associated with an overgrowth of bacteria in the stomach and an increased incidence of nosocomial pneumonia secondary to migration of these bacteria and gastric reflux.
    1. This is not a related occurence.
    3. This is not the primary cause of this process.
    4. This may also affect the respiratory system but is not related to ulcer therapy.

UNIT II   Principles of Perioperative Nursing

CHAPTER 7   Preoperative NursingAnalysis

Medicine/Surgery
Physiologic and Anatomic Equilibrium
Acute Care
Cardiovascular

1. During the preoperative history taking, a young client scheduled for a laparoscopic cholecystectomy tells the out-patient surgery nurse that she takes four to six aspirin tablets a day for relief of joint pain. The nurse should report this fact to the surgeon because aspirin use can:
   1. Delay wound healing
   2. Cause a potassium imbalance
   3. Increase operative blood loss
   4. Decrease the neuroendocrine response

RATIONALE

(3) Aspirin and anticoagulants should be discontinued or have the dosage adjusted before surgery, because their use can increase bleeding because of their effect on platelets.
   1. Wound healing is not directly affected.
   2. The potassium balance is unchanged by aspirin.
   4. Aspirin has no direct affect on the neuroendocrine system.

Analysis
Medicine/Surgery
Physiologic and Anatomic Equilibrium
Acute Care
Surgery

2. Nursing care of the client undergoing surgery requires aa understanding of which phase of surgical care:
   1. Intraoperative
   2. Preoperative

3. Postoperative
4. Perioperative

RATIONALE

(4) The term perioperative refers to nursing care delivered during the entire surgical experience including pre-, intra-, and postoperative phases. Nurses should have knowledge of all of them to ensure smooth, safe care.
   1. The intraoperative phase begins when the client arrives in the operating room and ends at the time of transport from the operating room.
   2. The preoperative period begins when the client arrives in the operating room holding area and ends at the time of transport to the specific operating room where the surgery will take place.
   3. The postoperative period begins when the client leaves the operating room and is transported to another location for aftercare. This period ends at the time of discharge from the facility.

Implementation
Medicine/Surgery
Psychosocial and Emotional
    Equilibrium
Acute Care
Emotional Needs Related to Health
    Needs

3. The parents of a 26-year-old woman who has severe brain damage after a motor vehicle accident are asked to sign a surgical consent form for a tracheostomy. They ask why the procedure is needed. The nurse explains that it is a palliative procedure, which means that it:
   1. Repairs, replaces, or removes defective tissue
   2. Minimizes the complications of a disease process
   3. Determines the origin or extent of a lesion
   4. Returns lost function or corrects deformities

RATIONALE

(2) Surgery is performed for a variety of reasons. Palliative surgery is done to slow the disease process and to relieve symptoms caused by disease. Severe brain injury often interferes with the client's ability to breathe spontaneously. A tracheostomy minimizes the damage that may occur from long-term oral or nasal intubation.
   1. This phrase defines curative surgery done in an attempt to eliminate disease.
   3. This phrase defines diagnostic or exploratory surgery that is done to obtain a biopsy or to visualize organs in order to obtain a medical diagnosis.
   4. The return of function is one goal of restorative surgery and includes repair of fractures and replacement of heart valves.

Analysis
Medicine/Surgery
Physiologic and Anatomic Equilibrium
Acute Care
Surgery

4. **Nursing staff in the preoperative holding area notice that an American Society of Anesthesiologists (ASA) classification has been included on the preoperative assessment sheet. The ASA Classification of Physical Status is a system used to:**
   1. Determine the length of hospital stay
   2. Simplify the outpatient assessment process
   3. Shorten the duration of the surgical procedure
   4. Estimate patient risk from anesthetic agents.

RATIONALE

(4) The anesthesia care provider reviews the client's medical history and performs a brief physical examination to determine the client's physical status and anesthesia risk. This enables anesthesia personnel to decide upon the appropriate anesthetic agents and techniques for the client.
   1. This system has no direct correlation to hospital length of stay.
   2. This process may be detailed and lengthy, depending upon the client's condition.
   3. Certain types of anesthetic techniques such as spinal and extremity blocks may actually prolong the total operating room time.

Analysis
Medicine/Surgery
Physiologic and Anatomic Equilibrium
Acute Care
Cardiovascular

5. **The intraoperative nurse monitoring a client who is receiving local anesthesia notices an increase in the heart rate. The change may be caused by the release of:**
   1. Norepinephrine
   2. Glucocorticoids
   3. Aldosterone
   4. Antidiuretic hormone

RATIONALE

(1) Norepinephrine is a stimulant that causes peripheral vasoconstriction and increased blood pressure and heart rate.
   2. This hormone causes gluconeogenesis, a negative nitrogen balance, decrease in the immune response and increased platelet activity. This results in an increase in the amount of available energy fuel, slowing of the tissue repair process, an increased risk of infection, and increased clot formation.
   3. Release of this hormone causes sodium and water resorption, leading to decreased urination and an increased circulatory volume.

4. The release of antidiuretic hormone causes the physiologic changes of sodium and water resorption.

Planning
Medicine/Surgery
Psychosocial
Acute Care
Emotional

6. **The surgical unit nurse is preparing a preoperative care plan for a client. The most common nursing diagnosis for surgical clients relates to:**
   1. Fear
   2. Infection
   3. Malignancy
   4. Social isolation

RATIONALE

(1) All clients fear the unknown, anesthesia, loss of control, pain, death, and mutilation.
   2. The risk of infection may not be experienced by everyone undergoing surgery.
   3. Cancer is not a concern of every client.
   4. Many clients have strong social support systems.

Planning
Medicine/Surgery
Physiologic and Anatomic Equilibrium
Acute Care
Respiratory

7. **Clients scheduled for general or regional anesthesia are not allowed to eat or drink for 6 to 8 hours before surgery. This is necessary to reduce the risk of:**
   1. Nausea
   2. Aspiration
   3. Stomach dilation
   4. Electrolyte imbalance

RATIONALE

(2) Aspiration of gastric contents into the lungs is a serious postoperative complication.
   1. Nausea is minimized through the use of antiemetics.
   3. Stomach dilation can occur and is relieved by the use of a nasogastric tube.
   4. Withholding food or fluids may increase the risk of electrolyte imbalance if prolonged.

Implementation
Medicine/Surgery
Education
Acute Care
Respiratory

8. **An obese client is counseled by an office nurse to lose weight before an upcoming surgery. Obesity places the client at greater risk for:**
   1. Vomiting
   2. Profuse bleeding
   3. Pulmonary complications
   4. Increased pain intensity

RATIONALE

(3) Hypoventilation and pneumonia are common in obese clients.

1. The risk of vomiting may not be increased.
2. Increased bleeding is not directly related to obesity. There are many factors involved.
4. Pain intensity is not automatically increased in these clients.

Implementation
Medicine/Surgery
Physiologic and Anatomic Equilibrium
Acute Care
Integumentary

9. **The presurgical unit nurse is asked to prepare a client's skin for an abdominal hysterectomy. The nurse would be expected to:**
   1. Shave the hair with a safety razor as far in advance of the surgery as possible.
   2. Shave the hair with an electric razor as far in advance of the surgery as possible.
   3. Shave the hair with an electric razor immediately before the client's being transported to the operating room.
   4. Shave the hair with a safety razor immediately before the client's being transported to the operating room.

RATIONALE

(3) Electric razors and depilatory creams cause fewer abrasions, nicks, lacerations or burns than safety razors. Research indicates an increase in infection rates as the time between the preoperative shave and the operation increase.

1. Safety razors can cause nicks that disrupt the mechanical barrier of the skin, and increasing the time between surgery and skin shave increases the risk of infection
2. Electric razors cause less skin damage, but the shave should be done as near to the time of surgery as possible.
4. Safety razors damage the mechanical barrier of the skin.

Evaluation
Medicine/Surgery
Education and Health Promotion
Acute Care
Respiratory

10. **An elderly client had bilateral total knee replacements under general anesthesia. The surgical procedure lasted 4 hours. Preoperatively, the client received instructions on deep breathing exercises to increase lung ventilation and gas exchange postoperatively. The postsurgical nurse observes correct technique when the client is able to:**
    1. Take quick, shallow breaths through the mouth, hold them, then cough deeply from the chest.

2. Take a slow, deep breath through the mouth, hold it, exhale and cough deeply from the throat.
3. Take a slow, deep breath through the nose, hold it, exhale and cough deeply from the chest.
4. Take a quick, deep breath through the nose, hold it, exhale and cough deeply from the throat

RATIONALE

(3) After surgery there is a decline in lung ventilation and gas exchange that varies with the individual client, length of anesthesia, and the surgical site. The client is taught this technique of sustained maximal inspiration to prevent collapse of alveoli and to mobilize secretions after surgery.

1. A deep breath through the nose is most effective.
2. Breathing in through the nose is recommended.
4. A slow breath through the nose and coughing from the chest is most effective.

Implementation
Medicine/Surgery
Physiologic and Anatomic Equilibrium
Surgery

11. **A graduate nurse completing an internship in perioperative nursing is asked to identify the correct statement about surgical consents on an examination. Indicate which one of these is correct:**
    1. The client's decision to have surgery can be revoked at any time.
    2. The consent form may be signed by the client if premedication has been given.
    3. A spouse, child, or friend may sign the consent form if the client asks them to.
    4. The perioperative nurse is required to inform the client of all of the surgical and anesthetic risks related to the procedure.

RATIONALE

(1) This statement is true. If a client should express a lack of understanding of the procedure or an unwillingness to continue with the surgery, this should be reported to the nursing supervisor and to the client's physician immediately.

2. No client should receive preoperative medication until the consent form has been signed. Mind-altering medication renders the client mentally incompetent. When the medication has been given, the drug effects should be allowed to wear off before the consent can be obtained.
3. Competent adults should sign their own consent forms. Spouses, children, and friends legally cannot.
4. The surgeon and the anesthesia care provider are required to inform the client of the risks of procedures that they will perform on the client, not the perioperative nurse.

Implementation
Medicine/Surgery
Physiologic and Anatomic Equilibrium
Acute Care
Neuromuscular

1. **The anesthesiologist asks the perioperative nurse to assist with the positioning of a client for anesthesia administration. This will involve injecting an anesthetic solution into the cerebrospinal fluid that surrounds the lower spinal cord and nerve roots and is referred to as:**
   1. Local anesthesia
   2. Spinal anesthesia
   3. General anesthesia
   4. Monitored anesthesia care

RATIONALE

(2) This technique blocks nerve transmission through the spinal nerve roots.
   1. A local anesthetic disrupts sensation at the level of the nerve endings.
   3. This is a drug-induced state in which analgesia, amnesia, muscle relaxation, and unconsciousness occur.
   4. This is type of local anesthetic technique.

Planning
Medicine/Surgery
Physiologic and Anatomic Equilibrium
Acute Care
Neuromuscular

2. **A perioperative nurse, completing an orientation to a new operating room, is shown the location of the emergency equipment within the department. The most common cause of anesthetic-induced death in North America is:**
   1. Cardiac arrest
   2. Respiratory arrest
   3. Malignant hyperthermia
   4. Toxic levels of anesthetic agents

RATIONALE

(3) Malignant hyperthermia is an inherited disorder of abnormal muscle metabolism, which causes an increase in heat production in response to stress and certain anesthetics.
   1. Cardiac arrest does occur as a result of anesthetic complications, but not as often as malignant hyperthermia.
   2. Respiratory arrest can also result from anesthesia complications.
   4. Toxic levels of anesthetic agents can cause serious complications.

Evaluation
Medicine/Surgery

Environmental Safety
Acute Care
Integumentary

3. **At the end of the surgical procedure, the perioperative nurse assesses the client's skin for burns that may be caused by:**
   1. Electrosurgery unit
   2. Irrigation fluids
   3. Positioning aids
   4. Skin preparation solution

RATIONALE

(1) Both thermal and electrical burns may be caused from improper grounding of the electrosurgery unit.
   2. The temperature of irrigation fluids is adjusted to match body temperature.
   3. A sheet or blanket is usually placed between the client's skin and the positioning aids. These may cause pressure points, but not burns.
   4. Skin preparation fluids can cause skin irritation, but not usually burns.

Assessment
Medicine/Surgery
Environmental safety
Acute Care
Surgery

4. **The person who reviews the client's chart before surgery and who is responsible for carrying out the nonsterile nursing functions within the operating room is the:**
   1. Surgeon
   2. Scrub nurse
   3. Anesthesiologist
   4. Circulating nurse

RATIONALE

(4) The circulating nurse is a registered nurse who ensures that the client is safely monitored and supported during the operation.
   1. The surgeon performs a surgical scrub and is considered sterile.
   2. The scrub nurse is responsible for supplying the surgeon with the needed sterile supplies.
   3. The anesthesiologist is a physician who administers the anesthetic agent.

Evaluation
Medicine/Surgery
Physiologic and Anatomic Equilibrium
Acute Care
Cardiovascular

5. **A middle-aged client has been placed in the prone position for a lumbar laminectomy. At the end of the procedure, the client is turned slowly to the supine position onto a stretcher for transport. The physiologic change that may occur from this activity is:**

1. Hypotension
2. Discomfort
3. Infection
4. Respiratory distress

RATIONALE

(1) Position changes in the anesthetized client should be made slowly to allow the circulatory system time to adjust to the changes in blood distribution.
2. The client remains anesthetized and cannot feel pain.
3. This change does not increase the risk of infection.
4. This should not occur because the client will have an endotracheal tube in place.

Assessment
Medicine/Surgery
Physiologic and Anatomic Equilibrium
Acute Care
Neuromuscular

6. The ambulatory surgery postanesthesia care unit nurse notices that an elderly man who has undergone a facial scar revision under local anesthesia appears to be exhibiting symptoms of toxicity. These symptoms include:
1. Anxiety, agitation
2. Tinnitus, slurred speech
3. Lethargy, cyanosis, muscle rigidity
4. Profuse sweating, skin mottling, fever

RATIONALE

(2) These are all central nervous system effects of local anesthetics. At low concentrations, these drugs have a stimulating effect on cardiac and vascular smooth muscle. At high concentrations, myocardial depression and vasodilation can occur. Bradycardia and cardiovascular collapse can also occur.
1. These symptoms may be caused by hypoxia and disorientation.
3. These symptoms may also be caused by hypoxia and/or oversedation.
4. These are symptoms associated with malignant hyperthermia, the most common anesthetic-related complication.

Implementation
Medicine/Surgery
Physiologic and Anatomic
    Equilibrium
Acute Care
Surgery

7. The perioperative nurse prepares to care for a trauma victim en route by helicopter from a nearby town. Nursing actions appropriate for this client include:

1. Obtaining a cooling blanket
2. Providing cool intravenous fluids
3. Preparing a warming mattress
4. Lowering the room temperature

RATIONALE

(3) Hypothermia is a serious complication for this client and can be prevented by the use of warming blankets, lights, and warmed inhaled anesthetic agents.
1. Further cooling is not indicated.
2. Warmed intravenous fluids are recommended.
4. Increasing the room temperature will provide more warmth.

Analysis
Medicine/Surgery
Physiologic and Anatomic Support
Acute Care
Neuromuscular

8. The most common client complication from laser use is:
1. Respiratory distress
2. Intense heat
3. Damage to the eyes
4. Itching of the skin

RATIONALE

(3) Lasers are used for cutting, coagulation, vaporizing, and welding tissue. The laser beam delivers energy directly to the tissue, which results in extremely high temperatures. The beam can cause severe burns to the eyes, which must be protected with moist pads or protective eyewear.
1. This is not a usual complication.
2. Intense heat may be generated, but the client usually does not feel the effects of it.
4. This is not a common complication. The skin can be burned if the laser beam is directed onto it.

CHAPTER 9   Postoperative Nursing

Implementation
Medicine/Surgery
Physiologic and Anatomic Equilibrium
Acute Care
Respiratory

1. The immediate priority of a postanesthesia care unit nurse admitting a client from the operating room after surgery under general anesthesia is:
1. Alleviate pain
2. Obtain vital signs
3. Provide warm blankets
4. Ensure a patent airway

(4) Airway patency, breathing, and circulation are assessed in this order. Oxygen is provided as indicated.

1. Pain relief is important once the stability of the client has been established.
2. Equipment to monitor blood pressure and pulse are placed once airway patency has been verified.
3. Hypothermia is a common problem after surgery and should be addressed after adequate ventilation has been assured.

> Implementation
> Medicine/Surgery
> Physiologic and Anatomic
> Acute Care
> Gastrointestinal

2. **After intestinal surgery, the surgical unit nurse might perform which one of these client interventions to stimulate peristalsis and relieve distention:**
   1. Encourage ambulation
   2. Apply an abdominal binder
   3. Offer a carbonated beverage
   4. Administer a tap water enema

RATIONALE

(1) Ambulation stimulates peristalsis and can help to prevent paralytic ileus caused by intestinal manipulation.

2. A binder may reduce gastrointestinal circulation.
3. Carbonated beverages increase intestinal distention.
4. Enemas can increase pressure on the suture line and cause rupture.

> Implementation
> Medicine/Surgery
> Physiologic and Anatomic Equilibrium
> Acute Care
> Gastrointestinal

3. **On the third day after abdominal surgery, the nurse notes that a client's incision has become separated and that the intestines are protruding through the incision. The most appropriate nursing action is to:**
   1. Raise the client's feet
   2. Instruct the client to take shallow, thoracic breaths.
   3. Cover the intestines with a warm, sterile saline dressing.
   4. Reinforce the abdominal dressing with a thick, sterile dressing

RATIONALE

(3) The intestines have eviscerated through the incision. The nurse should cover the intestines with a warm, sterile saline dressing and notify the surgeon.

1. Raising the feet is not a priority and may cause increased abdominal strain.
2. The emphasis should be on covering the intestines to prevent dryness and infection.
4. Warm, moist gauze prevents the intestines from heat loss through the open incision.

> Evaluation
> Medicine/Surgery
> Education
> Acute Care
> Integumentary

4. **A surgical clinic nurse notes that a client's incision is healing normally. It is explained to the client that this is called:**
   1. Scar formation
   2. Primary intention
   3. Tertiary intention
   4. Secondary intention

RATIONALE

(2) Healing by primary intention occurs when the wound edges are closely approximated and when there are no complications such as infection, necrosis, or abdominal scar formation.

1. Scar formation occurs when there is trauma to the wound edges or infection.
3. Tertiary intention occurs when there is a delay between the injury and wound closure.
4. Secondary intention occurs when the wound edges are not closely approximated, as in cases of infection, trauma, or tissue loss.

> Planning
> Medicine/Surgery
> Physiologic and Anatomic
> Equilibrium
> Acute Care
> Neuromuscular

5. **The nurse should offer prescribed analgesics to a client who is 24 hours postoperative:**
   1. Only when the client asks
   2. Only when the physician orders
   3. Regularly before the pain is severe
   4. Only when the client is in severe pain

RATIONALE

(3) Pain relief should be prompt and effective to avoid setting up a cycle of pain.

1. Clients may not request medication for fear of addiction.
2. If the pain is not adequately relieved, further physician's orders should be obtained.
4. Waiting until the pain is severe may result in the need for increased amounts of medication.

CHAPTER 10   Nursing Assessment of the
Respiratory System

Assessment
Medicine/Surgery
Physiologic and Anatomic Equilibrium
Acute Care
Respiratory

1. **A graduate nurse is reviewing the respiratory system in preparation for a new position on a pulmonary unit. The outline states that the process of respiration occurs only at:**
    1. Lungs
    2. Alveoli
    3. Capillaries
    4. Bronchioles

RATIONALE

(2) The alveoli form the mass of the lungs; ventilation of the alveoli results from alternately lowering and raising the air pressure within the lungs by alternately increasing and decreasing their volume, so that the air is drawn into and forced out of the alveoli.
1. The lungs contain all of the components needed for oxygenation to occur at the alveolar level.
3. Capillaries carry blood and interface with the alveoli, where gas exchange occurs.
4. Bronchioles branch into the alveoli, where respiration actually occurs.

Analysis
Medicine/Surgery
Physiologic and Anatomic Equilibrium
Long-term Care
Respiratory

2. **A home health nurse instructing client with chronic obstructive pulmonary disease about the disease explains that gas exchange from the pulmonary system to the blood occurs through:**
    1. Osmosis
    2. Diffusion
    3. Active transport
    4. Oncotic pressure

RATIONALE

(2) Gas diffuses from an area of high concentration to an area of low concentration.
1. Osmosis refers to the movement of particles in solution across a semipermeable membrane.
3. Active transport is the process in which substances move through a cell membrane in chemical combination with carrier substances against an energy gradient.
4. Oncotic pressure is pressure created by the concentration of particles in solution.

Analysis
Medicine/Surgery
Education
Acute Care
Respiratory

3. **A nurse educator explains to a group of nurse interns that normally ventilation is regulated by the central chemoreceptor response to levels of:**
    1. O_2
    2. pH
    3. CO_2
    4. PCO_2

RATIONALE

(4) An increase in the PCO_2, or arterial carbon dioxide level, is the most potent respiratory stimulant.
1. The oxygen level does not trigger the respiratory center.
2. This is the level of acidosis of the blood.
3. CO_2 is carbon dioxide gas. The arterial CO_2 (PCO_2) is the actual trigger for respiration.

Assessment
Medicine/Surgery
Physiologic and Anatomic Equilibrium
Acute Care
Respiratory

4. **A surgical intensive care unit nurse caring for a client with a closed head injury assesses for possible respiratory difficulties. Pulmonary ventilation is controlled in the brain by the:**
    1. Medulla
    2. Hypothalamus
    3. Chemoreceptors
    4. Cerebral cortex

RATIONALE

(1) Pulmonary ventilation is controlled by the respiratory centers in the medulla and pons of the brainstem, which receive sensory input from the brain.
2. The hypothalamus and its related structures control many internal conditions of the body as well as aspects of behavior.
3. Chemoreceptors in the carotid and aortic bodies transmit signals to the respiratory center in response to oxygen and carbon dioxide levels.
4. The cerebral cortex is a storage area for sensory information.

Assessment
Medicine/Surgery
Physiologic and Anatomic Equilibrium
Community-based Care
Respiratory

5. **A clinic nurse assessing a client for fremitus uses the technique of:**
    1. Inspection
    2. Percussion

3. Palpation
4. Auscultation

RATIONALE

(3) Palpation is used for the assessment of tactile fremitus.
1. Inspection is visual observation of a structure.
2. Percussion is tapping of a structure to elicit a sound.
4. Auscultation is listening to internal sounds with the aid of a stethoscope.

> Planning
> Medicine/Surgery
> Physiologic and Anatomic Equilibrium
> Acute Care
> Respiratory

6. The nurse is instructing a client on the best procedure to follow to obtain a sputum specimen. This includes:
1. "Spit whatever sputum you have in your mouth into this container."
2. "Take a deep breath and hold it, cough; now spit into this container."
3. "Cough and deep breathe first thing tomorrow morning and collect whatever you cough up."
4. "Limit the amount of fluids you drink today. Collect whatever you cough up in this container."

RATIONALE

(3) Collecting sputum when the client first awakens ensures that the sputum is not swallowed.
1. The client should cough to pull the secretions up from the lung.
2. Breath holding is not necessary.
4. Liberal intake of fluids facilitates specimen collection.

> Planning
> Medicine/Surgery
> Education
> Acute Care
> Respiratory

7. The nurse preparing a client for a diagnostic test explains, "The test you'll be having in the morning allows the doctor to view your trachea and bronchi by inserting an instrument down your throat." This partially explains the procedure for a:
1. Bronchoscopy
2. Bronchogram
3. Pulmonary angiography
4. Computerized tomography

RATIONALE

(1) The bronchoscope is introduced through the nose, mouth, tracheotomy tube, or endotracheal tube for the purpose of direct visualization of the larynx, trachea, and bronchi.

2. A bronchogram is rarely performed and involves introducing contrast medium into the tracheobronchial tree through a catheter.
3. Pulmonary angiography is used to visualize pulmonary vasculature and requires the use of radiopaque dye in a peripheral vein.
4. Computerized tomography is a special radiologic technique that may or may not involve the use of contrast medium.

> Planning
> Medicine/Surgery
> Physiologic and Anatomic Equilibrium
> Education
> Respiratory

8. A client about to undergo a thoracentesis is told by the nurse that a needle will be inserted into the:
1. Lungs
2. Thorax
3. Bronchi
4. Pleural space

RATIONALE

(4) During thoracentesis, the physician inserts a large-bore needle through the chest wall into the pleural space.
1. Lungs are not punctured directly except to obtain a biopsy.
2. The thorax or chest wall is rarely punctured.
3. The bronchi are examined and biopsied through a bronchoscope.

> Evaluation
> Medicine/Surgery
> Physiologic and Anatomic Equilibrium
> Acute Care
> Respiratory

9. If a client has followed the nurses' instructions, the post-thoracentesis position which the client should be in is:
1. Prone
2. Supine
3. Lying on unaffected side
4. Sitting up on the side of the bed

RATIONALE

(3) The client should be placed on the unaffected side for 1 hour to allow the puncture site to close.
1. The prone position would interfere with respiration.
2. Respiratory effort is reduced even in the supine position.
4. Sitting up immediately after a procedure may cause a client to have increased pain and dizziness.

> Evaluation
> Medicine/Surgery
> Physiologic and Anatomic Equilibrium

10. A client's nurse is asked to perform a Mantoux test to diagnose tuberculosis. The test should be read:
    1. Within 24 hours
    2. Within 48 hours
    3. Within 48 to 72 hours
    4. Within 3 to 4 days

RATIONALE

(3) The test helps to determine whether tuberculosis is present, and the test results need to be read in 48 to 72 hours.
    1. There may not be any change within 24 hours.
    2. This is the lower time limit for the test to be read.
    4. Within 3 to 4 days the amount of reactivity may have started to decrease.

Evaluation
Medicine/Surgery
Physiologic and Anatomic Equilibrium
Community-based Care
Respiratory

11. The nurse's correct interpretation of the Mantoux test is:
    1. 0 mm indicates the test did not take
    2. 5 mm is diagnostic of tuberculosis
    3. 4 mm indicates probability of tuberculosis
    4. 10 mm is highly significant for infection

RATIONALE

(4) Induration of 10 mm or more is a positive reaction.
    1. 0 to 4 mm of induration indicates a negative reaction.
    2. 5 mm is a doubtful reaction except in the case of persons who have been in close contact with persons with active tuberculosis.
    3. The range of doubtful reaction is 5 to 9 mm of induration.

Assessment
Medicine/Surgery
Physiologic and Anatomic Equilibrium
Community-based Care
Respiratory

12. The community clinic nurse auscultates breath sounds of medium pitch, heard on inspiration and expiration over the first and second intercostal spaces at the sternal border. These are:
    1. Adventitious
    2. Bronchial
    3. Vesicular
    4. Bronchovesicular

RATIONALE

(4) Bronchovesicular breath sounds are heard at this location and also over the upper right posterior lung field.

    1. Adventitious breath sounds are abnormal and include crackles and wheezes.
    2. Bronchial breath sounds are normally heard over the manubrium and are high pitched.
    3. Vesicular breath sounds are heard in the peripheral lung fields and are low pitched.

Assessment
Medicine/Surgery
Physiologic and Anatomic
    Equilibrium
Acute Care
Respiratory

13. The surgical intensive care unit nurse hears crackles bilaterally when assessing a client. These are caused by:
    1. Air flowing through moisture in air passages
    2. Air flowing through narrowed air passages
    3. Air flowing through abnormal fibrous tissue
    4. Air flowing through consolidated lung tissue

RATIONALE

(1) Crackles are caused by the movement of air through fluid in the airways and alveoli.
    2. Air flowing through narrowed passages produces wheezes.
    3. Air flow through fibrous tissue will diminish the sound and lead to a change in pitch.
    4. Air flow through consolidated lung tissue can be assessed by percussion.

Planning
Medicine/Surgery
Physiologic and Anatomic
    Equilibrium
Acute Care
Respiratory

14. The nurse preparing a client for a perfusion lung scan explains that the procedure includes the administration of:
    1. A xenon air mixture
    2. Intravenous radioactive particles
    3. Several endotracheal medications
    4. Bronchodilators and inhaled steroids

RATIONALE

(2) A perfusion scan of the lung assists in the screening and detection of thromboembolic and obstructive lung diseases and includes the use of macroaggregated albumin tagged with technetium 99m intravenously.
    1. Clients breathe air mixed with xenon through a mask for ventilation lung scans.
    3. Endotracheal medications are not routinely used.
    4. These drugs are used to treat asthma and are not routinely part of a lung scan.

CHAPTER 11 Nursing Interventions Common to Respiratory Disorders

Assessment
Medicine/Surgery
Physiologic and Anatomic Equilibrium
Acute Care
Respiratory

1. **The medical intensive care unit nurse auscultates the lungs of a client who is on ventilator support. One of the things that can be assessed is the placement of the endotracheal tube. This is necessary because:**
   1. It could become detached from the balloon
   2. It can slip out of place when the client turns
   3. When the client coughs, it can pull back up
   4. It could slip into the right main stem bronchus

   RATIONALE

   (4) The angle of the right mainstem bronchus is less acute than that of the left. An endotracheal tube that has been inserted too far will usually terminate in the right mainstem bronchus.
   1. Balloon detachment rarely occurs.
   2. The endotracheal tube in adults is usually cuffed to secure its placement in the trachea. It is also taped in place.
   3. Coughing rarely dislodges cuffed, taped endotracheal tubes.

Planning
Medicine/Surgery
Physiologic and Anatomic Equilibrium
Acute Care
Respiratory

2. **The intensive care unit nurse anticipates a tracheostomy when the client's endotracheal tube has been left in place for a maximum of:**
   1. 5 to 7 days
   2. 7 to 9 days
   3. 10 to 14 days
   4. 16 to 20 days

   RATIONALE

   (3) Concern regarding potential laryngeal damage usually begins around 10 to 14 days after insertion of an endotracheal tube.
   1. Permanent damage usually does not occur in this length of time.
   2. This is the time that concern begins about permanent damage, but it actually occurs after day 10.
   4. Permanent damage has usually occurred by this time.

Implementation
Medicine/Surgery
Physiologic and Anatomic
Equilibrium

Acute Care
Respiratory

3. **A nursing assessment of a ventilated client reveals that the lung sounds are not bilateral and chest expansion is not symmetric. The first nursing intervention is:**
   1. Suction cuffed tube immediately
   2. Check position of the cuffed tube
   3. Turn oxygen to 100% for two minutes
   4. Determine what is causing the obstruction

   RATIONALE

   (2) If the endotracheal tube has been inserted too far it will terminate in the right mainstem bronchus, which results in the movement of air in and out of the right lung, but no air movement in and out of the left lung.
   1. Suctioning may cause further displacement
   3. High concentrations of oxygen will be of no benefit if the endotracheal tube is misplaced.
   4. Possible tube dislodgement should be determined first.

Implementation
Medicine/Surgery
Physiologic and Anatomic Equilibrium
Acute Care
Respiratory

4. **When performing tracheal suctioning of a client with an artificial airway, the nurse should limit suctioning to periods of:**
   1. 3 to 5 seconds
   2. 6 to 10 seconds
   3. 15 to 20 seconds
   4. 20 to 25 seconds

   RATIONALE

   (2) Continuous suction may cause mucosal damage. The catheter should be withdrawn within 10 seconds.
   1. This short period of time usually does not cause damage, but suctioning time need not be this restricted.
   3. Longer suctioning periods can cause hypoxia and damage.
   4. This longer time period exceeds the maximum recommended suctioning time.

Implementation
Medicine/Surgery
Physiologic and Anatomic
Equilibrium
Acute Care
Respiratory

5. **When suctioning a ventilated client, the nurse will perform an intervention to decrease hypoxia. The nurse will:**
   1. Supply 100% oxygen
   2. Lubricate the suction catheter

3. Use a small catheter to suction
4. Suction for only 25 to 30 seconds

RATIONALE

(1) Preoxygenation with 100% oxygen will minimize the degree of deoxygenation and prevent atelectasis.
2. Lubrication of the catheter allows for ease of insertion.
3. Small catheters may prevent the removal of thick secretions.
4. This prolonged time may cause hypoxia and tracheal damage.

Implementation
Medicine/Surgery
Physiologic and Anatomic
    Equilibrium
Education
Respiratory

6. **The nurse caring for a client with reduced expiratory muscle ability teaches the client to perform the:**
   1. Huff cough
   2. Cascade cough
   3. Incisional cough
   4. Quad-assist cough

RATIONALE

(4) The quad-assist cough increases abdominal pressure and diaphragmatic movement upward to facilitate secretion clearance.
1. The huff cough requires the client to take a deep breath and then perform several "huffs." It is used for clients in pain.
2. The client with reduced muscle ability usually cannot perform this cough.
3. Incisional coughs are performed after splinting the surgical site.

Evaluation
Medicine/Surgery
Education
Acute Care
Respiratory

7. **After abdominal surgery the nurse evaluates a client's success in using the incentive spirometer. The correct procedure is:**
   1. Sit as upright as possible during the treatment
   2. Cough after each breath on the spirometer
   3. Use the "huff" cough before using the spirometer
   4. Keep a loose seal around the mouthpiece to prevent pressure buildup

RATIONALE

(1) The upright or high-Fowler's position allows for greater lung expansion.

2. The breath should be held after inhalation.
3. Inhalation should be slow and deep and does not include a "huff" cough.
4. Lips should be sealed around the mouthpiece.

Implementation
Medicine/Surgery
Physiologic and Anatomic Equilibrium
Long-term Care
Respiratory

8. **The intermediate care unit nurse is assigned a client with a tracheostomy tube. The part of the tube removed for cleaning is the:**
   1. Outer cannula
   2. Inner cannula
   3. Single lumen tube
   4. Double lumen tube

RATIONALE

(2) The inner cannula of the double-lumen tracheostomy tube should be inspected every shift and cleaned at least daily or as needed to remove excess secretions.
1. Removal of the outer cannula may result in the closing of the tracheostomy.
3. Single lumen tubes should not be removed.
4. Only the inner lumen should be removed.

Planning
Medicine/Surgery
Physiologic and Anatomic Equilibrium
Acute Care
Respiratory

9. **When weaning a client off ventilator support, the nurse analyzes the breathing difficulty. If the client cannot breathe easily the nurse will:**
   1. Call the physician immediately
   2. Increase humidified oxygenation
   3. Reconnect the ventilator as indicated
   4. Teach proper breathing techniques

RATIONALE

(3) If the client demonstrates signs or symptoms of tiring during the weaning process, the client is returned to total ventilator support.
1. The priority is supplying oxygen to the client.
2. The client may be unable to inhale humidified oxygen due to fatigue.
4. Breathing techniques will not be effective if the client has muscle wasting or fatigue.

Analysis
Medicine/Surgery
Physiologic and Anatomic Equilibrium
Acute Care
Respiratory

10. **A client has two chest tubes in place after resection of a lung lobe. The lower chest tube is to:**

1. Remove air
2. Prevent clots
3. Remove fluid
4. Facilitate "milking"

RATIONALE

(3) Fluid is pulled down by gravity and tends to pool in the base and posterior areas of the lung; pleural chest tubes are inserted to drain fluid.
1. Air removal is achieved by placing a chest tube in the anterior chest in the second intercostal space.
2. Chest tubes do not prevent clot formation.
4. "Milking" is the technique used to try to facilitate the movement of blood clots through the chest tubing.

Evaluation
Medicine/Surgery
Physiologic and Anatomic Equilibrium
Acute Care
Respiratory

11. **The nurse caring for a mechanically ventilated client who is receiving a paralytic agent should evaluate the effectiveness of the drug by observing the client's ventilatory effort and:**
1. Assessing capillary refill
2. Checking hand grip
3. Using a Wright's spirometer
4. Using a peripheral nerve stimulator

RATIONALE

(4) The response to electrical stimulation of peripheral nerves indicates the degree of nerve blockade.
1. Capillary refill assesses tissue perfusion
2. The paralyzed client will be unable to elicit a hand grasp.
3. The spirometer measures the client's inhaled volume of air.

Analysis
Medicine/Surgery
Physiologic and Anatomic
  Equilibrium
Acute Care
Respiratory

12. **A client receiving 100% oxygen by an endotracheal tube is monitored carefully by the nurse. High concentrations of oxygen can cause degenerative changes in the lung and:**
1. Hoarseness
2. Alveolar collapse
3. Airway dryness
4. Increased secretions

RATIONALE

(2) High concentrations of oxygen remove nitrogen, which results in collapse of the alveoli.

1. Hoarseness is a complication of prolonged endotracheal intubation.
3. High concentrations of oxygen are humidified.
4. This is a complication of various types of oxygen therapy.

CHAPTER 12 Nursing Management of Adults with Upper Airway Disorders

Analysis
Medicine/Surgery
Physiologic and Anatomic Equilibrium
Acute Care
Respiratory

1. **A client asks an office nurse about the new antihistamine drug that the physician has prescribed. The nurse explains that the newer drugs have the advantage of:**
1. Lower cost
2. Increased sedation
3. Moisten secretions
4. Longer duration of action

RATIONALE

(4) Newer drugs are longer lasting.
1. The newer drugs usually cost more than the older ones.
2. These drugs cause less sedation than the older drugs.
3. Antihistamines tend to dry secretions and impair clearance of purulent mucus.

Implementation
Medicine/Surgery
Physiologic and Anatomic Equilibrium
Acute Care
Respiratory

2. **In order to decrease edema in the head and neck after laryngectomy, the nurse carries out the following interventions:**
1. Keep the bed in a flat position
2. Elevate the head of the bed 30 degrees
3. Suction the tracheostomy frequently
4. Encourage the client to turn, cough and breathe deeply

RATIONALE

(2) Elevating the head facilitates drainage and reduces edema, which can compress major blood vessels and nerves.
1. This position would decrease drainage from the head.
3. Suctioning the tracheostomy clears the airway.
4. These actions mobilize secretions from the lungs.

Analysis
Medicine/Surgery

3. **Preoperatively, an elderly client about to undergo a total laryngectomy asks the nurse what effect the surgery will have on breathing. The nurse's response will be:**
   1. "You will be able to breathe normally."
   2. "You will have labored breathing through your nose."
   3. "You will breath through a temporary tube which will be removed later."
   4. "You will breathe through a permanent opening in your larynx."

RATIONALE

(4) Total laryngectomy involves the creation of a permanent tracheostomy. The trachea is sewn closed and does not communicate with the larynx.
   1. Normal breathing is interrupted by the tracheostomy.
   2. Inhalation through the nose is not conducted down to the lower airway.
   3. The tracheostomy is permanent.

Assessment
Medicine/Surgery
Physiologic and Anatomic Equilibrium
Acute Care
Respiratory

4. **A young man sustains a nasal fracture during a wrestling match. The fracture requires surgery and an overnight hospitalization for observation. The nurse's first assessment priority will be:**
   1. Pain severity
   2. Airway patency
   3. Placement of nasal packing
   4. Amount and color of the nasal drainage

RATIONALE

(2) Airway obstruction can occur as a result of accumulated blood in the nasopharynx and is the first focus of the nurse.
   1. Pain is treated with analgesics.
   3. Bleeding is observed, reported, and documented as appropriate and the nasal packing is removed in 72 hours.
   4. Clear fluid from the nose may indicate a cerebrospinal fluid leak.

Evaluation
Medicine/Surgery
Physiologic and Anatomic
    Equilibrium
Acute Care
Respiratory

5. **The otolaryngology unit nurse is evaluating the care that has been given to a client who had a laryngectomy 2 days earlier. If nursing interventions have been successful, the client would be expected to:**
   1. Speak in a weak hoarse voice
   2. Require only one dressing change per shift
   3. Have only a moderate level of pain
   4. Properly care for the feeding tube

RATIONALE

(4) Postoperative care of the tracheostomy, feeding tube, and suture line is taught preoperatively. The client should be encouraged to participate in this care as soon as possible.
   1. Laryngectomy clients lose their natural speaking voice and must communicate by using mechanical or electrical devices.
   2. Drainage from the incision site should be minimal, requiring only infrequent, if any, dressing changes.
   3. The goal for this client is full pain relief. Moderate pain requires further intervention.

Implementation
Medicine/Surgery
Physiologic and Anatomic Equilibrium
Acute Care
Respiratory

6. **A child with epistaxis, or nosebleed, is brought to the office of the school nurse after a schoolyard fight. The initial treatment of this problem should be:**
   1. Apply immediate pressure to the nose, have the client lie down in a supine position, and apply ice to the area
   2. Apply immediate pressure to the nose, have the client sit upright, apply ice to the area
   3. Apply direct pressure after determining fracture risk, have the client sit upright and swallow any drainage
   4. Have the client sit upright and lean forward

RATIONALE

(4) Epistaxis may result from nasal trauma. In this case, direct pressure should not be applied. Sitting upright and tilting the head forward decreases blood flow to the head and prevents drainage from accumulating in the nasopharynx and stomach.
   1. Direct pressure applied to a nasal fracture may worsen the injury. Lying in a supine position increases blood flow to the head.
   2. The upright position reduces blood flow to the head but may allow drainage into the nasopharynx.
   3. Nasal drainage will accumulate in the stomach and may cause vomiting.

Implementation
Medicine/Surgery
Education

7. **Home care instructions to a client with acute sinusitis might include:**
   1. Take the prescribed antibiotics until the symptoms subside; take ibuprofen, acetaminophen, or aspirin for pain
   2. Take all of the prescribed antibiotic; take ibuprofen, acetaminophen, or aspirin for pain; take over-the-counter antihistamines frequently.
   3. Take all of the prescribed antibiotic; take ibuprofen, acetaminophen, or codeine for pain; take decongestants as needed.
   4. Take all of the prescribed antibiotics; take ibuprofen, acetaminophen, and codeine for pain; take decongestants as needed and intranasal steroids once daily.

   RATIONALE

   (3) Antibiotics such as amoxicillin and clindamycin should be taken completely. The condition is usually painful and requires the use of the analgesics listed and occasionally narcotics. Decongestants relieve nasal mucosal edema.
   1. Taking part of a prescription may not completely eradicate the causative organism and superinfection may occur. Aspirin may cause polyposis.
   2. Over-the-counter antihistamines may dry secretions and impair the clearance of purulent mucus.
   4. Intranasal steroid sprays may impair the local immune response to infection.

8. **A client asks the nurse,"Why do I need penicillin? That seems like strong medicine for a sore throat." The nurse explains:**
   1. "Complications can occur without treatment."
   2. "Treatment is necessary to relieve the pain."
   3. "All sore throats can be cured by antibiotics."
   4. "Each physician has his own preferences."

   RATIONALE

   (1) Early diagnosis and the use of antibiotics have led to a lower incidence of complications related to untreated tonsillitis.
   2. Pain relief may be obtained by using gargles, analgesics, and humidified air.
   3. Antibiotics are not necessary in all cases.
   4. Antibiotics are used by physicians to stop the progression of tonsillitis to a peritonsillar abscess.

9. **The occupational health nurse in a large factory is conducting annual employee screening. One of the earliest symptoms of laryngeal cancer is:**
   1. Cough
   2. Hemoptysis
   3. Hoarseness
   4. Neck pain

   RATIONALE

   (3) Hoarseness or voice change that persists for longer than 2 weeks should be investigated to rule out cancer.
   1. This is a late symptom
   2. This is also a late sign.
   4. Pain within or around the thyroid or Adam's apple that radiates to the ear on the affected side is a late characteristic sign.

CHAPTER 13 Nursing Management of Adults with Lower Airway Disorders

1. **The emergency room nurse who is planning interventions for a client with a tension pneumothorax anticipates placement of a:**
   1. Chest tube
   2. Urinary catheter
   3. Endotracheal tube
   4. Central venous catheter

   RATIONALE

   (1) A tension pneumothorax must be treated immediately with a chest tube to decrease the intrapleural pressure.
   2. A urinary catheter is not always needed.
   3. An endotracheal tube is not usually required unless the client has other severe injuries.
   4. A central venous catheter is rarely used.

Assessment
Medicine/Surgery
Physiologic and Anatomic
    Equilibrium
Long-term Care
Respiratory

2. **An employee health nurse is asked to perform a physical assessment of a new employee who has a history of chronic obstructive pulmonary disease (COPD). The findings may include:**

1. Loud breath sounds
2. Hyperinflated chest
3. Distinct heart sounds
4. Hypotrophy of upper chest

RATIONALE

(2) A barrel shaped chest is visible on inspection and indicates an increase in the anteroposterior dimension of the chest.
1. Breath sounds are diminished.
3. Heart sounds are muffled.
4. The accessory muscles of inspiration in the upper chest and neck are hypertrophied.

Assessment
Medicine/Surgery
Physiologic and Anatomic Equilibrium
Long-term Care
Respiratory

3. The office nurse obtains the results of pulmonary function tests (PFTs) from the computer before the client's appointment with the pulmonologist. If the client has chronic obstructive pulmonary disease (COPD), the PFTs will indicate:
1. Increased expiratory volume
2. Decreased expiratory airflow
3. Increased vital capacity
4. Decreased total lung volume

RATIONALE

(2) FEV_1 indicates the expiratory airflow, which is decreased in clients with increased airway resistance such as COPD.
1. The expiratory volume is decreased because of airway collapse and air trapping.
3. The vital capacity or maximum volume of air exhaled after a maximum inhalation is normal or reduced.
4. The total lung volume is increased because of air trapping.

Analysis
Medicine/Surgery
Physiologic and Anatomic
Equilibrium
Acute Care
Respiratory

4. An arterial blood gas analysis of a client in the emergency room indicates:
   PO_2 50 mm Hg
   PCO_2 55 mm Hg
   O_2 saturation of 68%
Based on these data, the nurse makes a nursing diagnosis of:
1. Ineffective airway clearance related to increased secretions
2. Ineffective breathing patterns related to increased work of breathing

3. Impaired gas exchange related to ventilation-perfusion mismatch
4. Activity intolerance related to decreased oxygenation

RATIONALE

(3) The decreased PO_2 and increased PCO_2 are indicators of ineffective gas exchange. Arterial blood gas results in this range indicate respiratory failure, which will probably require mechanical ventilation.
1. The PO_2 and PCO_2 values indicate a problem with oxygenation at the alveolar level.
2. Increased work of breathing does not directly cause drastic changes in the PO_2 and PCO_2.
4. This may be a nursing diagnosis, but it is not the most significant one at this time.

Planning
Medicine/Surgery
Physiologic and Anatomic Equilibrium
Education
Long-term Care
Respiratory

5. A home health nurse preparing for the next visit to the home of a client with chronic obstructive disease (COPD) prepares a teaching plan for the client, including the following instructions:
1. Smoking limitations
2. Postural drainage techniques
3. Strict fluid and activity restrictions
4. Open mouth breathing techniques

RATIONALE

(2) Postural drainage and percussion help to loosen and mobilize secretions so that they can be expectorated.
1. Clients should cease smoking altogether.
3. Drinking 10 to 12 glasses of water a day is encouraged to liquefy secretions.
4. Pursed-lipped breathing and abdominal breathing techniques are most effective.

Assessment
Medicine/Surgery
Physiologic and Anatomic Equilibrium
Long-term Care
Respiratory

6. A home health nurse is sent to assess a new client with cor pulmonale. This term refers to:
1. Enlargement of the pulmonary artery
2. Enlargement of the right ventricle
3. Atrophy of the right ventricle
4. Giant bullae growth on the lung

RATIONALE

(2) This condition results when hypoxemia causes vasoconstriction of the pulmonary

vascular bed, which increases pulmonary vascular resistance. The right ventricle has to pump against increased pulmonary artery pressures, which leads to hypertrophy.

1. The pulmonary artery vasoconstricts because of hypoxemia.
3. Increased pulmonary vascular resistance causes hypertrophy, not atrophy.
4. Giant bullae are air-containing structures within the lung parenchyma. Cor pulmonale is a separate disease process.

> Implementation
> Medicine/Surgery
> Physiologic and Anatomic Equilibrium
> Acute Care
> Respiratory

7. **A middle-aged client with chronic obstructive pulmonary disease (COPD) is dyspneic and has low PO$_2$ levels. The nurse administers oxygen as ordered. Caution is used in administering oxygen because of:**
1. Carbon dioxide retention
2. Drying of mucous membranes
3. Dependency on oxygen
4. Long-term aminophylline use

RATIONALE

(1) The nurse should monitor for possible carbon dioxide retention caused by loss of the hypoxic stimulus to breathe.
2. Oxygen can be humidified to reduce the drying effect.
3. Most COPD clients already require O$_2$ therapy.
4. There is no direct correlation between O$_2$ use and aminophylline.

> Evaluation
> Medicine/Surgery
> Physiologic and Anatomic Equilibrium
> Long-term Care
> Respiratory

8. **The home health nurse caring for an elderly client with chronic obstructive pulmonary disease writes in the care plan that the client is responding favorably to therapy. This positive evaluation is made because of the client's:**
1. Clear vision
2. Elevated blood pressure
3. Infrequent theophylline level checks
4. Frequent use of over-the-counter bronchodilators

RATIONALE

(1) Anticholinergic bronchodilators such as theophylline often cause urinary retention and blurred vision.

2. Hypertension is a complication of drug therapy. Over-the-counter bronchodilators can aggravate preexisting health problems such as hypertension.
3. Theophylline levels should be checked more frequently in the elderly than in the young adult.
4. These drugs usually contain alpha- and beta-agonists that can increase the risk of hypertension and diabetes.

> Planning
> Medicine/Surgery
> Physiologic and Anatomic Equilibrium
> Acute Care
> Respiratory

9. **An emergency room nurse has received a call from an EMS unit that they are bringing in an asthma client who is dyspneic. In planning for the client's care, the first therapy usually provided is:**
1. Inhaled beta-agonists
2. Methylxanthines
3. Systemic corticosteroids
4. Mechanical ventilation

RATIONALE

(1) Inhaled or subcutaneous beta-agonists are given first in an attempt to open the bronchial airways.
2. Methylxanthines are not usually given in the emergency room.
3. Systemic corticosteroids are the second group of drugs used if the beta-agonists are ineffective.
4. Mechanical ventilation is used as a last resort for severe unrelieved dyspnea or respiratory failure.

> Evaluation
> Medicine/Surgery
> Education
> Long-term Care
> Respiratory

10. **As a school nurse teaches a class to elementary aged clients who have asthma. At the end of the session, the nurse conducts a return demonstration to ensure that each client can use a metered dose inhaler properly. Each child should:**
1. Place the mouthpiece in the mouth, empty the lungs, inhale quickly and deeply through the nose while pressing down on the canister, then exhale quickly.
2. Place the mouthpiece in the mouth, empty the lungs, inhale slowly and deeply through the nose while pressing down on the canister, exhale slowly.
3. Place the mouthpiece 1 1/2 to 2 inches from the mouth, empty the lungs, inhale quickly and deeply, press down on the canister, breath in slowly, exhale.

4. Place the mouthpiece 1 1/2 to 2 inches from the mouth, empty the lungs, inhale slowly and deeply, press down on the canister, breathe in slowly and hold the breath for 10 seconds.

RATIONALE

(4) This technique is necessary to administer the maximal amount of medication directly into the lungs.

1. The mouthpiece should be placed 1 1/2 to 2 inches from the mouth with slow, deep inhalation of medication and continued slow inhalation and brief breath holding to allow for maximum aerolization of the medication.
2. The mouthpiece should be placed 1 1/2 inches to 2 inches from the mouth to allow for aerolization of the medication.
3. The medicine should be inhaled slowly, and inhalation should be continued and the breath held briefly to ensure maximum distribution of the medication.

Analysis
Medicine/Surgery
Physiologic and Anatomic Equilibrium
Long-term Care
Respiratory

11. A nurse on a medical unit admits a client who has recently been diagnosed with a type of restrictive lung disease called interstitial pulmonary fibrosis. This disease is characterized by:
1. Increased lung volume
2. Decreased lung compliance
3. Decreased lung elasticity
4. Decreased work of breathing

RATIONALE

(2) Interstitial pulmonary fibrosis is caused by an idiopathic process that increases the stiffness of the lungs, making them less compliant.

1. The total lung volume is reduced because of decreased lung expansion.
3. The lungs become more elastic. Compliance and elastance are reciprocal.
4. The respiratory muscles must work harder to generate large changes in pressure, which results in only small volume changes.

Planning
Medicine/Surgery
Physiologic and Anatomic Equilibrium
Long-term Care
Respiratory

12. A home health nurse preparing to visit a client with interstitial pulmonary fibrosis reviews the care plan and gathers educational material that will outline the usual primary therapy of:
1. Antibiotics
2. Percussion

3. Bronchodilators
4. Corticosteroids

RATIONALE

(4) Steroid therapy slows the progression of the disease. Cytotoxic medication has also shown promise.

1. Antibiotics are not indicated unless an underlying infection is present.
2. Percussion is used to mobilize secretions, which are not the primary problem in this disease.
3. Bronchodilators do not have any effect on the changes in the lung tissue.

Evaluation
Medicine/Surgery
Physiologic and Anatomic Equilibrium
Acute Care
Respiratory

13. An emergency room nurse is doing follow-up telephone calls to clients seen in the department during the previous 24 hours. One client has a long history of Pickwickian syndrome. The nurse would assess the effectiveness of the client's recent therapy by inquiring about:
1. Sputum color
2. Fluid intake
3. Apnea episodes
4. Estrogen therapy

RATIONALE

(3) Pickwickian syndrome is another name for obesity hypoventilation syndrome. Persons with this syndrome seem to have a decreased central drive to breathe and have episodes of apnea and hypoventilation.

1. Sputum color is assessed when infection is present.
2. Fluid intake is not specifically restricted, although the client should be on an over-all weight reduction plan.
4. These clients are usually receiving progesterone. It is a respiratory stimulant discovered when it was noted that pregnant women tend to hyperventilate.

Evaluation
Medicine/Surgery
Physiologic and Anatomic Equilibrium
Acute Care
Respiratory

14. The medical intensive care unit nurse is reviewing the arterial blood gases of a client with chronic obstructive pulmonary disease to evaluate readiness for weaning from mechanical ventilation. The most significant value will be the:
1. PCO_2
2. PO_2

3. pH
4. Tidal volume

RATIONALE

(1) The goal of therapy in this client is to attain a P_{CO_2} equivalent to the client's baseline. The P_{CO_2} level is used to monitor gas exchange.
2. Arterial oxygen levels are important but the P_{CO_2} is a critical indicator of oxygenation in this client.
3. The pH value relates to the acidity of the blood.
4. Tidal volume is the amount of air delivered by the ventilator and inhaled by the client.

Analysis
Medicine/Surgery
Physiologic and Anatomic Equilibrium
Acute Care
Respiratory

15. **The medical intensive care unit nurse notes that a client who is mechanically ventilated has lipid emulsions added to his intravenous fluids. This solution:**
1. Lowers phosphate
2. Metabolizes quickly
3. Increases carbon dioxide production
4. Decreases carbon dioxide production

RATIONALE

(4) High carbon dioxide levels make weaning more difficult. Nonprotein calories in chronic obstructive pulmonary disease clients are composed of a higher proportion of lipids than carbohydrates, which results in a lower production of carbon dioxide.
1. High glucose levels from carbohydrates lower the phosphate level.
2. Lipids metabolize slowly.
3. The carbon dioxide production is lowered.

Analysis
Medicine/Surgery
Physiologic and Anatomic Equilibrium
Acute Care
Respiratory

16. **A near-drowning victim is rushed to the emergency room and mechanical ventilation is administered. Salt water in the lungs triggers adult respiratory distress syndrome, which causes:**
1. Alveolar space clearing
2. Pulmonary capillary permeability
3. Increased surfactant activity
4. Decreased hyaline membranes

RATIONALE

(2) Acute injury increases capillary permeability and allows movement of fluid and protein from the capillaries to the interstitial and alveolar spaces.

1. The alveolar spaces are flooded with debris.
3. Surfactant activity is reduced.
4. Hyaline membranes are formed from alveolar epithelial debris.

Evaluation
Medicine/Surgery
Physiologic and Anatomic Equilibrium
Acute Care
Respiratory

17. **A nurse examining the chest x-ray film of a client with adult respiratory distress syndrome (ARDS) expects to see:**
1. "White-out"
2. "Black-out"
3. "A water mark"
4. No significant change

RATIONALE

(1) ARDS produces diffuse alveolar infiltrates, which cause a "white-out" pattern. The film is covered with white areas.
2. "Black out" is seen on a film when a lung has been removed.
3. A "water mark" is a straight line that indicates a collection of fluid in the lung.
4. The radiographic changes produced by ARDS are wide-spread and easily visible.

Planning
Medicine/Surgery
Physiologic and Anatomic Equilibrium
Acute Care
Respiratory

18. **The medical intensive care unit nurse requests a medication order for sedation for a client who is receiving mechanical ventilation. This is done to prevent:**
1. Hypotension
2. Frequent suctioning
3. Asynchronous breathing
4. Decreased central venous pressure

RATIONALE

(3) Clients often "fight the ventilator" and attempt to exhale while the ventilator is delivering a breath. Sedatives and paralytic agents help to calm the client so that ventilation is maximized.
1. Sedation can cause hypotension.
2. Secretion production is not affected by sedation.
4. Sedation can cause vasodilation, which decreases central venous pressure.

Assessment
Medicine/Surgery
Physiologic and Anatomic Equilibrium
Acute Care
Respiratory

19. **Clients receiving positive end-expiratory pressure (PEEP) should be assessed frequently, particularly their:**
    1. Tidal volume
    2. Cardiac output
    3. Oxygen percentage
    4. Exhaled volume

RATIONALE

(2) PEEP increases intrathoracic pressure, which reduces venous return and thus cardiac output. Vital organ perfusion must also be monitored.
1. Tidal volume is a separate ventilator parameter.
3. Oxygen concentrations and PEEP levels are independent ventilator settings.
4. Exhaled volume is usually not significantly affected by PEEP.

> Assessment
> Medicine/Surgery
> Physiologic and Anatomic Equilibrium
> Long-term Care
> Respiratory

20. **An elderly nursing home client has been diagnosed with pneumonia. The nurse assesses the breathing pattern and lung fields. Expected findings include:**
    1. Barrel chest
    2. Cheyne-Stokes breaths
    3. Dullness on percussion
    4. Hyperresonance on percussion

RATIONALE

(3) Physical examination of the lungs reveals signs of consolidation such as dullness and crackles.
1. A barrel chest is characteristic of chronic obstructive pulmonary disease.
2. Cheyne-Stokes respirations are present in clients with central nervous system injury.
4. Hyperresonance is indicative of air-filled spaces.

> Analysis
> Medicine/Surgery
> Physiologic and Anatomic Equilibrium
> Older Adult Care
> Respiratory

21. **The geriatric nurse knows that most cases of pneumonia in the elderly are caused by:**
    1. Fungi
    2. Viruses
    3. Protozoa
    4. Bacteria

RATIONALE

(4) Less than one half of all reported pneumonias are caused by bacteria, but most pneumonias found in older people are bacterial in origin.
1. Fungal infections are common in areas where the soil is high in nitrogen and near bird droppings and compost heaps.

2. Influenza A commonly causes pneumonia in healthy clients; cytomegalovirus is the cause of viral pneumonia in the immunocompromised.
3. Protozoa rarely cause pneumonia in the elderly. Pneumocystis carinii, thought to be a unicellular protozoan, is common in AIDS clients.

> Planning
> Medicine/Surgery
> Education
> Long-term Care
> Respiratory

22. **The nurse in a clinic for the homeless is developing a care plan for a client with tuberculosis. The client will be instructed to prevent transmission of the bacilli by:**
    1. Use of ultraviolet lights in the clinic
    2. Covering the mouth and nose when coughing
    3. Instructing friends and family to wear masks
    4. Remaining in the homeless shelter until blood studies are negative

RATIONALE

(2) The most effective and practical way to prevent spread of the bacilli is to contain the client's droplets, which are highly contagious and transmitted by air.
1. Ultraviolet light does kill the bacillus but is not a practical solution.
3. Masks are expensive, are usually used incorrectly, and are of limited value.
4. This is not a practical or rational solution. Treatment effectiveness is proven by three negative sputum cultures.

> Implementation
> Medicine/Surgery
> Education
> Long-term Care
> Respiratory

23. **The nurse's instructions to a client about the use of drug therapy for tuberculosis will include:**
    1. "Take the medication until the Mantoux test is negative."
    2. "Take the medication for the rest of your life."
    3. "Have your family take the medication to prevent reinfection."
    4. "Follow the course of treatment consistently for 6 to 9 months."

RATIONALE

(4) Combinations of medication will be administered for 6 to 9 months because the TB bacilli are not all susceptible to the same drugs and drug-resistant mutants are common.
1. The effectiveness of drug therapy is tested by sputum examination.
2. The medication is taken until the bacilli no longer are evident in the sputum.

3. If the client follows the drug regimen carefully, and is careful to contain droplet transmission, others have little risk of infection.

Assessment
Medicine/Surgery
Education
Long-term Care
Respiratory

24. **An occupational health nurse preparing to conduct a class on the prevention of smoking will include information about the relationship of smoking to lung cancer. The most commonly reported symptom at the time of diagnosis of lung cancer is:**
    1. A cough
    2. Weight loss
    3. Hoarseness
    4. Purulent sputum

RATIONALE

(1) Most clients with lung cancer are heavy smokers with chronic obstructive pulmonary disease and long histories of a productive cough. For them, a change in cough is significant.
2. Weight loss is a late sign.
3. Hoarseness is a warning sign for laryngeal cancer.
4. Purulent sputum is a sign of infection.

CHAPTER 14 Nursing Assessment of the Peripheral Vascular System

Assessment
Medicine/Surgery
Physiologic and Anatomic Equilibrium
Acute Care
Cardiovascular

1. **A client comes into the clinic with the preliminary diagnosis of an enlarged spleen. The nurse gently palpates the area and feels a mass. When the client asks why the spleen is enlarged, the nurse explains:**
   1. "It is a routine occurrence."
   2. "You may have a malignancy."
   3. "We are doing tests to help us find out."
   4. "You probably have leukemia."

RATIONALE

(3) The spleen is an organ of the lymphatic system. It removes defective red cells from circulation, stores blood, and enlarges because of monocyte and lymphocyte production during infections. All diagnoses must be confirmed and discussed with the client by a physician before the nurse discusses it.
1. Spleen enlargement is not a routine situation and should be evaluated.
2. The nurse should never alarm a client with unsubstantiated information.

4. Leukemia does cause spleen enlargement, but all diagnoses must be confirmed and discussed with the client by a physician before the nurse discusses it.

Assessment
Medicine/Surgery
Physiologic and Anatomic
   Equilibrium
Acute Care
Cardiovascular

2. **When performing a cardiovascular assessment on an elderly client, the nurse will:**
   1. Proceed quickly and throughly
   2. Allow more time than for a younger adult
   3. Not repeat questions but explain them at length
   4. Speak loudly and pause during the assessment, allowing for interruptions

RATIONALE

(2) Consider that all elderly clients may have many physical impairments and that the assessment will probably take longer than it would on a younger person.
1. A slow, steady pace is best.
3. Questions need to be asked in simple language and may need to be rephrased and repeated.
4. The client may be able to hear normal voice tones; however, the environment should be kept free of distractions and interruptions.

Assessment
Medicine/Surgery
Physiologic and Anatomic Equilibrium
Acute Care
Integumentary

3. **The client's skin may give indications of poor circulation. One such sign is:**
   1. Bounding pulse
   2. Quick capillary refill
   3. Smooth moist texture
   4. Absence of hair growth

RATIONALE

(4) Absence of hair growth is an indication of decreased blood flow.
1. A strong pulse indicates increased circulation.
2. This is a sign of normal vascular blood flow.
3. This indicates adequate blood flow and hydration.

Assessment
Medicine/Surgery
Physiologic and Anatomic Equilibrium
Acute Care
Cardiovascular

4. **A bruit auscultated in the abdominal midline may indicate:**

1. An aortic aneurysm
2. Intestinal activity
3. Abdominal cavity fluid
4. Active internal bleeding

RATIONALE

(1) A bruit in this area may indicate an abdominal aortic aneurysm and should be further assessed.
2. This activity sounds like a rumble or growl.
3. The presence of fluid is assessed by percussion of the abdominal cavity.
4. This cannot be auscultated.

Assessment
Medicine/Surgery
Physiologic and Anatomic Equilibrium
Acute Care
Cardiovascular

5. **A client is scheduled for a Trendelenburg test. This noninvasive diagnostic technique is used in assessing:**
   1. Arterial occlusion
   2. Primary lymphedema
   3. Deep thrombophlebitis
   4. Superficial thrombophlebitis

RATIONALE

(4) The retrograde filling or Trendelenburg test is used in evaluating valvular competency in the superficial venous system.
1. The arterial system is not assessed with this test.
2. The lymphatic system is not evaluated.
3. This test involves superficial veins only.

Assessment
Medicine/Surgery
Physiologic and Anatomic Equilibrium
Acute Care
Cardiovascular

6. **A client may need a specimen for arterial blood gas analysis drawn from the radial artery. Before this, the nurse will perform an Allen test to assess:**
   1. Varicose veins
   2. Primary lymphedema
   3. Arterial supply to the hand
   4. Superficial thrombophlebitis

RATIONALE

(3) Allen's test is done is assess the arterial patency of the palmar arch. Intact ulnar circulation may protect the hand from ischemia and possible death if the radial artery should thrombose.
1. The arterial circulation is being assessed.
2. The lymph system is not evaluated.
4. This is not assessed.

Assessment
Medicine/Surgery

Physiologic and Anatomic Equilibrium
Acute Care
Cardiovascular

7. **After a client has had either a contrast venogram or arteriogram, an expected finding on assessment is:**
   1. Normal pulses
   2. Decreased pulses
   3. Decreased capillary refill
   4. Loss of function of the extremity

RATIONALE

(1) The pulses and vital signs are assessed frequently and should be within normal limits of the client's preprocedure baseline.
2. This is an abnormal finding.
3. This is also an abnormal finding.
4. This is an unexpected finding.

CHAPTER 15 Nursing Management of Adults with Arterial Disorders

Planning
Medicine/Surgery
Physiologic and Anatomic Equilibrium
Acute Care
Cardiovascular

1. **The new case manager for clients with arterial disorders is planning an educational program on atherosclerosis. One factor that clients can modify is:**
   1. Age
   2. Weight
   3. Gender
   4. Heredity

RATIONALE

(2) Controllable risk factors to reduce the incidence of atherosclerosis and hypertension include weight, smoking, stress, and diabetes.
1. This cannot be modified.
2. This is uncontrollable.
4. This is uncontrollable.

Evaluation
Medicine/Surgery
Physiologic and Anatomic Equilibrium
Acute Care
Cardiovascular

2. **A client has returned to be evaluated for the effectiveness of therapy for atherosclerosis. A serious manifestation of the disease is:**
   1. Sharp pain
   2. Rest pain
   3. Intermittent stabbing pain
   4. Intermittent claudication

RATIONALE

(2) Pain at rest indicates that the arterial circulation is inadequate to maintain tissue viability even at rest.

1. This may indicate acute injury
3. This may be associated with claudication.
4. This is indicative of stenosis or chronic occlusion and occurs when muscles without adequate blood supply are exercised.

> Planning
> Medicine/Surgery
> Physiologic and Anatomic Equilibrium
> Long-term Care
> Cardiovascular

3. **In planning for a client with atherosclerosis, the nurse's treatment goal will be:**
   1. Relieve symptoms
   2. Cure the disease
   3. Ignore major risks
   4. Slow disease progression

RATIONALE

(1) Relief of symptoms and prevention of the progression of disease are the treatment goals.
   2. Treatment, including surgery, does not cure the disease, an important client concept.
   3. Risk reduction is a goal.
   4. Preventing disease progression is a goal.

> Planning
> Medicine/Surgery
> Physiologic and Anatomic Equilibrium
> Long-term Care
> Cardiovascular

4. **A client has severe hyperlipidemia. The nurse anticipates that this high-risk individual will be treated with:**
   1. Vasodilators
   2. Anticoagulant therapy
   3. Intensive dietary restrictions
   4. Diet restriction and drug therapy

RATIONALE

(4) Strict reduction of ingested dietary fat and cholesterol alone may not be sufficient when lipid levels are severely elevated.
   1. This may be a part of the treatment but does not address the primary cause of the disease.
   2. This may be insufficient therapy.
   3. This may be partly effective.

> Assessment
> Medicine/Surgery
> Physiologic and Anatomic Equilibrium
> Long-term Care
> Cardiovascular

5. **An elderly client arrives in the emergency room in a wheelchair. Both lower legs and feet appear red. This is assessed to be a result of:**
   1. Blood cell destruction
   2. Increased temperature
   3. Venous dilation
   4. Arterial dilation

RATIONALE

(4) Arterial insufficiency may appear as pallor when the lower extremity is elevated. When it is placed in a dependent position, the skin becomes red as a result of arteriole dilation.
   1. This is not a cause of this condition.
   2. This is an unrelated occurrence.
   3. This is not the primary pathology.

> Assessment
> Medicine/Surgery
> Physiologic and Anatomic Equilibrium
> Acute Care
> Cardiovascular

6. **A nurse in the surgical intensive care unit is caring for a client who had surgery yesterday for an abdominal aortic aneurysm. The client complains of severe left lower-quadrant pain. One possible cause is:**
   1. Fat embolism
   2. Ischemic colitis
   3. Renal shutdown
   4. Retroperitoneal hemorrhage

RATIONALE

(2) Gastrointestinal complications such as colon ischemia occur because of graft thrombosis or thrombosis of the vessels past the graft. When the blood supply to the bowel is blocked, there is mucosal destruction within 30 minutes and gangrene within hours.
   1. This is unlikely.
   2. This is not related.
   4. Symptoms would appear elsewhere.

> Assessment
> Medicine/Surgery
> Physiologic and Anatomic Equilibrium
> Acute Care
> Cardiovascular

7. **A client in a surgical intensive care unit has had an abdominal aortic aneurysm resection. The nurse is aware that graft occlusion may occur at any time. An acronym that represents key assessment factors for this client is:**
   1. A, B, C, D
   2. P, Q, R, S, T
   3. The six Ps
   4. The seven Ps

RATIONALE

(3) Pain, pulselessness, pallor, paresthesias, paralysis, and polar sensation or cold are all signs of graft occlusion and must be reported immediately.
   1. These letters have no specific meaning.

2. These letters identify electrocardiogram waveforms.

4. This has no relevance to this situation.

CHAPTER 16 Nursing Management of Adults with Hypertension

Evaluation
Medicine/Surgery
Physiologic and Anatomic Equilibrium
Acute Care
Cardiovascular

1. **The nurse is evaluating the effects of a weight reduction program involving a client. A desired effect of this program is lowered blood pressure. On two different occasions, the client's blood pressure has been 150/95. The client is:**
   1. Hypertensive
   2. Normotensive
   3. Hypotensive
   4. Benign hypertensive

RATIONALE

(1) Hypertension or high blood pressure is identified when the systolic blood pressure exceeds 140 mm Hg or the diastolic blood pressure exceeds 90 mm hg with a sustained mean arterial blood pressure greater than 100 mm Hg at rest. It must be reconfirmed on two or more measurements at each of two or more follow-up visits.
2. This is not a normal blood pressure reading.
3. Hypotension is characterized by systolic blood pressures below 100 mm Hg.
4. The term benign and labile are no longer appropriate. Hypertension is classified in stages now.

Evaluation
Medicine/Surgery
Physiologic and Anatomic Equilibrium
Acute Care
Cardiovascular

2. **In evaluating the effectiveness of the therapy that has been given to a client in the emergency room who arrived in a hypertensive crisis, the nurse finds that the blood pressure is 165/105 mm Hg, despite treatment with four agents. This condition is referred to as:**
   1. Normotension
   2. Borderline hypertension
   3. Resistant hypertension
   4. Sustained hypertensive crisis

RATIONALE

(3) Resistant hypertension refers to hypertension that cannot be reduced to less than 160/100 mm hg with attempted treatment using three different agents.

1. This is not a normal blood pressure.
2. This term refers to blood pressure that is in the slightly elevated above normal range.
4. This is not the appropriate term for this condition.

Planning
Medicine/Surgery
Physiologic and Anatomic Equilibrium
Acute Care
Cardiovascular

3. **In planning a blood pressure screening program for the community, the nurse will target those at highest risk, which includes:**
   1. Black males
   2. White males
   3. White women
   4. Older adolescents

RATIONALE

(1) Hypertension is the most prevalent and serious health problem in black adults in the United States. It causes 30% of all deaths in black males and 20% of all deaths in black females.
2. White males are at less risk than black males.
3. White women are at less risk than men or black women.
4. Hypertension is rare in this segment of the population.

Planning
Medicine/Surgery
Physiologic and Anatomic Equilibrium
Acute Care
Cardiovascular

4. **The nurse administers a personality test as part of a class on hypertension. Further instructions will be given to those with personality types:**
   1. A and B
   2. A and E
   3. B and C
   4. C and D

RATIONALE

(2) Type As are hard-driven, ambitious, time-oriented persons with suppressed anger and hidden hostility. Type E is a recently identified type that describes persons with the "hot reactor" or explosive reactions when their goals have been thwarted.
1. Type B is less likely to develop cardiovascular disease.
3. These types are at reduced risk for heart disease.
4. These are irrelevant answers.

Evaluation
Medicine/Surgery
Physiologic and Anatomic Equilibrium

5. **A client returns for a follow-up appointment and tells the nurse that he has stopped taking his diuretic. It is causing impotence. His blood pressure is 130/88, and he has gained 2 pounds since his last visit. The nurse makes the following evaluation:**
   1. He does not understand the side effects of drug therapy
   2. He is noncompliant with the therapy because of the side effects
   3. He has taken the appropriate course of action in this situation
   4. He has severe fluid overload related to weight gain

RATIONALE

(2) Clients are often noncompliant because of the occurrence of side effects from medication such as impotence, ejaculation problems, gynecomastia, and decreased sex drive.
1. This client does understand the side effects.
3. Stopping the medication was inappropriate.
4. A 2-pound weight gain does not equate to fluid overload.

Implementation
Medicine/Surgery
Physiologic and Anatomic Equilibrium
Long-term Care
Cardiovascular

6. **To ensure accurate blood pressure measurement in the clinic the nurse would:**
   1. Record only the systolic reading
   2. Obtain a reading immediately upon the client's arrival
   3. Use the smallest blood pressure cuff possible
   4. Instruct the client not to smoke or drink coffee before measurement

RATIONALE

(4) These substances can cause vasoconstriction and tachycardia, which increase the heart rate.
1. Both systolic and diastolic readings should be obtained.
2. The measurement should be taken after 5 minutes of rest
3. The appropriate size cuff should be used and the rubber bladder should nearly or completely encircle the arm.

Implementation
Medicine/Surgery
Physiologic and Anatomic Equilibrium
Long-term Care
Education

7. **One of the examples of a nonpharmacologic intervention that the nurse might initiate to control hypertension is:**

1. Biofeedback
2. Phosphorus supplement
3. Minimize sodium restriction
4. Decrease dietary potassium

RATIONALE

(1) Stress management including the use of relaxation techniques such as yoga, meditation, and biofeedback have been found to decrease blood pressure.
2. This is not relevant.
3. Sodium is one of the primary causes of this disease and should be restricted.
4. Hypertensive persons usually have reduced potassium levels.

CHAPTER 17 Nursing Management of Adults with Venous or Lymphatic Disorders

Evaluation
Medicine/Surgery
Physiologic and Anatomic Equilibrium
Long-term Care
Cardiovascular

1. **A favorable outcome of the treatment of a client with lymphedema is measured by:**
   1. Mild chest pain
   2. Minimal dyspnea
   3. Decrease in limb size
   4. Localized area of infection

RATIONALE

(3) Evaluation of treatment is determined by a decrease (or lack of increase) in the size of the limb and patient satisfaction.
1. No chest pain should be present.
2. No dyspnea should be evident.
4. There should be no infection or injury.

Implementation
Medicine/Surgery
Physiologic and Anatomic Equilibrium
Long-term Care
Cardiovascular

2. **A home health nurse with a client who has lymphedema will monitor the treatment plan, which will include:**
   1. Oil-based lotions
   2. Supine position
   3. Limb dangling
   4. Elastic wraps

RATIONALE

(4) Elastic wraps in the daytime alternating with external pneumatic compression devices are helpful in moving the fluid.
1. Water-based skin lotions are recommended.
2. The limbs should be elevated on a foam wedge.
3. Limb dangling should be avoided.

3. **A client has a venous (stasis) ulcer on the medial aspect of his left ankle. Expected nursing observations at the site include:**
   1. Edema
   2. No edema
   3. Diminished pulses
   4. Pale and cool skin

RATIONALE

(1) Edema is common because of the venous stasis.
2. This is consistent with arterial ulcers.
3. This is characteristic of arterial ulcers.
4. This is a common finding with arterial ulcers.

4. **An expected outcome for a client with a pulmonary embolism is:**
   1. One transfusion only
   2. Mild to moderate pain
   3. Effective gas exchange
   4. Manageable coagulopathies

RATIONALE

(3) Effective gas exchange as evidenced by improved arterial blood gases is a goal of therapy.
1. No fall in hemoglobin or hematocrit is a desirable objective.
2. Complete pain relief is expected.
4. No ill effects from anticoagulants are planned.

5. **Anticoagulation therapy must be interrupted on a client with a pulmonary embolus. To prevent additional emboli from traveling to the lungs, the physician will use:**
   1. Sclerotherapy
   2. Vena cava interruption
   3. External pneumatic compression
   4. Ligation of peripheral pulmonary vessels

RATIONALE

(2) A filter placed in the vena cava traps the emboli.
1. Sclerotherapy is used on varicose veins.
3. These are used to relieve venous congestion.
4. This is not a logical therapy.

6. **A client in surgical intensive care is suspected of having a pulmonary embolism. A symptom that may be expected is:**
   1. Tachypnea
   2. Bradycardia
   3. Slow respirations
   4. Copious secretions

RATIONALE

(1) Pulmonary embolism commonly has no warning signs. The symptoms are related to the size of the clot and to the client's own cardiac reserve. Common symptoms are severe chest pain, dyspnea, and tachypnea.
2. Tachycardia usually occurs.
3. Fast respirations are common.
4. Hemoptysis is common.

UNIT V   Cardiac System

CHAPTER 18   Nursing Assessment of the Cardiac System

1. **In educating a client about coronary artery disease, the nurse explains that the coronary arteries branch from the aorta:**
   1. At the descending aorta
   2. At the aortic arch
   3. Behind the semilunar valve flaps
   4. In front of the semilunar valve flaps

RATIONALE

(3) The right and left coronary arteries branch just behind the semilunar valve. The heart supplies blood to itself first.
1. This is too far away.
2. This is impractical.
4. The blood could be pushed back into the ventricle.

Assessment
Medicine/Surgery
Physiologic and Anatomic
   Equilibrium
Acute Care
Cardiovascular

2. **On reviewing a client's chest radiograph, the nurse notices an enlarged heart. This is a sign of:**

1. Obesity
2. Increased fluid intake
3. An athletic lifestyle
4. A chronically overworked heart

RATIONALE

(4) An overworked or failing heart enlarges to increase the strength of the contraction and compensate for the extra workload.
1. Enlarged hearts may be present in clients who are not obese.
2. Short-term fluid intake will not cause enlargement.
3. Athletes may have only slightly enlarged hearts.

Evaluation
Medicine/Surgery
Physiologic and Anatomic Equilibrium
Acute Care
Cardiovascular

3. **In evaluating the severity of a client's cardiac disease, the nurse will calculate the amount of blood ejected from the left ventricle into the aorta per minute. This is called:**
1. Heart rate
2. Cardiac index
3. Cardiac output
4. Stroke volume

RATIONALE

(4) Stroke volume and heart rate are the two components of cardiac output.
1. This is the number of cardiac cycles per minute.
2. This is cardiac output in relation to body surface area.
3. This is the stroke volume times the heart rate per minute.

Assessment
Medicine/Surgery
Physiologic and Anatomic
Equilibrium
Acute Care
Cardiovascular

4. **In performing a physical examination on a client with a cardiac problem, the nurse determines the location and size of the apical impulse. It is found:**
1. Near the midsternal line
2. In the fifth left intercostal space
3. Near the apex of the heart
4. Above the third intercostal space

RATIONALE

(2) The apical impulse is generally located in the fifth left intercostal space at the midclavicular line.
1. It is normally in the midclavicular line.
3. This is not a specific response.
4. The location should be the fifth intercostal space.

Assessment
Medicine/Surgery
Physiologic and Anatomic
Equilibrium
Acute Care
Cardiovascular

5. **When auscultating heart sounds through the chest wall, the nurse should:**
1. Locate only the apical impulse
2. Listen on the anterior and posterior surfaces
3. Listen at one or two sites on the chest wall
4. "Inch" the stethoscope along the chest wall

RATIONALE

(4) This systematic approach enables the nurse to identify normal and abnormal heart sounds, pericardial friction rubs, and murmurs.
1. This would not be a comprehensive examination.
2. The posterior surface is auscultated for respiratory abnormalities.
3. There are at least five sites that should be auscultated.

Analysis
Medicine/Surgery
Physiologic and Anatomic
Equilibrium
Acute Care
Cardiovascular

6. **The nurse has a client who has a heart murmur. This is caused by:**
1. Increased activity
2. Turbulence of blood flow
3. Thinness of the chest wall.
4. Increased stress and fatigue

RATIONALE

(2) Murmurs can be caused by a high flow rate through a normal or abnormal orifice or backward flow through an incompetent valve.
1. This is not a usual cause.
2. In thin clients, the heart sounds may be more audible but not abnormal.
4. Murmurs are caused by abnormal movement of blood through the heart.

Evaluation
Medicine/Surgery
Physiologic and Anatomic
Equilibrium
Acute Care
Cardiovascular

7. **When establishing the diagnosis of myocardial infarction, the nurse will look specifically at the:**
1. CK-BB
2. CK-MB
3. Prothrombin time
4. Erythrocyte sedimentation rate

RATIONALE

(2) The pattern of total creatine kinase (CK) and CK-MB values is significant in identifying a myocardial infarction. These are enzymes that leak into the circulation after myocardial damage has occured.
1. This is present in brain and nervous tissue.
2. This is useful in monitoring anticoagulant therapy.
4. This is a nonspecific indicator of myocardial damage.

CHAPTER 19 Nursing Management of Adults with Common Complications of Cardiac Disease

Assessment
Medicine/Surgery
Physiologic and Anatomic Equilibrium
Acute Care
Cardiovascular

1. **The nurse is performing nursing assessments on a group of clients. A physician should be notified immediately when the nurse identifies:**
1. Dry skin and itching
2. Mild anxiety and irritability
3. Lung crackles and a respiratory rate of 38
4. A weight loss of three pounds in three weeks and anorexia

RATIONALE

(3) These are serious abnormal symptoms that may be signs of congestive heart failure, which may be life threatening.
1. These are not critical symptoms.
2. These are common symptoms among people who are hospitalized.
4. This does not require immediate attention.

Analysis
Medicine/Surgery
Physiologic and Anatomic Equilibrium
Acute Care
Cardiovascular

2. **A client on a telemetry unit has had a permanent demand pacemaker implanted. The purpose of this device is to:**
1. Establish normal atrioventricular synchrony
2. Prevent premature ventricular contractions
3. Obtain baseline data during exercise
4. Establish effective heart rate and rhythm

RATIONALE

(4) The pacemaker is used to provide electrical stimulation that maintains an effective heart rate and rhythm.
1. The device may only pace the ventricle.
2. These may occur even with a pacemaker.

3. This describes a stress test or Holter monitor.

Planning
Medicine/Surgery
Physiologic and Anatomic Equilibrium
Acute Care
Cardiovascular

3. **The nurse has a client who has a palpable pulse, a heart rate of 160, and decreasing cardiovascular stability. The nurse prepares to cardiovert. The defibrillator unit is synchronized to fire on the:**
1. R wave
2. T wave
3. P wave
4. ST segment

RATIONALE

(1) Delivery is timed to avoid the T wave to prevent ventricular fibrillation.
2. This could be life threatening.
3. This would be ineffective.
4. This could be dangerous if the impulse fired on the T wave.

Planning
Medicine/Surgery
Physiologic and Anatomic Equilibrium
Acute Care
Cardiovascular

4. **A client on a telemetry unit has recently developed atrial fibrillation. The nurse might anticipate a drop in blood pressure because of a loss of:**
1. Heart rate
2. Venous return
3. Atrial kick
4. Ventricular strength

RATIONALE

(3) In atrial fibrillation, the atria quiver and their contraction is not coordinated with the ventricles. This results in a loss of approximately 20% of the ventricular stroke volume.
1. The ventricular rate is often within normal limits in atrial fibrillation.
2. This is not affected.
4. The problem is within the atria.

Analysis
Medicine/Surgery
Physiologic and Anatomic Equilibrium
Acute Care
Cardiovascular

5. **Sluggish blood flow within the atria in a client with atrial fibrillation may cause:**
1. Mural thrombi
2. Slowed heart rate
3. Increased blood pressure
4. Increased pulse quality

(1) Turbulent blood flow triggers the clotting cascade and sets the stage for the formation of thrombi on the atrial walls. They can dislodge and travel to the brain, pulmonary circulation, or periphery.

2. The heart rate is not usually affected.
3. The blood pressure may decrease.
4. The pulse quality may also decrease.

> Implementation
> Medicine/Surgery
> Physiologic and Anatomic Equilibrium
> Acute Care
> Cardiovascular

6. The nurse identifies ventricular fibrillation on a client's electrocardiogram. The most effective treatment for this is:
   1. Epinephrine
   2. Defibrillation
   3. Lidocaine
   4. Bretylium

RATIONALE

(2) The most appropriate therapy is defibrillation, as soon as possible.

1. Epinephrine is used if electrical therapy is not successful.
3. Lidocaine is a recommended secondary treatment.
4. Bretylium is sometimes used in clients who do not respond to lidocaine.

> Planning
> Medicine/Surgery
> Physiologic and Anatomic Equilibrium
> Acute Care
> Cardiovascular

7. A client on the telemetry unit suddenly shows ventricular asystole on the cardiac monitor. The first treatment plan is:
   1. Cardioversion
   2. Defibrillation
   3. Transcutaneous pacing
   4. Transvenous pacing

RATIONALE

(3) The appropriate treatment protocol is to consider immediate transcutaneous pacing in order to generate cardiac output.

1. Cardioversion is inappropriate.
2. There is no electrical activity to defibrillate.
4. This is less accessible than transcutaneous pacing.

> Analysis
> Medicine/Surgery
> Physiologic and Anatomic Equilibrium
> Acute Care
> Cardiovascular

8. A third degree heart block or complete heart block in a client represents:
   1. Absent conduction between atria and ventricles
   2. Prolonged conduction between atria and ventricles
   3. Normal conduction between atria and ventricles
   4. Intermittent conduction between atria and ventricles

RATIONALE

(1) This represents a disturbance in conduction either at the atrioventricular node or within the bundle branches. The atria and ventricles fire independently of each other, so there is no relationship between the P waves and QRS complexes.

2. This describes first degree atrioventricular block.
3. This is not normal.
4. This describes second degree atrioventricular block.

> Evaluation
> Medicine/Surgery
> Physiologic and Anatomic Equilibrium
> Acute Care
> Cardiovascular

9. A client with a permanent pacemaker is experiencing "failure to capture." This implies that:
   1. The pacemaker is firing too rapidly
   2. The ventricles partially depolarize only
   3. The pacemaker is firing when it is not needed
   4. The heart does not respond to the pacemaker stimulus

RATIONALE

(4) Capture implies depolarization of the heart in response to the electrical stimulus. Failure to capture means that the pacemaker fires but the heart does not respond.

1. This is not the underlying problem. The pacemaker is working but the heart is not responding.
2. The ventricles depolarize completely or not at all.
3. This is called "failure to sense."

CHAPTER 20 Nursing Management of Adults with Disorders of the Coronary Arteries, Myocardium, or Pericardium

> Evaluation
> Medicine/Surgery
> Physiologic and Anatomic Equilibrium
> Acute Care
> Cardiovascular

1. A middle-aged construction worker arrives in the emergency room in the late afternoon of a summer's

day complaining of "heaviness in the chest." The 12-lead electrocardiogram shows ischemic changes, and the nurse is asked to start an intravenous infusion of nitroglycerin. In evaluating the effectiveness of the intervention the nurse might expect:

1. Absence ectopy
2. Relief of chest pain
3. Drop in blood pressure
4. Alteration in isoenzymes

RATIONALE

(3) Nitroglycerin acts to reduce myocardial oxygen demand by decreasing systemic vascular resistance, and causes vasodilation of the peripheral and coronary arteries, thereby decreasing chest pain.

1. Nitroglycerin does not affect ventricular irritability.
2. This is one usual action but does not always occur.
4. The cardiac isoenzymes are not affected.

> Planning
> Medicine/Surgery
> Physiologic and Anatomic Equilibrium
> Acute Care
> Cardiovascular

2. **An appropriate nursing goal for a client during the first 48 hours after a myocardial infarction is:**
   1. Relief of chest pain
   2. Maintaining minimal cardiac output
   3. Avoiding discussion of the extent of injury
   4. Increasing activities of daily living

RATIONALE

(1) Relieving chest pain also reduces anxiety, which decreases the myocardial oxygen demand.

2. Adequate cardiac output is a desired goal.
3. Allowing the client to verbalize fears, concerns and questions is a desired goal.
4. Activity should be limited to those required to meet basic hygiene needs only.

> Assessment
> Medicine/Surgery
> Physiologic and Anatomic Equilibrium
> Acute Care
> Cardiovascular

3. **A client who has had a recent myocardial infarction undergoes a percutaneous transluminal coronary angioplasty (PTCA). One of the most critical nursing actions during the 4 to 6 hours after the procedure is:**
   1. Assuring patency of the chest tubes
   2. Monitoring for signs of ischemia distal to the insertion site
   3. Monitoring urinary output for signs of renal damage
   4. Preventing infection of the insertion site and pain relief

RATIONALE

(2) Hematomas at the insertion site are potential complications of a PTCA and would be noted by signs of obstruction of blood flow distally.

1. Chest tubes are not needed for this procedure.
3. Renal damage is not a usual complication of this procedure.
4. The risk for infection at the insertion site and level of pain are usually minimal.

> Evaluation
> Medicine/Surgery
> Physiologic and Anatomic Equilibrium
> Long-term Care
> Cardiovascular

4. **After a percutaneous transluminal coronary angioplasty with stent placement, one aspect of care that will require on-going evaluation is:**
   1. Antibiotic levels
   2. Extremity pulses
   3. Coagulation levels
   4. Exercise tolerance levels

RATIONALE

(3) A stent is a device placed in the coronary artery to prevent plaque reocclusion. Stents cause thrombus formation and require long-term anticoagulation therapy.

1. Prolonged antibiotic therapy is not usual.
2. There should be no long-term need for this.
4. Pain after this procedure is usually minimal.

> Planning
> Medicine/Surgery
> Education
> Long-term Care
> Cardiovascular

5. **In planning long-term care for a client with coronary artery disease, the client should be told to take a dose of nitroglycerin:**
   1. Every 4 hours to prevent chest pain
   2. At bedtime to prevent nocturnal angina
   3. As soon as signs of pain are noticed
   4. Before beginning activities that cause pain

RATIONALE

(4) The client should be taught to reduce risk factors and avoid factors that precipitate angina.

1. This is unnecessary and potentially harmful.
2. Many clients do not have nocturnal angina.
3. It is best to take the medicine before symptoms begin if activities are known to cause angina.

> Evaluation
> Medicine/Surgery
> Physiologic and Anatomic Equilibrium
> Acute Care
> Cardiovascular

6. **In clients with diabetes mellitus, the nurse will evaluate the presence of a "silent" myocardial infarction by noting:**
   1. Levin's sign
   2. Shortness of breath
   3. Mild to moderate pain levels
   4. Increased activity levels

RATIONALE

(2) Some clients, such as the elderly and those with diabetes mellitus, do not experience chest pain. The nurse should observe for shortness of breath, decreased cardiac output, and changes in sensorium.
   1. This is a clinched fist over the left chest associated with severe pain.
   3. "Silent "refers to the absence of pain.
   4. Decreased activity levels and syncope may occur.

   Planning
   Medicine/Surgery
   Education
   Long-term
   Cardiovascular

7. **In teaching a client with hypertrophic cardiomyopathy about activities that may provoke chest pain, the nurse advises:**
   1. Squatting
   2. Lying supine
   3. Lying prone
   4. Walking quickly

RATIONALE

(1) Squatting or lying down with legs elevated will relieve dizziness.
   2. Legs should be elevated.
   3. Not a recommended therapy.
   4. Walking slowly and holding on to stable objects is recommended.

   Analysis
   Medicine/Surgery
   Physiologic and Anatomic Equilibrium
   Acute Care
   Cardiovascular

8. **After coronary artery bypass graft surgery, the nurse in the intensive care unit observes the chest tube drainage carefully for the first 2 to 6 hours. Output from the tubes should not exceed:**
   1. 50 ml /hr
   2. 75 ml/hr
   3. 100 ml/hr
   4. 200 ml/hr

RATIONALE

(4) Bloody drainage should not exceed 200 ml/hr and should steadily decrease. By the second or third postoperative day it becomes serous and stops.

   1. Drainage usually exceeds this because of the irrigation fluid used during the procedure.
   2. This is an acceptable level.
   3. This amount and higher should be assessed carefully and frequently.

CHAPTER 21   Nursing Management of Adults with Endocardial Disorders

   Evaluation
   Medicine/Surgery
   Physiologic and Anatomic
      Equilibrium
   Acute Care
   Cardiovascular

1. **In evaluating the progression of endocarditis, the nurse observes for:**
   1. Petechiae
   2. Flank nodules
   3. Eyelid lesions
   4. White spots on the tongue

RATIONALE

(1) A vascular manifestation of endocarditis is flat, red lesions that appear in groups within a few days in up to 50% of clients. They appear around the conjunctiva, mucous membranes, wrists, ankles, and neck.
   2. Nodules called Osler nodes may appear on the pads of the fingers and toes.
   3. Janeway lesions may appear on the fingertips, palms, soles or plantar surfaces of the feet.
   4. These are not usual findings.

   Implementation
   Medicine/Surgery
   Physiologic and Anatomic
      Equilibrium
   Acute Care
   Cardiovascular

2. **The most important nursing activity provided for clients with infective endocarditis is:**
   1. Temperature control
   2. Providing nutrients
   3. Administering antibiotics
   4. Reducing anxiety

RATIONALE

(3) Infective endocarditis is managed medically by the administration of antibiotics.
   1. Avoiding chills, using cooling measures and administering antipyretics are all important but treat the symptoms and not the cause of the problem.
   2. Adequate hydration with possible fluid restrictions is maintained.
   4. Increased client comfort and decreased anxiety are secondary goals of treatment.

Evaluation
Medicine/Surgery
Physiologic and Anatomic Equilibrium
Acute Care
Cardiovascular

3. **In evaluating the effectiveness of therapy for a client with infective endocarditis, the nurse will monitor the:**
   1. Anxiety level
   2. Blood culture reports
   3. Activity level
   4. Respiratory drainage

RATIONALE

(2) The blood cultures should show no growth of organisms.
   1. This is important, but the signs of infection such as temperature are more critical.
   3. This is also not a critical parameter.
   4. Respiratory drainage is usually minimal.

Implementation
Medicine/Surgery
Education
Acute Care
Cardiovascular

4. **While teaching a client about upcoming valve replacement surgery, the nurse explains that biologic tissue valves are used:**
   1. In sedentary clients
   2. In young, athletic clients
   3. In postmenopausal women
   4. In clients with no significant medical histories

RATIONALE

(2) These valves are used in clients in whom anticoagulation is not desirable, such as athletes, because the risk of thrombosis is reduced and anticoagulants are not needed.
   1. These valves are ideal for active clients.
   3. They are preferred for women of childbearing age.
   4. They are used successfully in clients with peptic ulcer or liver disease.

Implementation
Medicine/Surgery
Physiologic and Anatomic Equilibrium
Acute Care
Cardiovascular

5. **One successful nursing intervention to relieve pulmonary edema because of valvular disease is to place the client in:**
   1. Supine position
   2. Trendelenburg position
   3. Semi-Fowler's position with the knees bent
   4. High Fowler's position with the legs dangling

RATIONALE

(4) This prompt intervention should relieve severe shortness of breath because of decreased venous return and increased lung expansion.
   1. This position decreases respiratory function.
   2. This head-down position actually makes the situation much worse.
   3. This may help somewhat, but it is not the best position.

UNIT VI   Hematologic and Immune Systems

CHAPTER 22   Nursing Assessment of the Hematologic System

Implementation
Medicine/Surgery
Physiologic and Anatomic Equilibrium
Acute Care
Blood and immunity

1. **In performing a physical assessment of a client suspected of having a lymphatic disorder, the nurse will have the head:**
   1. Straight
   2. Bent forward
   3. Slightly flexed
   4. Turned to the side

RATIONALE

(3) When one is palpating lymph nodes in the neck, it is helpful to have the client's neck slightly flexed.
   1. This is appropriate for a visual inspection.
   2. This may be useful in a musculoskeletal examination.
   4. This may be used to determine range of motion.

Evaluation
Medicine/Surgery
Physiologic and Anatomic Equilibrium
Acute Care
Blood

2. **In evaluating the client who has recently undergone a bone marrow aspiration, the nurse will observe for:**
   1. Bleeding
   2. Restlessness
   3. Respiratory difficulty
   4. Nutritional status

RATIONALE

(1) When blood disorders are being diagnosed, clients often undergo aspiration of samples of bone marrow from the iliac crest or the sternum.
   2. This is not common after the procedure.
   3. This is not expected.
   4. Fluids can be resumed within a short period of time.

Implementation
Medicine/Surgery
Education
Acute Care
Blood and immunity

3. **When a client is to undergo a Schilling test, instructions that the nurse will give include:**
   1. Avoid strenuous exercise
   2. Drink 100 ml of water 1 hour before the test
   3. Eat a high carbohydrate meal 1 hour before the test
   4. Avoid oral intake for 8 to 12 hours before the test

RATIONALE

(4) The Schilling test is the definitive test for pernicious anemia and is useful in detecting several other diseases. Avoiding oral intake before the test is essential.
   1. This is not necessary.
   2. This is not required.
   3. The client should not eat or drink anything.

Analysis
Medical/Surgery
Education
Acute Care
Blood and immunity

4. **The educator on a hematologic unit will review facts about blood components for new employees. One thing that the nurse will include is that erythrocytes survive in circulation for:**
   1. 30-60 days
   2. 60-90 days
   3. 105-120 days
   4. 130-150 days

RATIONALE

(3) Erythrocytes survive in the circulation for approximately 105 to 120 days.
   1. This is less than the normal time frame.
   2. This is the incorrect time frame.
   4. This is more than the normal time frame.

Analysis
Medicine/Surgery
Education
Acute Care
Blood and immunity

5. **In explaining the process of erythrocyte production to a client, the nurse explains that it is regulated by the hormone:**
   1. Estrogen
   2. Androgen
   3. Testosterone
   4. Erythropoietin

RATIONALE

(4) Erythrocyte production is controlled by the renal hormone erythropoietin. It is secreted in

increased amounts when the partial pressure of oxygen in the blood is less than a critical amount.
   1. Estrogen is not correct; choose another answer.
   2. Androgen is not correct.
   3. Testosterone is not correct.

CHAPTER 23 Nursing Management of Adults with Hematologic Disorders

Implementation
Medicine/Surgery
Physiologic and Anatomic Equilibrium
Acute Care
Blood and immunity

1. **Nursing actions that might be implemented for a client with sickle cell anemia include:**
   1. Rest
   2. Exercise
   3. Fluid restriction
   4. Application of cold to joints

RATIONALE

(1) Clients with high concentrations of sickle hemoglobin and frequent painful crisis require rest, analgesics for pain, and treatment of infections.
   2. Exercise is not recommended.
   3. Hydration is important.
   4. Local application of heat for joint pain is recommended.

Implementation
Medicine/Surgery
Physiologic and Anatomic Equilibrium
Acute Care
Blood and immunity

2. **An appropriate nursing action for a client with a severely depressed leukocyte count is to:**
   1. Institute reverse isolation
   2. Avoid taking rectal temperatures
   3. Obtain a private room
   4. Enforce complete bed rest

RATIONALE

(3) The decreased leukocyte count places the client at increased risk for infection. A private room along with aseptic technique decreases the risk.
   1. This is unnecessary.
   2. This precaution is taken in clients with potential bleeding problems.
   4. This is not necessary.

Planning
Medicine/Surgery
Physiologic and Anatomic Equilibrium
Long-term Care
Blood and immunity

3. **A client with thalassemia may develop severe anemia. The nurse anticipates that which of the following will be given:**

1. Antibiotics
2. Fluid challenge
3. Blood transfusions
4. Iron rich foods

RATIONALE

(3) Thalassemia is a genetic disorder in which the synthesis of hemoglobin is decreased. This results in decreased red blood cell count production and a chronic hemolytic anemia that may require transfusion therapy.
1. This is not usually needed.
2. This is not an appropriate therapy.
4. This will not solve the underlying problem.

> Planning
> Medicine/Surgery
> Physiologic and Anatomic Equilibrium
> Long-term Care
> Blood and Immunity

4. **The nurse is developing a plan of care for a client who has recently been diagnosed with polycythemia vera. The nurse explains that treatment may involve periodic:**
   1. Blood transfusion
   2. Blood removal
   3. Anticoagulants
   4. Iron supplements

RATIONALE

(2) For clients with little or no clinical discomfort, the treatment is phlebotomy (the removal of blood at regular intervals).
1. This would worsen the problem.
3. Bleeding is already a risk.
4. This is not an appropriate therapy.

> Planning
> Medicine/Surgery
> Physiologic and Anatomic Equilibrium
> Long-term Care
> Blood and Immunity

5. **For the client with a red blood cell disorder, one planned nursing outcome would be:**
   1. No modifications to health practices
   2. Infection or injury will be minimal
   3. Completion of normal activities without fatigue
   4. Hemoglobin and hematocrit would not reach critically low levels

RATIONALE

(3) One successful nursing intervention should allow the client to complete desired activities without fatigue.
1. The client and family should modify some of their health practices and discuss family planning.

2. No occurrence of infection or injury is preferred.
4. Hemoglobin, hematocrit and red blood cell counts should be within normal limits.

> Evaluation
> Medicine/Surgery
> Physiologic and Anatomic Equilibrium
> Long-term Care
> Blood and Immunity

6. **In an evaluation of the care provided to a client with a red blood cell disorder, one favorable outcome would be:**
   1. Mild fatigue
   2. Moderate dyspnea
   3. Comfortable at rest
   4. Hemoglobin of 5 g/L

RATIONALE

(1) Changes in laboratory values will provide information about the success of the nursing interventions. Fewer reports of fatigue are desired.
2. Mild symptoms such as dyspnea are desired.
3. Little to no pain with activity is preferred.
4. Hemoglobin and hematocrit levels within normal limits are best.

> Evaluation
> Medicine/Surgery
> Physiologic and Anatomic Equilibrium
> Long-term Care
> Blood and Immunity

7. **Successful response to the plan of care for the client with a white blood cell (WBC) disorder would be:**
   1. WBC 100 mm^3
   2. Infection prevention
   3. Mild redness and tenderness
   4. Minimal purulent drainage

RATIONALE

(2) Prevention or rapid resolution of infectious episodes are desired.
1. This represents severe neutropenia. WBCs within normal limits are desired.
3. Normal body temperature and no redness or tenderness is preferred.
4. The goal is no infection or inflammation.

CHAPTER 24 Nursing Assessment of the Immune System

> Analysis
> Medicine/Surgery
> Physiologic and Anatomic Equilibrium
> Long-term Care
> Blood and Immunity

1. In reading for work on an immunology unit, the nurse learns that many organisms enter the body through the mouth but do not multiply because of:
   1. Normal flora
   2. Oxygen level
   3. Temperature
   4. Stomach acid

RATIONALE

(4) Organisms are destroyed by the hydrochloric acid secreted by the stomach.
   1. These usually do not interfere.
   2. This is ideal for bacterial growth.
   3. The warmth promotes growth.

Analysis
Medicine/Surgery
Physiologic and Anatomic Equilibrium
Acute Care
Blood and Immunity

2. The most important white blood cells (WBC) and the first to respond to tissue damage are:
   1. Neutrophils
   2. Monocytes
   3. Mast cells
   4. T lymphocytes

RATIONALE

(1) Neutrophils make up 50% to 70% of all circulating WBCs and respond to tissue damage or pathogen invasion first.
   2. These are macrophages that defend against pathogens.
   3. These cells are involved with the IgE-mediated inflammation associated with allergic reaction.
   4. Lymphocytes are antigen specific.

Analysis
Medicine/Surgery
Physiologic and Anatomic Equilibrium
Acute Care
Blood and Immunity

3. The primary site for T lymphocyte production is the:
   1. Liver
   2. Thymus
   3. Spleen
   4. Bone marrow

RATIONALE

(2) The thymus is a flat organ lying below the thyroid. It is the primary site for the production, maturation, and differentiation of T lymphocytes.
   1. The liver contains macrophages.
   3. The spleen contains macrophages and B lymphocytes.
   4. This is the site of red blood cell production.

Analysis
Medicine/Surgery
Physiologic and Anatomic Equilibrium
Acute Care
Blood and Immunity

4. When any injury occurs from an organism, trauma, or ischemia, the body first produces:
   1. Infection
   2. Inflammation
   3. Vasoconstriction
   4. Decreased vascular permeability

RATIONALE

(2) The nonspecific immune response termed inflammation occurs first.
   1. This may develop later as the inflammatory state progresses.
   3. Vasodilation of the small blood vessels occurs.
   4. There is increased vascular permeability.

Evaluation
Medicine/Surgery
Physiologic and Anatomic Equilibrium
Acute Care
Blood and Immunity

5. In evaluating a client with a traumatic injury, the nurse knows that the inflammatory response produces four cardinal signs, one of which is:
   1. Heat
   2. Coolness
   3. Paresthesia
   4. Vasoconstriction

RATIONALE

(1) Heat, or calor, is one of the signs that provide the basis for evaluating the extent of the inflammatory response.
   2. Rubor or redness is produced.
   3. Dolor or pain is another sign.
   4. Tumor or swelling occurs also.

Analysis
Medicine/Surgery
Physiologic and Anatomic Equilibrium
Acute Care
Blood and Immunity

6. A nurse on a transplant unit understands that the rejection of transplanted organs is a result of tissue damage by:
   1. Erythrocytes
   2. B lymphocytes
   3. Natural killer cells
   4. CD8 T lymphocytes

RATIONALE

(4) CD8 cytotoxic T lymphocytes are responsible for this process.
   1. Red blood cells do not cause rejection.

2. These cells are not involved.

3. These cells engage in "immune surveillance" and look for tumor cells.

CHAPTER 25   NURSING MANAGEMENT OF ADULTS WITH IMMUNE DISORDERS

> Evaluation
> Medicine/Surgery
> Physiologic and Anatomic Equilibrium
> Acute Care
> Blood and Immunity

1. **In evaluating the presence or extent of an immunodeficient state, the nurse will evaluate the:**
   1. Viral load
   2. Red blood cells
   3. White blood cells
   4. Nutritional status

RATIONALE

(3) The primary indicator of immunodeficient states is a decrease in the number of white blood cells or their chemical mediators in the blood. The absolute neutrophil count is the specific parameter.
   1. This indicates how fast a virus is replicating.
   2. This value does not relate to immunodeficiency.
   4. This can affect the health of the immune system.

> Planning
> Medicine/Surgery
> Physiologic and Anatomic Equilibrium
> Long-term Care
> Blood and Immunity

2. **The nurse's ultimate goal in caring for an immunodeficient client is to:**
   1. Eradicate the disease
   2. Maintain daily routine
   3. Increase coping skills
   4. Prevent and treat infection

RATIONALE

(4) All members of the health care team monitor for signs of infection and the side effects of antiinfective drug therapy.
   1. This is not possible in some cases.
   2. This may not be attainable.
   3. This is a valid secondary goal.

> Assessment
> Medicine/Surgery
> Physiologic and Anatomic Equilibrium
> Long-term
> Blood and Immunity

3. **In assessing a client in the immunology clinic, the nurse notices a "butterfly" rash over the cheek bones. The nurse would suspect:**

1. Myasthenia gravis
2. Pernicious anemia
3. Rheumatoid arthritis
4. Systemic lupus erythematous

RATIONALE

(4) This is a chronic, progressive inflammatory disease of multiple organ systems with remissions and exacerbations. The disease also produces joint pain and affects the red blood cell and platelet levels.
   1. This is a disease in which autoantibodies destroy acetylcholine receptors, which affects myoneural junction impulse transmission.
   2. Autoantibodies destroying cells in the gastric mucosa affecting absorption of vitamin B_{12} cause this disease.
   3. Autoantibodies create inflammation in the joint spaces here.

> Implementation
> Medicine/Surgery
> Physiologic and Anatomic Equilibrium
> Long-term Care
> Blood and Immunity

4. **In providing treatment for a client with systemic lupus erythematous (SLE), one primary intervention will be to provide drug therapy, specifically:**
   1. NSAIDs
   2. Antibiotics
   3. Corticosteroids
   4. Insulin or oral hypoglycemics

RATIONALE

(3) Treatment is focused on corticosteroid therapy to reduce the effects of inflammation on organ systems.
   1. These are used for symptom relief but will not slow the disease progression.
   2. Antibiotics are not effective SLE therapy.
   4. These drugs are used to treat diabetes, an autoimmune disorder of the pancreas.

> Evaluation
> Medicine/Surgery
> Physiologic and Anatomic Equilibrium
> Acute Care
> Drug-related response

5. **A client with AIDS is receiving zidovudine. One of its most serious side effects is:**
   1. Nausea
   2. Drug resistance
   3. Stomach cramps
   4. Bone marrow depression

RATIONALE

(4) Bone marrow depression leads to severe anemia, further compromising the client's state of health.

1. This is a common side effect of AIDS drug therapy.
2. This does not occur.
3. This is a side effect of many of the drugs used to treat AIDS.

Assessment
Medicine/Surgery
Physiologic and Anatomic Equilibrium
Acute Care
Blood and Immunity

6. **A homeless client has requested an AIDS test. The test that offers the most definitive confirmation of HIV is:**
   1. White blood cell count
   2. Complete blood cell count
   3. Wood's light test
   4. Western blot test

RATIONALE

(4) Diagnosis of HIV infection is made by detecting antibodies to HIV in the blood, using enzyme-linked immunosorbent assay (ELISA) confirmed by the more sensitive and specific Western Blot test.
   1. This test indicates the presence of infection.
   2. This test identifies blood components.
   3. This test is used to identify skin disorders.

UNIT VII   Renal and Urinary Systems

CHAPTER 26   Nursing Assessment of the Renal and Urinary Systems

Implementation
Medicine/Surgery
Physiologic and Anatomic Equilibrium
Acute Care
Fluid and Electrolyte

1. **A urine culture is needed in order to diagnose a urinary tract infection. In order to obtain accurate results, the nurse instructs the client to:**
   1. Clean the perineal area well
   2. Clean the inside of the container
   3. Void continually and fill the container
   4. Steady the container on clothing to avoid spills

RATIONALE

(1) Females should separate the labia and clean the perineum from front to back. Men should retract the foreskin, and both should wipe the urethra at least 3 times.
   2. The container should not be touched on the inside.
   3. The client should void, wipe the urethra, then void again.
   4. The container should not contact legs, genitalia, or clothing.

Implementation
Medicine/Surgery
Physiologic and Anatomic Equilibrium
Acute Care
Fluid and Electrolyte

2. **When instructing a client in obtaining a composite urine specimen, the nurse will specify that:**
   1. Both the first and the last specimens are discarded:
   2. Both the first and the last specimens are sent to lab
   3. First specimen is discarded, last specimen is sent to lab
   4. First specimen is sent to lab, last specimen is discarded

RATIONALE

(3) The client is instructed to void and discard the first urine specimen; at the end of the collection period, the nurse instructs the client to void and add the specimen to the container.
   1. Only the first is discarded.
   2. The first is not sent to the lab.
   4. The first is discarded while the last is included.

Implementation
Medicine/Surgery
Physiologic and Anatomic Equilibrium
Acute Care
Fluid and Electrolyte

3. **After obtaining a routine urinalysis specimen, the nurse must:**
   1. Test with reagent strip
   2. Send immediately to lab
   3. Test urine with reagent tablets
   4. Leave specimen out for 6 hours

RATIONALE

(2) The specimen should be sent to the laboratory immediately or be refrigerated if it must be kept longer than I hour.
   1. This is not done routinely.
   3. This is not standard practice.
   4. Leaving a specimen standing at room temperature longer than 5 hours will invalidate the results.

Planning
Medicine/Surgery
Physiologic and Anatomic Equilibrium
Acute Care
Fluid and Electrolyte

4. **The nurse is asked by a physician to obtain a creatinine clearance specimen. The care plan will indicate that the urine specimen required is:**
   1. 24-hour urine
   2. Clean catch
   3. Sterile specimen
   4. Early morning urine

(1) A 24 hour specimen is usually collected, although 2-, 6-, or 12-hour specimens may also be obtained.

2. This is important for an accurate urine culture.
3. This is obtained by catheterizing the client.
4. This is best for a routine urinalysis.

Planning
Medicine/Surgery
Education
Acute Care
Fluid and Electrolyte

5. The nurse is developing a care plan for a client who is to have a renal scan. The client is told that:
    1. Oral intake is avoided
    2. Scans take 1½ hours
    3. The supine position is used
    4. Radioactive material remains in the body for 1 month

RATIONALE

(2) Renal scans are used in monitoring rejection of transplanted kidneys and in disease detection. They last approximately 1½ hours.

1. No dietary restrictions are required.
3. The client will be in the prone position.
4. Radioactive material is completely excreted in 24 hours.

Evaluation
Medicine/Surgery
Physiologic and Anatomic Equilibrium
Acute Care
Fluid and Electrolyte

6. In evaluating a client after a renal biopsy, the nurse will observe for:
    1. Bleeding
    2. Activity
    3. Mental status
    4. Bowel movement

RATIONALE

(1) The biopsy site is checked frequently for bleeding.

2. The client should lie still for 4 to 12 hours.
3. This should not be affected by the procedure.
4. Voidings are checked for gross and microscopic hematuria.

CHAPTER 27 Nursing Management of Adults with Renal Disorders

Evaluation
Medicine/Surgery
Physiologic and Anatomic Equilibrium

Long-term Care
Fluid and Electrolyte

1. An adult client with renal failure should be evaluated on an on-going basis for the effectiveness of care. One desired finding is:
    1. Partial diet compliance
    2. Stable "dry" weight
    3. Moderate hypertension
    4. Minimal leakage from dialysis site

RATIONALE

(2) This is the weight of the client after dialysis.

1. The client should be compliant with dietary and fluid restrictions.
3. The blood pressure should be within normal limit.
4. The dialysis access site should be dry and free of infection.

Evaluation
Medicine/Surgery
Physiologic and Anatomic Equilibrium
Acute Care
Fluid and Electrolyte

2. Postoperative evaluation of a client who has received a kidney transplant focuses on signs of graft rejection. A favorable evaluation should reveal:
    1. Edema
    2. Weight gain
    3. Normal urine output
    4. Increased blood pressure

RATIONALE

(3) The client is monitored carefully for changes in fluid and electrolyte levels and graft rejection. If the graft is functioning normally, there should be no change in the urine output, fever, pain at the graft site, or increased white blood cell count or lymphocyte count.

1. There should be no edema.
2. This is an ominous sign.
4. The blood pressure should remain within normal limits.

Planning
Medicine/Surgery
Physiologic and AnatomicEquilibrium
Acute Care
Fluid and Electrolyte

3. In planning long-term care and expected outcomes for a client with renal failure after a kidney transplant, one goal would be:
    1. No longer requires dialysis
    2. Fluid and electrolyte balance within normal limits
    3. Restricts calories to spare protein breakdown
    4. Resumes a normal schedule with minimal rest or sleep

RATIONALE

(2) The fluid and electrolyte level is monitored carefully because dialysis may be required after transplantation until the graft begins to function adequately.
1. Dialysis may be needed after transplant.
3. Sufficient calories should be ingested to spare protein breakdown.
4. Normal activities should be resumed, but the client should obtain sufficient sleep and rest to prevent undue stress or fatigue.

Evaluation
Medicine/Surgery
Physiologic and Anatomic Equilibrium
Long-term Care
Fluid and Electrolyte

4. When a client with chronic renal failure is evaluated, one of the hallmarks of renal disease is:
1. Metabolic acidosis
2. Metabolic alkalosis
3. Respiratory acidosis
4. Respiratory alkalosis

RATIONALE

(1) The diseased kidneys are unable to excrete metabolic acids and to conserve bicarbonate.
2. Bicarbonate is lost; alkalosis does not occur.
3. This is not related to renal disease.
4. This occurs because of changes within the respiratory system.

Planning
Medicine/Surgery
Physiologic and Anatomic
Equilibrium
Long-term Care
Fluid and Electrolyte

5. Two weeks after the onset of renal failure, a client is in the diuretic phase of renal failure. The primary nursing goal at this time is to:
1. Restrict fluids
2. Maintain electrolyte balance
3. Decrease excretion of wastes
4. Increase loss of electrolytes

RATIONALE

(2) As the client recovers from acute renal failure, the kidneys are not healed yet. The blood urea nitrogen and creatinine continue to rise and act as an osmotic diuretic. Sodium and potassium are lost.
1. Dehydration may occur; fluids and electrolytes may need to be replaced in the later phases of diuresis.
3. The excretion of waste products is desired.
4. This is not an appropriate goal.

Evaluation
Medicine/Surgery
Physiologic and Anatomic Equilibrium
Long-term Care
Fluid and Electrolyte

6. As clients enter the recovery phase of acute renal failure, an expected outcome is:
1. Chronic kidney infections
2. Total recovery of injured nephrons
3. Long-term use of a catheter
4. Long-term electrolyte imbalance

RATIONALE

(4) The recovery phase continues for up to 12 months. Usually the client is left with some residual impairment in renal function.
1. This is not an automatic outcome of acute renal failure.
2. Total recovery usually does not occur.
3. This is usually not necessary.

Evaluation
Medicine/Surgery
Physiologic and Anatomic Equilibrium
Long-term Care
Fluid and Electrolyte

7. An expected outcome for a client with renal obstruction is:
1. Pain relief
2. Unrestricted diet
3. Low-grade fever
4. Positive urine cultures

RATIONALE

(1) Pain control evidenced not only by statements made by the client but also by relaxed body posture and facial expression is a desired goal.
2. Diet adherence and meal planning with specific dietary restrictions are important.
3. The absence of fever is expected.
4. Negative urine cultures are desired.

CHAPTER 28   Nursing Management of Adults with Urinary Tract Disorders

Planning
Medicine/Surgery
Physiologic and Anatomic Equilibrium
Long-term Care
Fluid and Electrolyte

1. An expected postoperative outcome of a client after urinary diversion for bladder cancer is:
1. Sexual abstinence
2. Pink, moist stoma
3. Mild systemic infection
4. Denial of urinary diversion

(2) A urinary diversion stoma should be moist and pink-red, and urine should drain freely from any stents or catheters.

1. Sexual intercourse and alternative methods of sexual expression are possible.
3. No systemic infection should be evident.
4. Acceptance of urinary diversion and accompanying changes is expected.

> Implementation
> Medicine/Surgery
> Physiologic and Anatomic Equilibrium
> Acute Care
> Fluid and Electrolyte

2. **One nursing action for a client who has had urinary diversion for bladder cancer is:**
   1. Potassium restriction
   2. Alkaline diet
   3. Encouraging fluids
   4. Restricting fluids

RATIONALE

(3) The client is encouraged to take in between 2500 ml and 3000 ml of fluid daily to flush the urinary tract and decrease the risk of infection.

1. Potassium intake is increased through foods and medication because potassium is lost because of acidosis.
2. An acid-ash diet is encouraged to ensure acidic urine to decrease bacterial growth.
4. Fluids should be encouraged.

> Evaluation
> Medicine/Surgery
> Physiologic and Anatomic Equilibrium
> Acute Care
> Fluid and Electrolyte

3. **A client who was involved in a motor vehicle accident has sustained a ruptured bladder, requiring surgical repair. Postoperatively, the nurse will evaluate the effectiveness of the treatment by monitoring:**
   1. Urinary output
   2. Mental status
   3. Anxiety level
   4. Urine color

RATIONALE

(1) The quality and quantity of the urinary output is observed closely.

2. This is important but does not relate to normal urinary function.
3. This is a secondary concern.
4. Color changes are anticipated because of the trauma and repair.

> Implementation
> Medicine/Surgery
> Physiologic and Anatomic Equilibrium
> Acute Care
> Fluid and Electrolyte

4. **One important nursing intervention for a client with urethral trauma is:**
   1. Monitoring edema
   2. Applying heat to scrotum
   3. Removing the catheter
   4. Monitoring intake and output

RATIONALE

(4) Treatment for clients with lower urinary tract injury focuses on maintenance of adequate urinary output.

1. This is unnecessary unless the client has renal or cardiac failure or other problems which might cause fluid retention.
2. Ice packs to relieve edema and scrotal suspension may be necessary to alleviate pain.
3. A catheter of some kind is used until the traumatic injury has had time to heal.

> Evaluation
> Medicine/Surgery
> Physiologic and Anatomic Equilibrium
> Acute Care
> Fluid and Electrolyte

5. **A client in the emergency room has been diagnosed with renal calculi. In evaluating the results of nursing actions, the nurse would expect the following client response:**
   1. Oliguria
   2. Pain relief
   3. Moderate pain
   4. Decreased nausea

RATIONALE

(2) Renal calculi can be very painful. Complete relief or a reduction to an acceptable level is expected.

1. The urinary pattern present before the obstruction should be regained.
3. Mild pain only is acceptable.
4. This is not a common symptom.

> Planning
> Medicine/Surgery
> Physiologic and Anatomic Equilibrium
> Acute Care
> Fluid and Electrolyte

6. **The nurse caring for a young woman in the emergency room who has a urinary tract infection explains that the symptoms that may be expected with this disease include:**
   1. Temperature above 100° F
   2. Urinary frequency

3. Clear, yellow voided urine
4. Pain and burning on urination

RATIONALE

(3) Effective treatment should produce clear, odorless urine.
1. Temperature below 100° F are expected.
2. This should not occur.
4. This should be eliminated.

Planning
Medicine/Surgery
Physiologic and Anatomic Equilibrium
Long-term Care
Fluid and Electrolyte

7. **An evaluation of a postsurgical client with urinary retention should indicate:**
1. Partial bladder emptying
2. Mild urine bacteriuria
3. Proper self-catheterization technique
4. Proper catheterization by a family member

RATIONALE

(3) The client should be able to perform intermittent self-catheterization if needed.
1. Complete bladder emptying is expected.
2. No evidence of a urinary tract infection such as a negative urine culture is expected.
4. The client should be able to perform this task.

UNIT VIII   Neurologic System

CHAPTER 29   Nursing Assessment of the Neurologic System

Implementation
Medicine/Surgery
Physiologic and Anatomic Equilibrium
Acute Care
Neuromuscular

1. **When the physician obtains a specimen of spinal fluid from lumbar puncture, it is important that the nurse:**
1. Collect it in three labeled tubes
2. Dispose of the first specimen drawn
3. Dispose of the last specimen drawn
4. Combine all fluid into one sterile container

RATIONALE

(1) Samples are collected in three labeled tubes for protein and glucose determination, blood cell counts, and culture.
2. None of the specimen is disposed of.
3. All of the sample is saved.
4. The fluid should be divided.

Planning
Medicine/Surgery
Physiologic and Anatomic Equilibrium
Acute Care
Neuromuscular

2. **A client is scheduled for an echoencephalogram. The care plan includes teaching the client that the test is:**
1. Long
2. Painless
3. Loud
4. Painful

RATIONALE

(2) In this test, a sound transducer/receiver is placed against the skull, which transmits and receives sound waves. The sound waves are converted to electrical impulses and displayed on an oscilloscope. It is painless.
1. The test takes 10 minutes.
3. There is minimal sound involved.
4. The test is painless.

Implementation
Medicine/Surgery
Physiologic and Anatomic
    Equilibrium
Acute Care
Neuromuscular

3. **A client is scheduled for a magnetic resonance imaging test. The nurse explains that this test is useful in identifying abnormalities of:**
1. Bone
2. Conduction
3. Soft tissue
4. Electricity

RATIONALE

(3) This test uses an electromagnetic echo to produce images of soft tissue.
1. Bone is not visualized.
2. Conduction defects are not identified.
4. Electricity is not measured.

Evaluation
Medicine/Surgery
Physiologic and Anatomic
    Equilibrium
Acute Care
Neuromuscular

4. **A client has had cerebral angiography using a carotid artery. In evaluating for possible complications, the nurse will monitor for signs of:**
1. Pallor
2. Nausea
3. Fatigue
4. Dysphagia

RATIONALE

(4) Dysphagia, respiratory distress, and arterial spasms may all be symptoms of transient ischemic attacks.
1. Blood loss and associated pallor are not expected.
2. This is not common.
3. This is not expected.

> Evaluation
> Medicine/Surgery
> Physiologic and Anatomic Equilibrium
> Acute Care
> Neuromuscular

5. A client who has had a myelogram with an oil-based dye is being observed for complications, which may include:
   1. Headache
   2. Nausea
   3. Neck stiffness
   4. Pressure

RATIONALE

(3) Headache is relatively common after this procedure, but neck stiffness and pain should be reported because they may signal meningeal irritation.
1. This is a common occurrence.
2. This is not common complication.
4. This is not a usual finding.

> Assessment
> Medicine/Surgery
> Physiologic and Anatomic Equilibrium
> Acute Care
> Neuromuscular

6. A client is suspected of having a disorder of proprioception. The test that is used to evaluate this disorder is:
   1. Achilles reflex
   2. Patellar reflex
   3. Babinski's reflex
   4. Romberg's sign

RATIONALE

(4) The client should be able to stand with eyes closed and feet together without swaying for approximately 5 seconds.
1. This tests plantar flexion of the foot when the Achilles tendon is tapped.
2. This tests for extension of the lower leg as the patellar tendon contracts.
3. This is an abnormal reflex which is present when the client has severe brain stem injury.

> Assessment
> Medicine/Surgery
> Physiologic and Anatomic Equilibrium
> Acute Care
> Neuromuscular

7. A nurse is conducting a neurologic assessment of a client. The client is asked to stick out the tongue and move it from side to side. This tests cranial nerve XII or:
   1. Hypoglossal
   2. Trigeminal
   3. Spinal accessory
   4. Glossopharyngeal

RATIONALE

(1) This nerve innervates the muscles that are responsible for movement of the tongue; any deviation of the tongue to one side is normal.
2. This tests facial movement.
3. This tests shoulder strength.
4. This tests the gag reflex and the ability of the client to swallow.

CHAPTER 30 Nursing Management of Adults with Common Neurologic Problems

> Assessment
> Medicine/Surgery
> Physiologic and Anatomic Equilibrium
> Acute Care
> Neuromuscular

1. The nurse on a neurosurgical unit knows that the most critical indicator of central nervous system dysfunction is:
   1. Pattern of breathing
   2. Level of consciousness
   3. Oculomotor responses
   4. Pupillary changes

RATIONALE

(2) Change in level of consciousness can indicate clinical improvement or deterioration. It is usually an early sign.
1. This indicates the level of brain dysfunction.
3. Eye position and oculomotor responses are controlled by brain stem and higher brain centers. They are used to assess the level of brain function.
4. Brain stem areas controlling arousal are adjacent to areas controlling pupils. Pupillary changes are a quick guide to the present level of brain stem dysfunction.

> Assessment
> Medicine/Surgery
> Physiologic and Anatomic Equilibrium
> Acute Care
> Neuromuscular

2. A neurosurgical client is exhibiting an unusual breathing pattern. The nurse observes a pause at the end of respiration. This is called:
   1. Apneusis
   2. Cluster breathing

3. Ataxic breathing
4. Gasping breathing pattern

RATIONALE

(1) This brain stem breathing pattern indicates damage to the respiratory control mechanism located at the pontine level.

2. These are breaths in a disordered sequence.
3. This is a completely irregular breathing pattern.
4. These are deep breaths accompanied by a slow respiratory rate.

Analysis
Medicine/Surgery
Physiologic and Anatomic Equilibrium
Acute Care
Neuromuscular

3. In performing a physical assessment on a client, the nurse notices that both pupils are greater than 5 mm in diameter and fixed. This condition may be caused by:
   1. Opiates
   2. Anoxia
   3. Temporal lobe herniation
   4. Cerebral dysfunction

RATIONALE

(2) Low oxygen levels, atropine, scopolamine, amphetamines, and mydriatics all can cause this.

1. Opiates will cause small, pin-point pupils.
3. Temporal lobe herniation compressing the ipsilateral oculomotor nerve against the posterior communicating area will cause a sluggish-responding pupil that is gradually dilating.
4. This causes small reactive pupils (1 to 2.5 mm), regularly shaped.

Planning
Medicine/Surgery
Physiologic and Anatomic Equilibrium
Acute Care
Neuromuscular

4. An expected outcome for the client with an altered level of consciousness is:
   1. Minimal oral mucosal damage
   2. Minimal corneal abrasions
   3. Lower Glasgow coma scale
   4. Higher Glasgow coma scale

RATIONALE

(4) Progression to a higher level of responsiveness as evidenced by a higher Glasgow coma scale is expected.

1. Intact, clean oral and nasal mucosa is desired.
2. Intact corneas are expected.
3. The client's scale value should be increasing or maximized.

Implementation
Medicine/Surgery
Physiologic and Anatomic Equilibrium
Acute Care
Neuromuscular

5. A young adult client has sustained head injuries as a result of driving under the influence of drugs. The client is in a coma. One appropriate intervention at this time is:
   1. Oral care every 8 hours
   2. Lower head of bed
   3. Elevate head of bed
   4. Provide liquids by mouth

RATIONALE

(3) Elevating the head improves cerebral blood flow and respiratory effort.

1. This should be done at least every 4 hours.
2. The head should be elevated approximately 30 degrees.
4. The client should be given nothing by mouth because the swallowing and cough reflexes are often impaired.

Implementation
Medicine/Surgery
Physiologic and Anatomic Equilibrium
Acute Care
Neuromuscular

6. A client has sustained blunt trauma to the head during a fight. To reduce the cerebral edema, the nurse will be asked to administer:
   1. Analgesics
   2. Fluid boluses
   3. Antibiotics
   4. Corticosteroids

RATIONALE

(4) Corticosteroids and osmotic diuretics are used to reduce edema and thus the intracranial pressure.

1. Analgesics are used cautiously in clients with head injuries.
2. Fluids are monitored carefully and are often restricted in these clients.
3. These decrease the risk of infection.

Evaluation
Medicine/Surgery
Physiologic and Anatomic Equilibrium
Acute Care
Neuromuscular

7. Evaluation of a client with intracranial hypertension is critical. One expected outcome of treatment is:
   1. Normal ICP
   2. CPP < 50 mm Hg
   3. PCO_2 < 70 mm Hg
   4. Absent DTRs

RATIONALE

(1) An intracranial pressure less than 15 mm Hg is expected.
2. A cerebral perfusion pressure greater than 50 mm Hg is desired.
3. Arterial oxygen levels greater than 70 mm Hg is expected.
4. Normal deep tendon reflexes are desired.

CHAPTER 31 Nursing Management of Adults with Degenerative Disorders

Analysis
Medicine/Surgery
Physiologic and Anatomic Equilibrium
Long-term Care
Neuromuscular

1. **Alzheimer's disease is the most common type of cerebral disorder that is characterized by a diffuse progressive loss of mental function because of an organic disturbance. Another name for this disorder is:**
   1. Confusion
   2. Dementia
   3. Delirium
   4. Asterixis

RATIONALE

(2) Alzheimer's disease is the most common type of dementia.
   1. This affects attention and the speed, clarity, and amount of mental activity.
   3. This is short-lived disorientation, restlessness, hyperirritability, fear and hallucinations.
   4. This is a flapping motion of the hand.

Planning
Medicine/Surgery
Physiologic and Anatomic Equilibrium
Long-term Care
Neuromuscular

2. **In developing a care plan for a client with dementia, the nurse identifies an appropriate outcome of:**
   1. Unrestricted diet
   2. Full-time assistance with ADLs
   3. Reduced focus on cognitive abilities
   4. Minimal physical and mental family stress

RATIONALE

(4) Long-term care of a client with dementia such as Alzheimer's disease can be very stressful to the family. They must be taught appropriate coping strategies.
   1. Sufficient nutrients should be ingested to maintain weight and provide energy for daily activities.

2. Clients should live in a safe environment that fosters cognitive and functional abilities.
3. Emphasis should be placed on the clients' participation in daily activities.

Implementation
Medicine/Surgery
Physiologic and Anatomic Equilibrium
Long-term Care
Neuromuscular

3. **In implementing a plan of care for a client with dementia, the nurse will:**
   1. Encourage activity
   2. Use memory enhancers
   3. Stimulate all of the senses
   4. Focus on mental capabilities

RATIONALE

(2) Calendars, clocks, posted schedules and notebooks with specific references seem to enhance memory.
   1. Proper amounts of rest and sleep to avoid fatigue are important.
   3. Overstimulation should be avoided.
   4. The client has important physical needs as well.

Analysis
Medicine/Surgery
Physiologic and Anatomic Equilibrium
Long-term Care
Neuromuscular

4. **In understanding the pathophysiology of Parkinson's disease, the nurse is aware that this degenerative process is caused by a loss of:**
   1. Dopamine
   2. Zona incerta
   3. Acetylcholine
   4. Gamma aminobutyric acid

RATIONALE

(1) There is a loss of the pigmented cells in the substantia nigra and a depletion of the monoamine neurotransmitter dopamine.
   2. This is an area of the brain not affected by this disease.
   3. This neurotransmitter has increased dominance in this disease.
   4. This is a neurotransmitter that is not involved in this process.

Assessment
Medicine/Surgery
Physiologic and Anatomic Equilibrium
Long-term Care
Neuromuscular

5. **Parkinsonism has several characteristic symptoms. When assessing a client with this disease, the nurse may observe:**

1. Normal speech
2. Facial tremor
3. Shuffling gait
4. Fast body movement

RATIONALE

(3) This shuffling or "festination" gait occurs when the client moves faster to keep the center of gravity balanced to compensate for a flexed postural deformity.
1. The speech is usually rapid, slurred, or soft.
2. Tremors of the distal extremities are common, the face has a characteristic "mask."
4. Bradykinesia or slowness of body movement is common.

CHAPTER 32 Nursing Management of Adults with Infectious, Inflammatory, or Autoimmune Disorders

Assessment
Medicine/Surgery
Physiologic and Anatomic Equilibrium
Acute Care
Neuromuscular

1. **The nurse has completed the assessment of a client with meningitis. An expected nursing diagnosis might be:**
1. Alteration in nutrition
2. Cardiac output compromise
3. Altered peripheral tissue perfusion
4. Risk for injury related to seizures

RATIONALE

(4) Altered intracranial fluid dynamics may cause motor and cognitive neurologic deficits.
1. This is not a critical concern.
2. This is usually not a treatment problem.
3. Cerebral tissue perfusion may be compromised.

Planning
Medicine/Surgery
Physiologic and Anatomic Equilibrium
Acute Care
Neuromuscular

2. **A client is admitted to the intensive care unit with a diagnosis of possible pneumococcal meningitis. The nurse should admit the client to:**
1. An open unit with other clients
2. A private room with respiratory isolation
3. A private room with reverse isolation
4. A private room where the lights can be dimmed

RATIONALE

(2) Clients with bacterial meningitis should be placed in respiratory isolation until 24 hours after antimicrobial therapy has been instituted.
1. This would expose others to the bacteria

3. The reverse isolation is not needed
4. The light intensity is not the critical factor to be considered.

Evaluation
Medicine/Surgery
Physiologic and Anatomic Equilibrium
Acute Care
Neuromuscular

3. **In evaluating the effects of drug therapy on a client with meningitis, the nurse observes for opisthotonos. The presence of this sign of meningeal irritation is indicated by:**
1. Curling in a fetal position
2. Tonic spasms of the legs
3. Arching of the neck and back
4. Flexion of the hip and knee when the neck is flexed

RATIONALE

(3) Opisthotonos is caused by extensor muscle spasm.
1. This is not an abnormal finding.
2. Deep tendon reflexes may be increased.
4. This is Brudzinski's sign, also associated with meningitis.

Implementation
Medicine/ Surgery
Physiologic and Anatomic
   Equilibrium
Acute Care
Neuromuscular

4. **The nurse establishes a goal of ensuring safety for a client with encephalitis. The nursing action that will contribute to this goal is:**
1. Pad the side rails
2. Administer sedative
3. Move the client often
4. Position client on side

RATIONALE

(1) Padding ensures safety in case the client should have a seizure.
2. This is rarely done.
3. Bed rest and sleep are important.
4. This is not critical.

Evaluation
Medicine/Surgery
Physiologic and Anatomic
Acute Care
Neuromuscular

5. **An indication that the nurse's teaching to a client with multiple sclerosis has been successful might be the statement:**
1. "The laxatives aren't necessary."
2. "Sex is not important to me anymore."
3. "I will be able to care for myself soon."
4. "I am turning often and using my cushion."

(4) Maintaining skin integrity requires vigilance in preventing problems.

1. Bowel dysfunction will be an on-going problem.
2. Sexual enjoyment can be regained by these clients.
3. The deficits will be long-term.

CHAPTER 33 Nursing Management of Adults with Cerebrovascular Disorders

> Analysis
> Medicine/Surgery
> Physiologic and Anatomic Equilibrium
> Acute Care
> Neuromuscular

1. **A client returns from CAT scan with a diagnosis of subarachnoid hemorrhage. This is most commonly caused by:**
   1. Hypertension
   2. Lacunar brain infarction
   3. Intracranial aneurysm rupture
   4. Atrial wall thrombus emboli

RATIONALE

(3) This may also be caused by an intracerebral hemorrhage that dissects into the subarachnoid space.

1. This is the main cause of intracerebral hemorrhage.
2. This causes an ischemic cerebrovascular accident.
4. These cause ischemic cerebrovascular accidents.

> Implementation
> Medicine/Surgery
> Physiologic and Anatomic Equilibrium
> Acute Care
> Neuromuscular

2. **In acute stroke, protecting the brain from further damage is essential. One drug that the nurse might expect to administer to improve cerebral blood flow is:**
   1. Nimodipine
   2. Nitroprusside
   3. Dipyridamole
   4. Ticlopidine

RATIONALE

(1) This is a calcium channel agonist that has been used effectively in acute ischemic stroke to improve cerebral blood flow around infarcts.

2. This causes hypertension and will worsen the situation.
3. This causes platelet inhibition and may increase bleeding.
4. This may also cause bleeding.

> Evaluation
> Medicine/Surgery
> Physiologic and Anatomic Equilibrium
> Acute Care
> Neuromuscular

3. **An expected outcome during the acute phase for the client with a stroke includes:**
   1. Airway patent
   2. Contractures treated
   3. Minimal cerebral perfusion
   4. Lowered fluid and electrolyte levels

RATIONALE

(1) The airway should be patent and the client should be free of aspiration.

2. The client should be free of contractures.
3. Cerebral tissue perfusion should be adequate.
4. These should remain within normal limits.

> Planning
> Medicine/Surgery
> Physiologic and Anatomic Equilibrium
> Long-term Care
> Neuromuscular

4. **The nurse makes a nursing diagnosis of impaired verbal communication related to aphasia and establishes a plan to help the client communicate effectively. The nursing action that will contribute to this plan is:**
   1. Provide frequent correction of mispronounced words
   2. Read to the client to provide sensory input for commonly used words
   3. Provide flash cards with words and pictures of commonly used items
   4. Limit sensory stimuli until the client indicates a readiness to attempt speech

RATIONALE

(3) Communication is stimulated by providing pictures of needed items and supporting and encouraging attempts at speech.

1. Constant correction increases the client frustration level.
2. Stimulating conversation is encouraged. Communicate in short phrases.
4. The client should be encouraged to speak and any attempts to speak should be praised.

> Implementation
> Acute Care
> Physiologic and Anatomic Equilibrium
> Long-term Care
> Neuromuscular

5. **The nurse makes a nursing diagnosis of sensory perceptual alteration related to hemianopsia and establishes a plan to manage the visual field deficits. An appropriate nursing intervention is:**

1. Approach the client on the affected side
2. Use artificial tears twice a day to prevent drying
3. Cover the eyes with a patch to prevent corneal damage
4. Teach the client to turn the head and eyes in the direction of the deficit

RATIONALE

(4) The client has difficulty seeing out of the affected field of vision; scanning the environment in the direction of the affected visual field allows the client to see objects in the environment.
1. The nurse should approach from the unaffected side so that the client can see him or her.
2. These will be needed more frequently during the day.
3. This will further limit the visual field.

CHAPTER 34 Nursing Management of Adults with Intracranial Disorders

> Planning
> Medicine/Surgery
> Physiologic and Anatomic Equilibrium
> Acute Care
> Neuromuscular

1. **A client arrives in the emergency room having sustained a head injury at a soccer match. There was a momentary loss of consciousness at the site. The client is now confused and lethargic. An appropriate plan of care for this client includes:**
   1. Immediate discharge
   2. Hospitalization
   3. Observation and release
   4. Surgery in 1 week

RATIONALE

(2) The altered level of consciousness indicates a grade II head injury, which requires hospitalization, generally in an intensive care unit.
1. These clients need observation.
3. Hospitalization is required.
4. Immediate surgery may be needed.

> Evaluation
> Medicine/Surgery
> Physiologic and Anatomic Equilibrium
> Acute Care
> Neuromuscular

2. **In monitoring a client with a head injury, the nurse anticipates a possible disruption of fluid balance. One physical finding that indicates syndrome of inappropriate antidiuretic hormone (SIADH) is:**
   1. Increased urinary output
   2. Decreased urinary output
   3. Increased serum sodium concentrations
   4. Decreased levels of antidiuretic hormone

RATIONALE

(2) SIADH causes antidiuretic hormone to be released when it is not needed, resulting in decreased urinary output.
1. The urinary output is decreased.
3. This level is decreased because of the ratio of sodium to the actual fluid amounts. This is referred to as dilutional hyponatremia.
4. The antidiuretic hormone levels are increased.

> Evaluation
> Medicine/Surgery
> Physiologic and Anatomic Equilibrium
> Acute Care
> Drug-related response

3. **The physician prescribes mannitol for a client with a head injury. The expected therapeutic outcome of using this drug is:**
   1. Decreased cerebral edema
   2. Decreased urinary output
   3. Increased intracranial pressure
   4. Dissolution of the hematoma

RATIONALE

(1) Mannitol is an osmotic diuretic that pulls fluid from the intravascular to the extravascular space, thus decreasing cerebral edema.
2. The urinary output is increased.
3. This lowers the intracranial pressure.
4. This drug does not affect clots.

> Assessment
> Medicine/Surgery
> Physiologic and Anatomic Equilibrium
> Acute Care
> Neuromuscular

4. **When the nurse is assessing a client with a head injury, the first priority of nursing management is to:**
   1. Assess pupillary changes
   2. Assess motor function
   3. Assess level of consciousness
   4. Stabilize cervical injuries

RATIONALE

(4) Stabilizing the neck to prevent further injury and ensuring protection of the airway are primary interventions.
1. These are ongoing assessments done after a baseline has been established.
2. This is a secondary assessment criteria.
3. This should be done continuously.

> Analysis
> Medicine/Surgery
> Physiologic and Anatomic Equilibrium
> Acute Care
> Neuromuscular

5. Three days after a client has had surgery to remove a brain tumor, the nurse notices crying. The client asks what deficits will remain after surgery. The nurse recognizes this behavior as:
   1. Pain related to postsurgical headache
   2. Potential ineffective coping related to surgery
   3. Personality changes expected after brain surgery
   4. Body image changes related to the bulky head dressing

RATIONALE

(2) After brain surgery, there is potential for ineffective coping. The nurse should encourage verbalization of thoughts and feelings.
   1. Postoperative pain is usually manageable and will not precipitate this response.
   3. This is not expected.
   4. These are only temporary.

CHAPTER 35 Nursing Management of Adults with Spinal Cord Disorders

Planning
Medicine/Surgery
Physiologic and Anatomic Equilibrium
Long-term Care
Neuromuscular

1. A client from a local moving company has recently been diagnosed with intervertebral disk disease. One important goal of care for this client is:
   1. Minimal skin breakdown
   2. Freedom from pain
   3. Able to perform self-catheterization
   4. Moderate reduction in activity level

RATIONALE

(2) Pain management is important to allow for activity to resume.
   1. No loss of skin integrity should occur.
   3. This should not be necessary.
   4. The client should be able to resume normal activities.

Implementation
Medicine/Surgery
Physiologic and Anatomic Equilibrium
Long-term Care
Neuromuscular

2. The nurse has identified pain related to nerve root compression as a nursing diagnosis for a client with a spinal cord tumor. One intervention that may help to control the pain is:
   1. Medicate with corticosteroids
   2. Apply heat to the area
   3. Encourage range of motion exercises
   4. Apply the transcutaneous electrical nerve stimulator (TENS) unit

RATIONALE

(4) The electrical unit blocks pain transmission.
   1. Analgesics are administered as needed depending on the type of pain.
   2. This is not recommended.
   3. All movement must be done carefully and may produce more pain.

Assessment
Medicine/Surgery
Physiologic and Anatomic Equilibrium
Long-term Care
Neuromuscular

3. A common sequela to spinal cord injury is heterotopic ossification. A common presentation of this disorder is:
   1. Hypothermia
   2. Proprioception disappearing
   3. Decreasing range of motion
   4. Inflammation of leg muscles

RATIONALE

(3) These ossifications are bony tissue that forms in muscle and fascia around joints, interfering with movement
   1. Fever is often present.
   2. This usually does not occur.
   4. Inflammation involves the joint space.

Analysis
Medicine/Surgery
Physiologic and Anatomic Equilibrium
Long-term Care
Neuromuscular

4. During the acute phase of care of a client with a spinal cord injury, one appropriate nursing diagnosis is:
   1. Social isolation
   2. Altered tissue perfusion
   3. Alteration in thought processes
   4. Alteration in comfort related to pain

RATIONALE

(2) Altered tissue perfusion to the central nervous system related to spinal instability is possible.
   1. Many clients have adequate social support.
   3. Cerebral functioning may not be affected.
   4. Often there is complete or partial loss of sensation.

Implementation
Medicine/Surgery
Physiologic and Anatomic Equilibrium
Acute Care
Neuromuscular

5. Four hours after a motor vehicle accident that caused spinal cord injury, a client in the neurologic intensive care unit is scheduled to

receive a drug to control central nervous system tissue edema. The nurse expects to administer:

1. Aspirin
2. Demerol
3. Mannitol
4. Solu-Medrol

RATIONALE

(4) Although somewhat controversial, high-dose corticosteroid treatment of acute spinal cord injury is now recommended within 8 hours of injury.

1. This may cause further complications.
2. Narcotics are rarely administered.
3. This is used for cerebral edema.

CHAPTER 36 Nursing Management of Adults with Peripheral or Cranial Nerve Disorders

Analysis
Medicine/Surgery
Physiologic and Anatomic Equilibrium
Long-term Care
Neuromuscular

1. A homeless client with a history of alcoholism comes to the clinic with complaints of a burning sensation in both the feet and the hands and tenderness of the calf muscles. These symptoms are consistent with:

1. Tarsal tunnel syndrome
2. Tic douloureux pain
3. Charcot-Marie Tooth disease
4. Nutritional deficiency neuropathy

RATIONALE

(4) This is a secondary nerve condition usually caused by vitamin B deficiency caused by alcoholism and anorexia.

1. This results in pain in the ankles and feet.
2. This is a disorder resulting in cheek pain.
3. This results in atrophy of the hands and feet.

Planning
Medicine/Surgery
Physiologic and Anatomic Equilibrium
Long-term Care
Neuromuscular

2. A home health nurse is monitoring the care of a client with Charcot-Marie-Tooth disease. One aspect of care will be:

1. Vitamin B complex therapy
2. Anticonvulsant therapy
3. Application of range of motion exercise to extremities
4. Immobilizing the extremities

RATIONALE

(3) This disease involves chronic degeneration of peripheral nerves and roots, resulting in distal muscle atrophy of the legs and feet.

1. This is not part of the usual therapy.
2. These are not effective for this disease.
4. Exercise is recommended.

Assessment
Medicine/Surgery
Physiologic and Anatomic Equilibrium
Acute Care
Neuromuscular

3. A client arrives in the clinic complaining of an intense pain in the lips and cheek that does not involve the teeth. These symptoms describe:

1. Bell's palsy
2. Sciatic nerve injury
3. Trigeminal neuralgia
4. Carpal tunnel syndrome

RATIONALE

(3) This disorder of cranial nerve V is also referred to as tic douloureux and produces excruciating pain in the lips, gums, cheeks, or chin.

1. Bell's palsy is a unilateral facial paralysis of sudden onset affecting the motor component of the cranial nerve VII.
2. This involves pain in the leg.
4. This causes pain and numbness in the hands.

Evaluation
Medicine/Surgery
Physiologic and Anatomic Equilibrium
Long-term Care
Neuromuscular

4. While evaluating the recovery of a client with Bell's palsy, the nurse observes a symptom that indicates a good chance of full recovery of motor function. It is:

1. Recovery of taste
2. Eye does not close
3. Drooling of the mouth
4. Paralysis of lower face

RATIONALE

(1) Recovery of taste within the first week signals a good chance for full recovery of motor function.

2. This is a presenting symptom.
3. This is a common symptom.
4. This occurs on one side of the face.

Planning
Medicine/Surgery
Physiologic and Anatomic Equilibrium
Long-term Care
Neuromuscular

5. A travel agent who frequently uses a computer has developed carpal tunnel syndrome. The nurse informs the client that therapy will include:
   1. Splinting
   2. Aspirin
   3. Vitamin K
   4. Increased fluids

RATIONALE

(1) Splinting of the hand is used initially and is most effective if begun early in the course of symptoms.
   2. This is not indicated.
   3. B vitamins are often prescribed.
   4. Diuretics can be given to decrease fluid retention.

UNIT IX   The Eye and Ear

CHAPTER 37   Nursing Assessment of the Eye

Assessment
Medicine/Surgery
Physiologic and Anatomic Equilibrium
Acute Care
Neuromuscular

1. In an examination of the eye, one potential symptom related to eye disorders that the nurse may observe is scotoma, which refers to:
   1. Drooping eyelid
   2. Abnormal light intolerance
   3. Blind spots in visual field
   4. Loss of peripheral vision

RATIONALE

(3) The visual field should be clear in all quadrants.
   1. This is ptosis.
   2. This is photophobia.
   4. This is tunnel vision.

Analysis
Medicine/Surgery
Physiologic and Anatomic Equilibrium
Acute Care
Neuromuscular

2. The Snellen chart is used to assess distance vision. The ability of the client to read letters is assessed at a distance of:
   1. 2 feet
   2. 20 inches
   3. 20 feet
   4. 30 feet

RATIONALE

(3) The client stands at a point 20 feet from the chart. Each eye is tested separately.
   1. This distance is too short.
   2. This is not far enough away from the chart.
   4. This distance is too far.

Evaluation
Medicine/Surgery
Physiologic and Anatomic Equilibrium
Acute Care
Neuromuscular

3. The nurse has provided an overview of the electroretinogram that a client is about to undergo. The client confirms understanding of the test by the statement:
   1. "Those needles in my eye won't hurt."
   2. "I am going to miss drinking my morning coffee."
   3. "I'll only have to lie still for 15 minutes."
   4. "I shouldn't feel anything after they put the drops in my eye."

RATIONALE

(4) This test evaluates the response of the eye to darkness and to light. Topical anesthetic is placed in the eye and contact lenses with electrodes incorporated into them are applied to the eye.
   1. There are no needles involved.
   2. There are no dietary restrictions before the test.
   3. The test lasts for about 1 hour.

Implementation
Medicine/Surgery
Physiologic and Anatomic Equilibrium
Acute Care
Neuromuscular

4. In preparing to perform an eye examination on an elderly client, the doctor asks that the nurse obtain equipment for measuring intraocular pressure. The device most commonly used for this purpose is a:
   1. Snellen eye chart
   2. Schiøtz tonometer
   3. Ocular ultrasonogram
   4. Internal direct ophthalmoscope

RATIONALE

(2) This instrument provides indirect measurement of intraocular pressure.
   1. This tests visual acuity.
   3. This is used to identify tissue masses inside the eye.
   4. This is used to evaluate retinal structures.

CHAPTER 38   Nursing Management of Adults with Eye Disorders

Implementation
Medicine/Surgery
Physiologic and Anatomic Equilibrium
Acute Care
Drug-related response

1. The nurse is caring for a client with AIDS who has developed cytomegalovirus retinitis. Without treatment, this can lead to blindness. To treat the

infections, the nurse is asked to administer a medication called:

1. Gancyclovir
2. Hydrogen peroxide
3. Phenylephrine
4. Tropicamide

RATIONALE

(1) Gancyclovir and foscarnet sodium are two drugs that have been approved by the FDA for intravenous use in the treatment of this disease.
2. This is not used intravenously or topically in the eye.
3. This causes pupillary dilation.
4. This causes temporary paralysis of the ciliary muscle.

> Analysis
> Medicine/Surgery
> Physiologic and Anatomic
>   Equilibrium
> Acute Care
> Neuromuscular

2. **In caring for ophthalmology clients, nurses has often been asked about the legal definition of blindness. It is:**
   1. Vision of 20/200 or less
   2. Vision of 20/200 or more
   3. Loss of all light perception
   4. Severe visual impairment

RATIONALE

(1) This means that the client cannot read letters smaller than the 20/200 line on the Snellen chart with the best eye.
2. This is not considered legal blindness.
3. This defines total blindness.
4. This defines low vision.

> Implementation
> Medicine/Surgery
> Physiologic and Anatomic Equilibrium
> Acute Care
> Drug-related response

3. **A nurse working on an American Indian reservation has several clients who have trachoma. The primary intervention in treating this disease is to teach the client to administer topical:**
   1. Silver nitrate
   2. Furosemide
   3. Salicylic acid
   4. Tetracycline

RATIONALE

(4) This disease is caused by the microorganism *Chlamydia trachomatis* and is easily treated with oral or topical tetracycline or erythromycin.
1. This is used in the eye for the treatment of neonatal gonorrhea

2. This is a diuretic.
3. This is an analgesic.

> Assessment
> Medicine/Surgery
> Physiologic and Anatomic Equilibrium
> Acute Care
> Neuromuscular

4. **A school nurse has seen a young person in the clinic who appears to have "acute bacterial conjunctivitis." This condition is more commonly called:**
   1. Infection
   2. Tearing
   3. Pinkeye
   4. Color blindness

RATIONALE

(3) Symptoms of conjunctivitis or pinkeye include a reddened conjunctiva (hyperemia) and serous or mucous discharge from the eyes.
1. This is an inflammatory process.
2. This is excess tear production.
4. This is the inability to identify different colors.

> Planning
> Medicine/Surgery
> Physiologic and Anatomic Equilibrium
> Acute Care
> Neuromuscular

5. **For a client with retinal detachment, the plan of care will include:**
   1. Enucleation
   2. Scleral buckling
   3. Antibiotic therapy
   4. External pressure

RATIONALE

(2) The treatment of this disease involves reattachment of the retina through the use of cryotherapy, buckling, or banding.
1. This is rarely necessary.
3. This will not remedy the problem.
4. Internal pressure to the retina is the appropriate treatment.

CHAPTER 39   Nursing Assessment of the Ear

> Analysis
> Medicine/Surgery
> Physiologic and Anatomic Equilibrium
> Acute Care
> Neuromuscular

1. **In a client with bacterial rhinitis, the nurse is aware that an infection may occur in the ear because of the connection between the inner ear and the nasopharynx. This structure is the:**
   1. Tragus
   2. Cochlea

3. Acoustic meatus
4. Eustachian tube

RATIONALE

(4) This tube provides a route for nasal and throat infections to spread up into the middle ear or even up into the mastoid sinuses of the meninges.
1. This is a structure of the outer ear.
2. This is a structure in the inner ear that is part of a membranous labyrinth.
3. This structure conducts sound waves through the temporal bone of the skull to the tympanic membrane.

> Assessment
> Medicine/Surgery
> Physiologic and Anatomic Equilibrium
> Acute Care
> Neuromuscular

2. **In assessing a client with a possible ear disorder, the nurse notices involuntary rhythmic oscillations of the eyes. This is called:**
1. Dizziness
2. Nystagmus
3. Dysphagia
4. Mastoiditis

RATIONALE

(2) The static and dynamic equilibrium receptors in the utricle, saccula, and semicircular canals initiate the reflex activity called nystagmus. It allows persons to see objects clearly as they go by.
1. This refers to disequilibrium.
3. This is difficulty in swallowing.
4. This is inflammation of the mastoid bone.

> Evaluation
> Medicine/Surgery
> Education
> Long-term Care
> Neuromuscular

3. **In evaluation of the success of a class the nurse has conducted to promote ear health, a favorable health practice that might be observed would be:**
1. Headsets worn in high-risk work areas
2. Examinations at onset of hearing difficulties
3. Minimal contact with persons with infections
4. Complete evacuation of water from the ear after swimming

RATIONALE

(1) Protective devices to preserve hearing in high-risk occupations and activities are critical in avoiding ear damage.
2. Periodic ear and hearing examinations and screening should be conducted.
3. Avoidance of communicable disease, particularly people with upper respiratory infections is important.

4. Ears should be protected from water when swimming.

> Evaluation
> Medicine/Surgery
> Physiologic and Anatomic Equilibrium
> Acute Care
> Neuromuscular

4. **In conducting the Rinne test to evaluate cranial nerve VIII function, a normal finding would be:**
1. No lymphadenopathy
2. Tympanic membranes pearly gray
3. Air conduction greater than bone conduction
4. Bone conduction greater than air conduction.

RATIONALE

(3) This test involves the use of a tuning fork placed on the mastoid and in front of the ear to determine conduction of sound waves.
1. This is a finding found on neck examination.
2. This is a finding seen with an otoscope, which is beyond the scope of the bedside nurse.
4. The air conduction should be twice that of the bone.

> Planning
> Medicine/Surgery
> Physiologic and Anatomic Equilibrium
> Acute Care
> Neuromuscular

5. **Prior to the performance of a caloric test, the nurse should plan for:**
1. Rinne test
2. Weber test
3. Otoscopic examination
4. Spondee threshold test

RATIONALE

(3) This test involves instillation of cold and warm water into the ear to determine labyrinth disease. An otoscopic examination should be performed first to ensure that the tympanic membrane is intact.
1. This determines sound wave conduction and tests cranial nerve VIII function.
2. This is not needed. It also tests cranial nerve VIII function
4. This test measures the client's ability to detect and correctly repeat a set of two-syllable words presented through earphones.

CHAPTER 40 Nursing Management of Adults with Ear Disorders

> Planning
> Medicine/Surgery
> Education
> Acute Care
> Neuromuscular

1. **A client who is receiving an ototoxic drug should receive adequate teaching about the possible complication of the therapy, which is:**
   1. Noise damage
   2. Presbycusis
   3. Conduction hearing loss
   4. Sensorineural hearing loss

RATIONALE

(4) A loss of the sensory or neural components in the inner ear can be caused by drugs, trauma, neuromas, and complications from infections.
   1. This is caused by exposure to loud noises.
   2. This is caused by degenerative changes bilaterally in the supporting cells of the organ of Corti.
   3. This caused by trauma, infection, and a foreign body in the ear.

> Assessment
> Medicine/Surgery
> Physiologic and Anatomic Equilibrium
> Acute Care
> Neuromuscular

2. **A client tells the nurse that conversation in restaurants has become difficult to understand. This is a symptom of:**
   1. Tinnitus
   2. Ototoxicity
   3. Presbycusis
   4. Psychogenic hearing loss

RATIONALE

(3) People with this disorder commonly complain of not understanding what has been said to them, especially in noisy environments. This is a degenerative disease of the inner ear.
   1. This is a ringing in the ear.
   2. This is ear damage caused by drugs.
   4. This is hearing loss for which no organic reason can be found.

> Analysis
> Medicine/Surgery
> Education
> Long-term
> Neuromuscular

3. **An elderly client, who is part of a home health case load, explains that both hearing aids make a squealing sound when they are placed in the ears. The nurse suspects that:**
   1. They are wet
   2. The battery is low
   3. The volume is too high
   4. They are in the wrong ear

RATIONALE

(4) Elderly clients often cannot tell the nurse in which ear the aid goes. The bore is inserted into the ear first, so the mold shape indicates the correct ear. Aids will squeal or not function if they are improperly placed.
   1. This usually causes them to not function.
   2. This also prevents functioning.
   3. This usually results in a loss of sound.

> Implementation
> Medicine/ Surgery
> Physiologic and Anatomic Equilibrium
> Long-term Care
> Neuromuscular

4. **A client is unable to clean the hearing aid, which was recently fitted. The nurse will clean the device by:**
   1. Avoiding soap
   2. Clearing the ear mold once a month
   3. Using a pipe cleaner to clean the cannula
   4. Protecting the transmitter under several layers of clothing

RATIONALE

(3) The aid is cleaned according to the manufacturer's instructions. Most detachable ear molds can be washed in warm, soapy water and dried. Plastic tubing can be cleaned with a pipe cleaner.
   1. Soapy water is safe.
   2. Daily cleaning is more appropriate.
   4. This is not necessary.

> Evaluation
> Medicine/Surgery
> Education
> Long-term
> Neuromuscular

5. **On a postoperative clinic visit, a client who has received a cochlear implant is evaluated for understanding of the device. An accurate perception is reflected in the statement:**
   1. "I will hear everything right away."
   2. "I can hear sounds but not spoken words."
   3. "I don't understand why everyone sounds like Mickey Mouse."
   4. "I don't need to use sign language or lip reading anymore."

RATIONALE

(2) The implant may help the client to hear sounds but not spoken words.
   1. Hearing does not usually magically begin after the implant.
   3. Voices through the implant have been described as sounding like the cartoon character Mickey Mouse.
   4. These tools,as well as written material, may be necessary to communicate with the client.

> Planning
> Medicine/Surgery
> Physiologic and Anatomic Equilibrium
> Long-term Care
> Neuromuscular

6. **A nurse preparing to practice at a summer camp will make certain that the clinic is stocked with drug therapy for swimmer's ear, which is:**
   1. 70% alcohol
   2. Clotrimazole
   3. Acyclovir
   4. Lidocaine

RATIONALE

(1) Swimmer's ear can be prevented by placing 70% alcohol or an over-the-counter solution for swimmer's ear in the ear immediately after swimming.
   2. This is an antifungal agent.
   3. This is used to treat herpes zoster.
   4. This is not appropriate.

> Implementation
> Medicine/Surgery
> Physiologic and Anatomic Equilibrium
> Long-term Care
> Neuromuscular

7. **A client with an upper respiratory infection laughs when the nurse explains the proper way to blow the nose. To prevent movement of infected material into the middle ear, the client should:**
   1. Keep the mouth closed when blowing
   2. Blow gently with both nostrils open
   3. Let nasal contents drain by gravity
   4. Hold one nostril shut while blowing

RATIONALE

(2) Keeping both nostrils open as well as the mouth decreases pressure and prevents movement into the middle ear.
   1. The mouth should be open.
   3. This is not hygienic.
   4. Both nostrils should be open.

> Assessment
> Medicine/Surgery
> Physiologic and Anatomic Equilibrium
> Acute Care
> Neuromuscular

8. **A client is complaining of vertigo. This is a symptom commonly associated with:**
   1. Trauma
   2. Meniere's disease
   3. Motion sickness
   4. Neoplastic disorders

RATIONALE

(2) Meniere's disease is a dilation of the scala media of the cochlea and saccule and is characterized by tinnitus, sensorineural hearing loss on the involved side, and severe vertigo with nausea and vomiting.

   1. This produces numbness, pain and paresthesia.
   3. Symptoms of this disease include nausea, vomiting, headache, and dizziness.
   4. Tinnitus and intermittent vertigo are symptoms of this disease.

UNIT X   Musculoskeletal System

CHAPTER 41   Nursing Assessment of the Musculoskeletal System

> Analysis
> Medicine/Surgery
> Physiologic and Anatomic Equilibrium
> Acute Care
> Skeletal

1. **The nurse is assisting a physician who is performing an examination on a client who has a torn meniscus. One possible test that is diagnostic of this condition is:**
   1. Tinel's test
   2. Patrick's test
   3. Lachmann's test
   4. McMurray's test

RATIONALE

(4) This involves extension and external rotation of the leg.
   1. This is diagnostic for carpal tunnel syndrome of the wrist.
   2. This is used to assess hip function.
   3. This is used to indicate injury to the anterior cruciate ligament.

> Planning
> Medicine/Surgery
> Physiologic and Anatomic Equilibrium
> Acute Care
> Skeletal

2. **The physician orders a joint aspiration to assess the presence of inflammation in the synovial fluid. The nurse prepares for a procedure that will be performed using:**
   1. Aseptic technique
   2. Clean technique
   3. Enteric isolation
   4. Sanitary conditions

RATIONALE

(1) Synovial fluid is obtained through arthrocentesis. Local anesthetic is injected with aseptic technique. Medications may also be injected into the joint capsule.
   2. The procedure requires sterility.
   3. This applies to gastrointestinal disorders.
   4. The joint space is sterile. Clean conditions are not adequate.

Evaluation
Medicine/Surgery
Physiologic and Anatomic Equilibrium
Acute Care
Skeletal

3. In evaluating the laboratory results of a client on an orthopedic unit, the nurse notices that the uric acid level is elevated. The client may possibly have:
   1. Gout
   2. Synovitis
   3. Meniscal tear
   4. Systemic lupus erythematosis (SLE)

RATIONALE

(1) Uric acid is an end product of purine metabolism that may be elevated with gout, chronic renal failure, chronic myeloid leukemia, and polycythemia vera.
2. This does not cause increased uric acid levels.
3. This is not related to the uric acid level.
4. This test is not diagnostic for SLE.

Implementation
Medicine/Surgery
Physiologic and Anatomic Equilibrium
Acute Care
Skeletal

4. The nurse in the ambulatory surgery unit is preparing a client for discharge after arthroscopy. The instructions will include:
   1. Avoid twisting the knee
   2. Exercise the extremity to avoid stiffness
   3. Keep the leg in a dependent position to increase circulation
   4. Some fever, swelling, and pain at the incision site are to be expected

RATIONALE

(1) Ice can be applies to the affected joint to relieve pain and swelling and the client should avoid twisting the knee.
2. Excessive use of the joint should be avoided for several days.
3. The knee should be elevated while the client is sitting.
4. These are symptoms of infection and should be reported to the physician immediately.

Analysis
Medicine/Surgery
Physiologic and Anatomic Equilibrium
Acute Care
Skeletal

5. The synovial fluid analysis of a client's knee yields pale yellow fluid. This is consistent with:
   1. Gout
   2. Normal fluid

3. Septic arthritis
4. Rheumatoid arthritis

RATIONALE

(2) Normal synovial fluid is colorless to pale yellow.
1. Gout produces yellow fluid
3. This causes a bloody colored fluid.
4. This also causes a yellowish discoloration.

Assessment
Medicine/Surgery
Physiologic and Anatomic Equilibrium
Long-term Care
Skeletal

6. In assisting an elderly client to the bathroom, the nurse hears a dry crackling sound and feels a grating sensation over the knee joint. This is:
   1. Atrophy
   2. Tremors
   3. Crepitus
   4. Fasciculations

RATIONALE

(3) This can be heard over joints, skin, and lungs.
1. This is loss of muscle mass.
2. These are involuntary movements of the extremities.
4. These are fine muscle twitches.

Assessment
Medicine/Surgery
Physiologic and Anatomic Equilibrium
Long-term Care
Skeletal

7. A school nurse conducts scoliosis screening. If the nurse is to perform an accurate assessment, the client should:
   1. Disrobe
   2. Crouch
   3. Bend to the side
   4. Expose the back

RATIONALE

(4) Scoliosis is a lateral curvature of the spine. Only the shoulders, scapula and iliac crest need to be viewed.
1. This will be embarrassing and unnecessary for school-aged children.
2. The client should stand erect and bend forward.
3. This is not necessary.

Analysis
Medicine/Surgery
Physiologic and Anatomic Equilibrium
Long-term Care
Skeletal

8. **The nurse notices an excessive anterior curvature of the lumbar spine of a client. This is indicative of:**
   1. Lordosis
   2. Scoliosis
   3. Kyphosis
   4. Parkinson's disease

RATIONALE

(1) This is an excessive anterior curvature of the lumbar spine.
   2. This is lateral curvature of the spine.
   3. This is excessive posterior curvature of the thoracic spine.
   4. This disease involves involuntary muscle movement.

CHAPTER 42 Nursing Management of Adults with Musculoskeletal Trauma

Evaluation
Medicine/Surgery
Physiologic and Anatomic Equilibrium
Long-term Care
Skeletal

1. **A client who had a traumatic amputation of the leg as the result of a motor vehicle accident is going home. The client has demonstrated the capability for self-care by:**
   1. Keeping both legs still
   2. Washing the incision with soap
   3. Rewrapping the elastic bandage loosely
   4. Putting petroleum jelly on the incision

RATIONALE

(2) The incision line should be cleaned daily with mild soap and a soft cloth.
   1. The unaffected extremities should be exercised regularly with range-of-motion exercises.
   3. The elastic wrap should be secure to prevent edema.
   4. No ointment, antiseptic, or other creams should be applied.

Evaluation
Medicine/Surgery
Physiologic and Anatomic Equilibrium
Long-term Care
Skeletal

2. **A client is in pelvic traction to relieve low back pain. When the nurse evaluates the placement of the traction, the correct position for the client is:**
   1. The side straps are even and clear the bed for a straight line of pull
   2. The belt is secured around the waist and the skin is protected from irritation
   3. The head of the bed is elevated 30 degrees and the knees are gatched at 45 degrees

   4. The weights are hanging free of the bed and the legs are flat in bed with the heels free of the foot of the bed.

RATIONALE

(3) Countertraction on the pelvis is maintained when the hips and knees are flexed and the head of the bed is slightly elevated.
   1. The pelvic belt is placed around the hips.
   2. The belt should be in place around the hips.
   4. The legs should be flexed.

Planning
Medicine/Surgery
Physiologic and Anatomic
   Equilibrium
Acute Care
Skeletal

3. **In planning the management of a client with an ankle sprain, the nurse will prepare for primary treatment, which includes:**
   1. Heat
   2. Rest
   3. Exercise
   4. Aspirin

RATIONALE

(2) The acronym RICE stands for rest, ice, compression, and elevation.
   1. Ice is recommended intermittently for the first 36 hours.
   3. Rest is important.
   4. Nonsteroidal antiinflammatory drugs are given to manage the pain.

Implementation
Medicine/Surgery
Physiologic and Anatomic
   Equilibrium
Acute Care
Skeletal

4. **An important nursing intervention for the client with soft tissue trauma of the ankle is:**
   1. Teaching pin care
   2. Discouraging crutch use
   3. Encouraging continued rest
   4. Instituting range of motion exercises

RATIONALE

(4) Ensuring that the client maintains the extremity in proper alignment and begins range of motion and stretching exercises is essential to a complete recovery from the injury.
   1. This is not necessary.
   2. Crutches are valuable until the area has had time to heal.
   3. Too much rest may produce complications.

Assessment
Medicine/Surgery
Physiologic and Anatomic Equilibrium
Acute Care
Skeletal

5. **A client comes into the emergency room and states "I think that I dislocated my shoulder playing tennis." The nurse's assessment confirms this by:**
   1. Absence of swelling
   2. Mild pain in arm
   3. Bruising at the joint
   4. Change in length of the arm

RATIONALE

(4) There is usually a noticeable change in the length of the extremity because the bone is not in the socket.
   1. Swelling is usually present.
   2. There is usually severe pain in the affected area.
   3. Bruising may or may not be present.

Analysis
Medicine/Surgery
Physiologic and Anatomic Equilibrium
Acute Care
Skeletal

6. **The five Ps is an appropriate method to determine neurologic and circulatory status. One of the Ps stands for:**
   1. Purple
   2. Pressure
   3. Pallor
   4. Pooling

RATIONALE

(3) The five P's are Pain, Pallor, Paralysis, Paresthesia, and Pulselessness.
   1. This is not a part of the assessment.
   2. This is not one of the five P's.
   4. This has no significance to this assessment tool.

Planning
Medicine/Surgery
Physiologic and Anatomic Equilibrium
Acute Care
Skeletal

7. **In the care plan of a client with a fracture, one treatment principle that should be followed is:**
   1. Restoration of function
   2. No realignment of bone fragments
   3. Discouraging immobilization
   4. Exercising as soon as possible

RATIONALE

(1) This is one of the primary treatment goals of fracture care.

2. Realignment of bone fragments or reduction is also essential.
3. Maintenance of the realignment by immobilization is essential.
4. Exercise is delayed until the fracture has healed.

Implementation
Medicine/Surgery
Physiologic and Anatomic Equilibrium
Acute Care
Skeletal

8. **Compartment syndrome is a progressive degeneration of muscles and nerves that results from a severe interruption of blood flow to a muscle compartment. One nursing intervention to prevent this syndrome from occurring is:**
   1. Keep the extremity in a dependent position
   2. Ensure that the cast or ace wrap is tight
   3. Elevate the extremity on 3 or 4 pillows
   4. Elevate the extremities on 1 or 2 pillows

RATIONALE

(4) This lessens venous pressure.
   1. This increases venous pressure.
   2. This can cause compartment syndrome.
   3. Elevation higher than 5 inches impedes venous return by interfering with arterial blood flow.

CHAPTER 43 Nursing Management of Adults with Degenerative, Inflammatory, or Autoimmune Disorders

Assessment
Medicine/Surgery
Physiologic and Anatomic Equilibrium
Acute Care
Skeletal

1. **When a client rises from the floor to an upright position using the hands to climb up the legs, this is a classic sign of muscular dystrophy known as:**
   1. Gower's sign
   2. Weber's sign
   3. Homan's sign
   4. Williams' sign

RATIONALE

(1) This is one way for the nurse to assess the client's muscle strength and degree of mobility.
   2. The Weber test is used to evaluate deafness.
   3. This has no significance to physical assessment.
   4. Williams' position is used for pelvic traction.

Evaluation
Medicine/Surgery
Physiologic and Anatomic Equilibrium
Acute Care
Skeletal

2. A client who has had a total hip replacement is preparing for discharge. The nurse knows that there is understanding of the correct position for optimal healing when the statement is made:
   1. "I will keep my knee bent."
   2. "I can't extend my leg at anytime."
   3. "I can't move my legs to the side."
   4. "I won't cross one leg over the other."

RATIONALE

(4) After total hip replacement the client should not adduct the hip until the prosthesis has healed completely.
   1. The knee can be bent.
   2. The leg can be straightened.
   3. The leg can be abducted.

> Planning
> Medicine/Surgery
> Physiologic and Anatomic Equilibrium
> Long-term Care
> Skeletal

3. In planning an educational program for clients with low back pain, the nurse will include prevention guidelines such as:
   1. Exercise vigorously
   2. Avoid lumbar supports
   3. Modify the environment or workplace
   4. Stand straight with both feet on the floor.

RATIONALE

(3) Adjusting the height of work surfaces; and when sitting the client should rest the feet on the floor or a stool to relieve back strain.
   1. Exercise should begin slowly and increase gradually.
   2. Lumbar supports are helpful.
   4. When standing, rest one foot on a low stool.

> Evaluation
> Medicine/Surgery
> Physiologic and Anatomic Equilibrium
> Long-term Care
> Skeletal

4. Successful therapeutic interventions for the client with Paget's disease can be evaluated by:
   1. Decreased muscle pain
   2. Decreased bone pain
   3. Decreased fracture formation
   4. Minimal alteration in body image

RATIONALE

(2) Bone pain is the most common symptom and may manifest in areas close to the joints.
   1. The pain is located in the bone.
   3. No pathologic fractures are desired.
   4. There should be no alteration in body image.

> Implementation
> Medicine/Surgery
> Physiologic and Anatomic Equilibrium
> Acute Care
> Skeletal

5. The nurse is asked to provide therapy for a client with Paget's disease. One component of drug therapy may be:
   1. Lithium
   2. Antibiotics
   3. Narcotics
   4. Calcitonin

RATIONALE

(4) This is a disease of excessive bone breakdown and altered bone formation treated with calcitonin, alendronate sodium, and bisphosphonates.
   1. This is used to treat mania.
   2. These are not routinely used.
   3. Aspirin and nonsteroidal antiinflammatory drugs are given for pain.

> Analysis
> Medicine/Surgery
> Physiologic and Anatomic Equilibrium
> Acute Care
> Skeletal

6. A client has osteomyelitis or infection of the bone. The most common cause of this disease is;
   1. Salmonella
   2. *Escherichia coli*
   3. *Staphylococcus aureus*
   4. *Pseudomonas aeruginosa*

RATIONALE

(3) Osteomyelitis may be bacterial, fungal or viral. The most common infecting organism is *Staphylococcus aureus*.
   1. This is also a causative agent.
   2. This also causes the disease.
   4. This can be an infecting organism as well.

> Implementation
> Medicine/Surgery
> Physiologic and Anatomic Equilibrium
> Long-term Care
> Skeletal

7. A client asks if osteoporosis can be prevented. The nurse's reply is based on the fact that:
   1. Currently there is no way to prevent or retard bone resorption in women over 60.
   2. Osteoporosis is preventable if women engage in weight bearing exercises.
   3. Calcium and vitamin D supplements after age 30 will prevent bony demineralization.
   4. Calcium loss is slowed by dietary supplements, estrogen replacements, and exercise.

RATIONALE

(4) Loss of bone density occurs with aging but can be slowed by diet, estrogen replacement, and exercise.

1. Exercise and dietary supplements retard the process.
2. It is a normal part of aging.
3. These slow the process but do not prevent it.

> Planning
> Medicine/Surgery
> Physiologic and Anatomic Equilibrium
> Acute Care
> Skeletal

8. **In planning care for a client who has undergone a total hip arthroplasty, one scheduled intervention will be:**
   1. Clean technique dressing changes
   2. Monitoring for positive Homan's sign
   3. Monitoring for positive Trousseau's sign
   4. Maintaining the joint aligned in adduction

RATIONALE

(2) This is pain in the calf when the foot is dorsiflexed and indicates thrombophlebitis.

1. Sterile technique should be used.
3. This is a test for hypocalcemia.
4. The joint should be maintained in abduction.

UNIT XI   Endocrine System

CHAPTER 44   Nursing Assessment of the Endocrine System

> Analysis
> Medicine/Surgery
> Physiologic and Anatomic
>   Equilibrium
> Acute Care
> Endocrine

1. **Melatonin is a hormone of the posterior pituitary gland. One of its actions is:**
   1. Increases cell replication
   2. Enhances immune system function
   3. Decreases immune system function
   4. Affects the color of the skin

RATIONALE

(2) Melatonin modulates the metabolic activities to ensure that their timing is synchronized with the environmental light cycle, including boosting the immune system.

1. It has been found to impede cell replication.
3. It enhances immune system function
4. It has no affect on the skin.

> Assessment
> Medicine/Surgery
> Physiologic and Anatomic Equilibrium
> Long-term Care
> Endocrine

2. **One of the signs of an endocrine disorder that may be visible on a physical examination is:**
   1. Tremors
   2. Oliguria
   3. Voice change: higher
   4. Increased hair growth

RATIONALE

(1) The client may have tremors and memory loss as well as changes in deep tendon reflexes and vibratory sensation.

2. Polyuria or increased amounts of urine are common.
3. The voice change is usually lower.
4. Decreased hair growth or alopecia is common.

> Planning
> Medicine/Surgery
> Physiologic and Anatomic Equilibrium
> Acute Care
> Endocrine

3. **For routine screening for hypofunction and hyperfunction of the thyroid, the nurse anticipates that the first test that the physician will order is:**
   1. Serum T4
   2. TSH test
   3. T3U levels
   4. Serum cholesterol

RATIONALE

(1) This test measures the total serum level of thyroxine; it is useful as a basic screening tool for thyroid disease and in monitoring responses to therapy.

2. This assay measures thyroid-stimulating hormone levels.
3. This is useful in confirming an elevated T4.
4. This test is not related to thyroid function.

> Implementation
> Medicine/Surgery
> Physiologic and Anatomic
>   Equilibrium
> Acute Care
> Endocrine

4. **When the nurse is assisting a physician with a thyroid biopsy, one nursing intervention may be to obtain:**
   1. Pillow
   2. Warming lights
   3. Radioactive dyes
   4. Test tubes for blood

(1) The client is placed in a supine position with a pillow under the shoulders to hyperextend the neck.

2. These are not necessary.
3. These are used in thyroid scans.
4. Slides are used to analyze cells.

Analysis
Medicine/Surgery
Physiologic and Anatomic Equilibrium
Acute Care
Endocrine

5. **Hormones are divided into three categories. An example of one of those is:**
   1. Hormones secreted by the liver
   2. Hormones secreted by bone
   3. Hormones secreted by the kidneys
   4. Hormones secreted by the neurohypophysis

RATIONALE

(4) Hormones are divided according to the way in which endocrine glands that secrete them are controlled by the nervous system.

1. The liver is not an endocrine gland.
2. Bone is not considered an endocrine gland.
3. The kidneys are not considered endocrine glands. They are target sites for hormones.

Implementation
Medicine/Surgery
Physiologic and Anatomic Equilibrium
Acute Care
Endocrine

6. **The nurse will obtain blood levels for a serum cortisol level at:**
   1. 8 AM
   2. 8 AM and 4 PM
   3. 4 PM and 12 AM
   4. Anytime during a 24-hour period

RATIONALE

(1) Normally cortisol levels are highest in the morning and lowest in the evening.

2. The afternoon testing is not necessary.
3. These times are inappropriate.
4. 8 AM is the correct testing time.

Evaluation
Medicine/Surgery
Physiologic and Anatomic Equilibrium
Acute Care
Endocrine

7. **When the nurse is evaluating the client's response to a glucose tolerance test, one symptom that might cause discontinuation of the test is:**
   1. Fever
   2. Tremors

3. Excitability
4. Blotching of the skin

RATIONALE

(2) The client may experience sweating, tremors, excessive nausea, or vomiting.

1. This is not a usual symptom.
3. Dizziness and faintness may occur.
4. This is not a common adverse reaction to the test.

Assessment
Medicine/Surgery
Physiologic and Anatomic Equilibrium
Acute Care
Endocrine

8. **In an assessment of a client who may have diabetes, the most specific, sensitive, and complete test is:**
   1. Glucose tolerance
   2. Fasting blood glucose
   3. Glycosylated hemoglobin
   4. Two-hour postprandial glucose

RATIONALE

(1) This test evaluates a client's ability to tolerate an oral glucose load.

2. This helps detect and evaluate diabetes mellitus, but a normal level does not rule out the disease.
3. This test gives a true indication of the degree of hyperglycemia present 2 or 3 months before the test.
4. This test measures the level of glucose in a client's body 2 hours after a meal.

CHAPTER 45 Nursing Management of Adults with Hypothalamus, Pituitary, or Adrenal Disorders

Assessment
Medicine/Surgery
Physiologic and Anatomic Equilibrium
Acute Care
Endocrine

1. **Hypopituitarism, or underactivity of the anterior pituitary gland, is a rare disorder that can cause deficiency of adrenocorticotrophic (ACTH) hormone. One physical finding of this is:**
   1. Facial flushing
   2. Hyperglycemia
   3. Postural hypotension
   4. Excessive energy

RATIONALE

(3) This means that if the client sits or stands quickly, fainting may occur.

1. Pallor is common.
2. Hypoglycemia is produced.
4. Weakness and tiredness are evident.

Planning
Medicine/Surgery
Physiologic and Anatomic Equilibrium
Acute Care
Neuromuscular

2. In developing a care plan for a client with hypopituitarism, the nurse arrives at a nursing diagnosis of body image disturbance related to changes in physic appearance and body functioning. One undesired change could be:
   1. Weight loss
   2. Loss of hair
   3. Enlarged genitalia
   4. Puffiness of the skin

RATIONALE

(2) Hair may be lost in the axilla, pubic area, and scalp.
   1. Weight gain is expected because of thyroid-stimulating hormone deficiency.
   3. These atrophy because of gonadotrophin deficiency.
   4. There is usually fine wrinkling of the skin.

Evaluation
Medicine/Surgery
Physiologic and Anatomic
   Equilibrium
Acute Care
Endocrine

3. Postoperative care of a client who has had transsphenoidal microsurgery for removal of a benign pituitary tumor requires the nurse's evaluation for surgical side effects such as:
   1. Scalp edema
   2. Facial scarring
   3. Cerebrospinal fluid leakage
   4. Bilateral arm weakness

RATIONALE

(3) Bleeding, meningitis, optic nerve damage, and hypopituitarism may also occur.
   1. There is no scalp incision.
   2. There should be no facial trauma involved. The procedure is done through the nose.
   4. There should be no loss of function.

Implementation
Medicine/Surgery
Physiologic and Anatomic Equilibrium
Acute Care
Drug-related Response

4. Special diagnostic tests are used to differentiate the various forms of diabetes insipidus. To facilitate the process, the nurse may be asked to administer a drug called:
   1. Morphine
   2. Nicotine
   3. Phenytoin
   4. Vasopressin

RATIONALE

(4) Dehydration and water deprivation tests are done along with tests of serum osmolality and sodium and vasopressin levels.
   1. This is an analgesic.
   2. This is found in cigarettes.
   3. This is an antiseizure drug.

Analysis
Medicine/Surgery
Physiologic and Anatomic Equilibrium
Acute Care
Endocrine

5. A simple treatment for syndrome of inappropriate antidiuretic hormone (SIADH) is fluid restriction. Drug therapy may include:
   1. DDAVP
   2. Lithium
   3. Carbamazepine
   4. Erythromycin

RATIONALE

(2) Lithium carbonate is effective because of its inhibition of cAMP synthesis in the renal tubule.
   1. Desmopressin is used in the treatment of diabetes insipidus.
   3. This drug is also used to treat diabetes insipidus.
   4. Demeclocycline, a tetracycline analog, is used to treat SIADH because of its inhibition of cAMP synthesis in the renal tubule.

Evaluation
Medicine/Surgery
Physiologic and Anatomic Equilibrium
Acute Care
Endocrine

6. One of the most important things to evaluate in clients with syndrome of inappropriate antidiuretic hormone is:
   1. Pain level
   2. Skin condition
   3. Blood pressure
   4. Fluid intake and output

RATIONALE

(4) Expected client responses to treatment include fluid intake not to exceed urinary output.
   1. This is usually not a concern.
   2. This is not a priority.
   3. This is a secondary consideration.

Planning
Medicine/Surgery
Physiologic and Anatomic Equilibrium
Acute Care
Endocrine

7. **The care plan for a client with pheochromocytoma will include:**
   1. Exercise
   2. Gancyclovir
   3. Propranolol
   4. Epinephrine

RATIONALE

(3) This is a tumor that arises from the adrenal medulla or sympathetic ganglion tissue and produces catecholamines causing hypertension. Propranolol is a beta-adrenergic blocking drug that interferes with this process.
   1. Bed rest is recommended.
   2. Antibiotic drugs such as this are not routinely used.
   4. This would cause a worsening of the hypertension.

> Evaluation
> Medicine/Surgery
> Physiologic and Anatomic Equilibrium
> Acute Care
> Endocrine

8. **Adrenalectomy may be required to reduce cortisol levels in clients with Cushing's syndrome. In developing a postoperative care plan, the nurse anticipates frequent monitoring for:**
   1. Infection
   2. Weight loss
   3. Hyperactivity
   4. Hypertension

RATIONALE

(1) Fluctuating cortisol and catecholamine levels put clients at risk for infection and thrombosis.
   2. This is an anticipated outcome.
   3. Weakness and mental status changes may occur.
   4. Hypotension may result from adrenal insufficiency.

CHAPTER 46 Nursing Management of Adults with Thyroid or Parathyroid Disorders

> Assessment
> Medicine/Surgery
> Physiologic and Anatomic Equilibrium
> Acute Care
> Endocrine

1. **In assessing a client who has undergone thyroid surgery for hypoparathyroidism, the nurse will observe for:**
   1. Finger nodules
   2. Serum calcium of 11 mg/dl
   3. The absence of Chvostek's sign
   4. The presence of Trousseau's sign

RATIONALE

(4) This is a spasm of the hand indicative of hypoparathyroidism.
   1. Numbness and tingling are present in the lips and fingertips but not nodules.
   2. This indicates hyperparathyroidism.
   3. This is a twitching of the facial nerve and is present in cases of hypocalcemia and hypoparathyroidism.

> Assessment
> Medicine/Surgery
> Physiologic and Anatomic Equilibrium
> Acute Care
> Endocrine

2. **For the client with hypoparathyroidism, the nurse is focusing on decreasing neuromuscular excitability. In particular, the nurse is observing for signs of:**
   1. Acidosis and hypokalemia
   2. Alkalosis and hypocalcemia
   3. Acidosis and hyponatremia
   4. Alkalosis and hypercalcemia

RATIONALE

(2) Symptoms of hypocalcemia are more severe in clients with alkalosis because alkalosis causes more of the dissolved calcium to bind to serum albumin, reducing the ionized calcium level and producing symptoms of hypocalcemia.
   1. Acidosis does not cause the problem. Hypoparathyroidism affects calciumnot potassium.
   3. This condition is not precipitated by acidosis or lowered sodium levels.
   4. Low calcemia levels cause tetany and the other symptoms common with this disease.

> Implementation
> Medicine/Surgery
> Physiologic and Anatomic Equilibrium
> Acute Care
> Drug-related Response

3. **Nursing strategies for a client with hypoparathyroidism focus on the prompt identification and treament of tetany. One aspect of therapy is the administration of calcium gluconate. The drug must be given:**
   1. Quickly
   2. Slowly
   3. Orally
   4. Topically

RATIONALE

(2) The drug is given slowly intravenously because it is extremely irritating to the veins. The client should also be connected to a cardiac monitor. Clients receiving digoxin are at additional risk.
   1. This could cause cardiac dysrhythmias.
   3. The drug is given intravenously.

    4. This route is not available for the administration of this drug.

Planning
Medicine/Surgery
Physiologic and Anatomic Equilibrium
Acute Care
Endocrine

4. **The goal of maintaining adequate nutritional intake for the client with hypercalcemia secondary to parathyroid gland dysfunction can best be met by:**
   1. Encouraging activity
   2. Encouraging large, high fiber diet
   3. Fluid restrictions of 1500 ml per 24 hours
   4. Encouraging client to stay in bed after meals

RATIONALE

(2) Small frequent meals and snacks with bulk and fiber added are best.
   1. Activities should be scheduled throughout the day with uninterrupted rest periods.
   3. Ensure that at least 2 to 3 liters of fluid are drunk each day.
   4. Activity is encouraged.

Implementation
Medicine/Surgery
Physiologic and Anatomic Equilibrium
Acute Care
Endocrine

5. **In delivering care to a client in myxedema coma, the nurse's actions may include providing:**
   1. Sedatives
   2. Cooling mattress
   3. Hydrocortisone
   4. Saline solution

RATIONALE

(3) Myxedema coma is the most severe manifestation of hypothyroidism. Hydrocortisone is given to support the stress response.
   1. These are contraindicated because clients often have depression.
   2. The core body temperature can fall to as low as 75° F. Heating mattresses are indicated.
   4. Glucose solutions are given to combat hypoglycemia.

Evaluation
Medicine/Surgery
Physiologic and Anatomic Equilibrium
Acute Care
Endocrine

6. **In evaluating the effects of nursing interventions for the client with hypothyroidism, an expected result should be:**
   1. Decreased activity

   2. Decreased edema
   3. Increased weight
   4. Decreased diarrhea

RATIONALE

(2) The client should demonstrate a reduction of the edematous state.
   1. The energy and activity tolerance level should improve.
   3. The client's weights should decrease or stabilize along with the edema.
   4. Clients usually have problems with constipation.

Assessment
Medicine/Surgery
Physiologic and Anatomic Equilibrium
Acute Care
Endocrine

7. **The nurse is caring for a client who has had a thyroidectomy and observes symptoms that indicate that the client may be experiencing a thyroid storm. The nurse notices:**
   1. Hyperthermia
   2. Hypothermia
   3. Bradycardia
   4. Listlessness

RATIONALE

(1) Fever, hypertension, dysrhythmias, and increased respiratory rate are visible signs of this crisis.
   2. Hyperthermia is produced by the hypermetabolic state.
   3. Tachycardia is evident.
   4. Agitation is noted first, progressing to a coma state.

Assessment
Medicine/Surgery
Physiologic and Anatomic Equilibrium
Acute Care
Endocrine

8. **The nurse anticipates being able to respond to potential emergencies after thyroid surgery by placing the following near the bedside:**
   1. 59% glucose
   2. Sodium bicarbonate
   3. Tracheostomy set
   4. Padded tongue blade

RATIONALE

(3) Respiratory obstruction is a potential complication because of hemorrhage.
   1. This is used to treat hypoglycemia.
   2. This is used in known cases of acidosis.
   4. This is needed for the client who is at risk for seizures

Analysis
Medicine/Surgery
Physiologic and Anatomic Equilibrium
Acute Care
Endocrine

1. **Insulin-dependent diabetes mellitus (IDDM) is common in persons under age 30 who produce:**
   1. No insulin
   2. Ketoacids
   3. Minimal insulin
   4. Increased insulin

RATIONALE

(1) IDDM is also called Type I and usually develops in childhood. Persons with this disease produce no insulin (insulinopenic).
   2. These are by-products of altered glucose metabolism common in diabetics.
   3. Clients who produce some insulin are included in the non–insulin-dependent diabetes mellitus (NIDDM) or Type II category.
   4. Type II diabetics may produce high insulin levels.

Analysis
Medicine/Surgery
Physiologic and Anatomic Equilibrium
Acute Care
Endocrine

2. **An autoimmune mechanism is responsible for one type of diabetes, called:**
   1. Impaired glucose metabolism
   2. Gestational diabetes mellitus
   3. Insulin-dependent diabetes mellitus
   4. Non–insulin-dependent diabetes mellitus

RATIONALE

(3) Type I diabetes is thought to be caused by the production of islet cell antibodies that attack the immune system and destroy the body's insulin-producing beta cells.
   1. This term describes persons with a fasting glucose level of between 140 and 200 mg/dl. It was formally called borderline diabetes.
   2. This is glucose intolerance, which develops during pregnancy.
   4. In type II diabetics, there is impaired insulin secretion, insulin resistance, and abnormally elevated glucose produced by the liver.

Evaluation
Medicine/Surgery
Education
Long-term Care
Endocrine

3. **The nurse who has conducted a class on nutritional considerations for diabetics knows that instruction has been understood when the comment is heard:**
   1. "I don't have to worry about being overweight."
   2. "I'll sell my roller blades right away. I shouldn't exercise anymore."
   3. "I don't need to stick my finger if I eat the same food every day."
   4. "I will monitor my blood glucose levels frequently throughout the day."

RATIONALE

(4) Blood glucose levels should be monitored frequently and the insulin doses adjusted for the amount of food eaten.
   1. Body weight should be maintained at desired levels.
   2. Exercise and activity are important to overall health. They need to be balanced with food intake and insulin dosing.
   3. Regular monitoring of blood glucose and lipid levels is critical, as is eating a balanced diet.

Implementation
Medicine/Surgery
Education
Long-term Care
Endocrine

4. **As part of a teaching plan for new diabetics, the nurse has included meal planning with the 1500 calorie ADA diet. The principles used in the exchange system are based on the fact that clients:**
   1. Must weigh all foods before determining serving size
   2. May eat any food as long as the calories are limited to 1500 and three meals
   3. May substitute foods between exchange lists to accommodate food preferences
   4. May eat any food on each exchange list as long as it does not exceed the serving size

RATIONALE

(4) The ADA exchange list system is designed so that foods on each list have comparable calories, carbohydrates, proteins, and fats.
   1. This may not be necessary, but serving size should be accurately measured.
   2. The meal plan should be nutritionally sound.
   3. Foods may only be exchanged within the same group.

Planning
Medicine/Surgery
Education
Long-term Care
Endocrine

5. **In discussing the goal of insulin therapy with Type I diabetics, the nurse explains that they**

should strive to maintain plasma glucose concentration at:

1. Below normal
2. Normal range
3. Above normal
4. Fluctuating levels to accommodate exercise

RATIONALE

(2) Euglycemia is the goal for these clients.

1. This may produce symptoms of hypoglycemia.
3. This may produce long-term adverse effects.
4. This is not desired.

> Analysis
> Medicine/Surgery
> Physiologic and Anatomic Equilibrium
> Long-term Care
> Endocrine

6. One type of oral hypoglycemic agent that Type II clients receive is the sulfonylureas. They act by:

1. Decreasing insulin production
2. Stimulating insulin secretion
3. Decreasing beta cell sensitivity to glucose
4. Decreasing hepatic production of glucose

RATIONALE

(2) Insulin secretion is increased and the beta cell sensitivity to glucose is increased.

1. The production is increased.
3. The sensitivity is increased.
4. This is one of the actions of a new oral agent called metformin.

> Analysis
> Medicine/Surgery
> Physiologic and Anatomic Equilibrium
> Long-term Care
> Drug-related Response

7. In screening clients for oral hypoglycemic therapy, the nurse knows that metformin is used with caution in clients with:

1. Obesity
2. Glaucoma
3. Liver disease
4. Nausea and vomiting

RATIONALE

(3) Metformin is used cautiously in clients with liver disease, heart failure, chronic lung disease, and heavy alcohol consumption.

1. This is not a contraindication.
2. There is no interaction with this eye disorder.
4. These are side effects of the drug.

> Evaluation
> Medicine/Surgery
> Physiologic and Anatomic Equilibrium

> Acute Care
> Endocrine

8. In evaluating therapy for a client with hyperglycemic hyperosmolar nonketotic coma (HHNC), the nurse would expect to see resolution of:

1. Potassium excess
2. Insulin excess
3. Fluid depletion
4. Metabolic acidosis

RATIONALE

(3) Correction of volume depletion is critical, usually with a 0.9% saline solution.

1. Potassium must be replaced.
2. The insulin deficiency is the underlying cause of the problem.
4. The distinction between HHNC and diabetic ketoacidosis is the absence of ketoacidosis in HHNC.

UNIT XII   The Gastrointestinal System

CHAPTER 48   Nursing Assessment of the Gastrointestinal System

> Analysis
> Medicine/Surgery
> Physiologic and Anatomic Equilibrium
> Acute Care
> Gastrointestinal

1. Most gastrointestinal absorption occurs in the:

1. Stomach
2. Small intestine
3. Large intestine
4. Sigmoid colon

RATIONALE

(2) Most of the nutrients from the ingested food is absorbed here through the villi.

1. The stomach stores partly digested food and controls the rate at which it enters the small intestine.
3. Contents are mixed, nutrients are absorbed, and waste is moved along for excretion.
4. Fecal matter is held here before defecation.

> Assessment
> Medicine/Surgery
> Physiologic and Anatomic Equilibrium
> Acute Care
> Gastrointestinal

2. In performing a physical assessment on a client with pancreatic cancer, the nurse is aware that one of the sites of referred pain is:

1. Neck
2. Sacrum

3. Left scapula
4. Right scapula

RATIONALE

(3) Many diseases cause referral of pain to others areas. This is the typical location for referred pancreatitic pain.
1. This is not the location for referred pancreatitic pain.
2. This is a referral site for rectal lesions.
4. This is a site for referred pain from a perforated duodenal ulcer.

Implementation
Medicine/Surgery
Physiologic and Anatomic Equilibrium
Acute Care
Gastrointestinal

3. **In an assessment of the abdomen, the first thing that the nurse will do after observing the abdominal wall is to:**
1. Percuss
2. Palpate
3. Inspect
4. Auscultate

RATIONALE

(4) This is done first to prevent disruption of auscultatory sounds.
1. This follows auscultation.
2. This follows percussion.
3. This is the same and is done before any of the other steps.

Planning
Medicine/Surgery
Physiologic and Anatomic Equilibrium
Acute Care
Gastrointestinal

4. **When a client is scheduled for scintigraphy for gallbladder disease, the client will:**
1. Have barium studies first
2. Have a nuclear scan first
3. Be radioactive for 48 hours
4. Receive a high carbohydrate meal 1 hour before the test

RATIONALE

(2) The scan should be done first because barium opacifies sites and blocks the exit of protons from the radionuclides
1. This is done after the scan.
3. After the scan only minimal amounts of radiation are excreted. Only universal precautions should be used in disposing of body waste.
4. The client will be required to fast for 3 to 4 hours before the test.

Evaluation
Medicine/Surgery
Physiologic and Anatomic Equilibrium
Acute Care
Gastrointestinal

5. **To ensure that no complications have developed after a barium swallow test, the nurse would expect:**
1. Diarrhea
2. Light colored stool
3. No stool for 5 days
4. Dark, tarry stools

RATIONALE

(2) Barium may cause constipation and obstruction. The client should have a bowel movement within 2 or 3 days. The stool will appear chalky and light colored.
1. This is not an expected finding.
3. A bowel movement should occur within 3 days.
4. This may indicate bleeding.

Implementation
Medicine/Surgery
Physiologic and Anatomic Equilibrium
Acute Care
Gastrointestinal

6. **After undergoing an esophagogastroduodenoscopy, a client will be monitored for:**
1. Fever
2. Nausea
3. Diarrhea
4. Vomiting

RATIONALE

(1) This test involves direct visualization of the lining of the upper gastrointestinal tract with a flexible fiberoptic endoscope. The client's temperature is monitored every 15 minutes for 4 hours. A sudden temperature spike may indicate perforation.
2. This is a secondary concern.
3. This is unlikely to occur.
4. Monitoring for throat discomfort and changes in vital signs is most important.

Planning
Medicine/Surgery
Physiologic and Anatomic Equilibrium
Acute Care
Gastrointestinal

7. **When planning the nursing care of a client who is to undergo small-bowel biopsy, the nurse includes instruction about the test. The specimen is obtained by:**
1. Direct puncture through the skin.
2. Small incision in the abdomen
3. Inserting a tube through the rectum
4. Inserting a tube through the mouth

RATIONALE

(4) The tube is passed through the mouth, and the area for biopsy is identified under fluoroscopy. The intestinal mucosa is then suctioned into a capsule for analysis.
1. This is not done.
2. This is unnecessary.
3. This is not part of the procedure.

Assessment
Medicine/Surgery
Physiologic and Anatomic
    Equilibrium
Acute Care
Gastrointestinal

8. In assessing a client for abdominal pain, one test that may be conducted is:
1. Iliopsoas test
2. Nonobturator test
3. Abdominal biopsy
4. Percussion of abdomen

RATIONALE

(1) A positive response to this test is abdominal pain or an increase in abdominal pain.
2. The obturator test also identifies abdominal pain.
3. This is not part of a routine assessment.
4. This evaluates the tone over various structures in the abdominal cavity

---

CHAPTER 49 Nursing Management of Adults with Disorders of the Mouth or Esophagus

Planning
Medicine/Surgery
Physiologic and Anatomic Equilibrium
Acute Care
Gastrointestinal

1. A client is to undergo treatment for esophageal stricture from reflux esophagitis. The nurse prepares the client for:
1. Resection
2. Dilation
3. Biopsy
4. Radiation

RATIONALE

(2) When the esophageal lumen has narrowed to the degree that dysphagia is a problem, dilation with a mechanical dilator is necessary.
1. This is done only if other treatment methods fail.
3. This is a diagnostic tool, not a treatment tool.
4. This may cause constriction.

Analysis
Medicine/Surgery
Physiologic and Anatomic Equilibrium
Acute Care
Gastrointestinal

2. A client is complaining of weight loss, substernal chest pain at mealtime, and regurgitation of food. These are symptoms associated with:
1. Achalasia
2. Hiatal hernia
3. Oral cancer
4. Esophageal diverticulum

RATIONALE

(1) Achalasia is a disorder of the upper and lower esophageal sphincter as well as the body of the esophagus, in which the client is unable to propel solids or liquids from the pharynx to the esophagus.
2. Most clients with hiatal hernia are asymptomatic.
3. This produces white patches on the mouth and tongue.
4. This causes a sour taste and a foul odor in the mouth.

Assessment
Medicine/Surgery
Physiologic and Anatomic Equilibrium
Acute Care
Gastrointestinal

3. In assessing a client for possible carcinoma of the esophagus, the most common clinical symptom is:
1. Diarrhea
2. Weight gain
3. Progressive dysphagia
4. Referred pain to the neck

RATIONALE

(3) Progressive dysphagia over a 6-month period with the sensation of food sticking in the throat is the most common symptom. Chronic cough and iron-deficiency anemia are two others.
1. Vomiting and regurgitation are common.
2. Weight loss is expected.
4. A steady, substernal, boring pain radiating to the back is characteristic.

Evaluation
Medicine/Surgery
Physiologic and Anatomic Equilibrium
Acute Care
Gastrointestinal

4. A client has had a surgical resection of an esophageal tumor. The nurse will evaluate carefully for:
1. Pain
2. Leakage

3. Hypothermia
4. Weight loss

RATIONALE

(2) Leakage of the incision site within the first week may occur, with serious consequences.
1. This is important and manageable.
3. Low grade temperature may occur with leakage.
4. Fluid accumulation after surgery may occur.

Implementation
Medicine/Surgery
Education
Acute Care
Gastrointestinal

5. When dietary management is taught to a client with gastroesophageal reflux, foods that are recommended include:
   1. Pastries
   2. Chocolate
   3. Caffeine drinks
   4. Unseasoned meats

RATIONALE

(4) The standard reflux diet restricts spicy and acidic foods.
1. Low-fat foods are recommended.
2. This is restricted along with spearmint and peppermint.
3. Coffee, tea, and colas are restricted.

Evaluation
Medicine/Surgery
Physiologic and Anatomic Equilibrium
Acute Care
Gastrointestinal

6. In addition to a nasogastric tube, a client who has undergone a fundoplication may have a:
   1. Chest tube
   2. Gastrostomy
   3. Tracheostomy
   4. Feeding catheter jejunostomy

RATIONALE

(1) An abdominal or thoracic approach may be used for this procedure.
2. This is usually not needed.
3. This is not necessary.
4. This is not routinely placed.

Assessment
Medicine/Surgery
Physiologic and Anatomic Equilibrium
Acute Care
Gastrointestinal

7. When the client is being assessed for possible oral cancer, the cardinal symptoms to be aware of are:
   1. Hoarseness
   2. Surface patches

3. Swelling in the cheek
4. Irritations that heal in 5 days

RATIONALE

(1) Mouth cancer has no reliable early signs or symptoms. The most common finding is that of a painful, indurated ulcer. Hoarseness is also a sign.
2. White or red surface patches are visible.
3. Lumps or swelling in the neck are common.
4. Irritations in the mouth that do not heal in 1 to 2 weeks are significant symptoms.

Analysis
Medicine/Surgery
Physiologic and Anatomic Equilibrium
Acute Care
Gastrointestinal

8. A client who is HIV positive has white plaques in the mouth that look like milk curds. This is characteristic of:
   1. Gingivitis
   2. Dental caries
   3. Trench mouth
   4. Candidiasis

RATIONALE

(4) Persons who are immunocompromised are at risk as well as those receiving long-term antibiotic therapy. This disrupts the balance of mucosal flora, allowing Candida to flourish.
1. Pain in the teeth and bleeding of gums may occur.
2. Pain and abscess are common with this disease.
3. Pain, fetid mouth odor, gingival erosion, and ulceration are common with this disease.

CHAPTER 50   Nursing Management of Adults with Disorders of the Stomach or Duodenum

Planning
Medicine/Surgery
Physiologic and Anatomic Equilibrium
Acute Care
Gastrointestinal

1. When the nurse is planning the care of a client with gastritis, one expected outcome will be:
   1. Drug rest
   2. Decreased hydration
   3. Relief of epigastric pain
   4. Relief of throat pain

RATIONALE

(3) Relief of epigastric discomfort and related symptoms is an appropriate goal.
1. Antiemetics and H2 receptor antagonists are frequently needed.
3. Adequate hydration and nutrition are needed.
4. This is usually not a symptom.

Implementation
Medicine/Surgery
Physiologic and Anatomic Equilibrium
Acute Care
Gastrointestinal

2. **In providing care to a client with chronic gastritis, the nurse will administer:**
   1. Vitamin C
   2. Vitamin B$_{12}$
   3. Antihistamines
   4. Large, infrequent meals

RATIONALE

(2) Pernicious anemia may occur with gastritis. This is treated with vitamin B$_{12}$.
   1. This is not usually prescribed.
   3. Antacids are given after meals.
   4. Small frequent bland feedings are given.

Analysis
Medicine/Surgery
Physiologic and Anatomic Equilibrium
Acute Care
Gastrointestinal

3. **In counseling a client with peptic ulcer disease, the nurse includes the statement that this disease is associated with:**
   1. *Pseudomonas*
   2. *Mycobacterium*
   3. *Helicobacter pylori*
   4. *Staphylococcus aureus*

RATIONALE

(3) This pathogen is present in clients who have peptic ulcer disease. It produces an enzyme that breaks down the mucosal defense barrier.
   1. This is not a causative pathogen.
   2. This is not associated with this disease.
   4. This bacteria is not related to peptic ulcer disease.

Evaluation
Medicine/Surgery
Physiologic and Anatomic Equilibrium
Acute Care
Gastrointestinal

4. **The dumping syndrome occurs in up to 50% of clients who have had a pyloroplasty. The nurse's instruction about the disease will be positively validated by the client's statement:**
   1. "I will avoid spicy foods."
   2. "I will eat as quickly as possible."
   3. "I will eat only 3 meals a day."
   4. "I will drink plenty of water with my meal."

RATIONALE

(1) Spicy or gas-forming foods contribute to the dumping syndrome.
   2. Eating slowly is encouraged.

3. Eating six meals a day that are high in protein is recommended.
4. Fluids should be taken between meals, not with meals.

Assessment
Medicine/Surgery
Physiologic and Anatomic Equilibrium
Acute Care
Gastrointestinal

5. **Clients with peptic ulcers are at risk for perforation. The nurse should assess for signs of perforation, which include:**
   1. Confusion
   2. Sudden diarrhea
   3. Palmar erythema
   4. Sharp abdominal pain

RATIONALE

(4) Midepigastric or upper right quadrant pain of sudden onset is a sign of perforation.
   1. This may develop later if the client develops peritonitis.
   2. This is not an associated symptom.
   3. This is not a sign of peptic ulcer disease.

Implementation
Medicine/Surgery
Physiologic and Anatomic Equilibrium
Gastrointestinal

6. **In treating a client with active peptic ulcer disease, the nurse will administer the mucosal healing agent sucralfate:**
   1. Seven times daily
   2. 1 hour before meals
   3. 10 minutes before meals
   4. 2 hours after breakfast and dinner

RATIONALE

(2) It is taken 1 hour before each meal and at bedtime.
   1. This is the schedule for antacid therapy.
   3. If taken immediately before eating, it binds with food in the stomach.
   4. This would be ineffective.

Planning
Medicine/Surgery
Physiologic and Anatomic Equilibrium
Acute Care
Gastrointestinal

7. **One expected outcome of a client undergoing therapy for gastrointestinal bleeding is:**
   1. Slight hematemesis
   2. Hemoglobin of 8 g/dl
   3. Potassium level of 4.2
   4. Mild dehydration

(3) Serum electrolytes should be within normal range.

1. This should not be present.
2. Hemoglobin and hematocrit should be within normal limits.
4. The client should be well hydrated, with serum electrolytes within normal limits.

> Evaluation
> Medicine/Surgery
> Physiologic and Anatomic Equilibrium
> Acute Care
> Gastrointestinal

8. After a client has had surgery for gastric cancer, effective therapy will be evident by:
   1. Dumping syndrome
   2. Nasogastric tube patent
   3. Moderate levels of edema
   4. Redness and swelling at the incision site

RATIONALE

(2) All tubes must be identified and patency and drainage should be recorded daily.

1. This should not occur.
3. Edema should not be present
4. These are signs of infection and should not be present.

CHAPTER 51 Nursing Management of Adults with Intestinal Disorders

> Assessment
> Medicine/Surgery
> Physiologic and Anatomic Equilibrium
> Acute Care
> Gastrointestinal

1. A client complaints of abdominal pain and diarrhea after the ingestion of milk and milk products. These are symptoms associated with:
   1. Peptic ulcer
   2. Gastric cancer
   3. Osteoporosis
   4. Lactose intolerance

RATIONALE

(4) Abdominal pain and diarrhea after drinking milk, abdominal bloating and increased flatulence are all symptoms of this disorder.

1. These symptoms are not associated with this disease.
2. These are not signs of this disease.
3. This disorder results from lactose intolerance.

> Analysis
> Medicine/Surgery
> Physiologic and Anatomic Equilibrium

> Acute Care
> Gastrointestinal

2. The nurse has a client who has been diagnosed as having celiac sprue. This is a disease characterized by intolerance for:
   1. Gluten
   2. Fruit juices
   3. Skim milk
   4. Organ meats

RATIONALE

(1) Diminished intestinal villi contribute to the malabsorption of fat, carbohydrates, iron, vitamins and water as well as gluten intolerance.

2. These do not cause the problem.
3. Initially, the diet should be low in lactose because of the villi damage.
4. These are not associated with the disease.

> Implementation
> Medicine/Surgery
> Physiologic and Anatomic Equilibrium
> Acute Care
> Gastrointestinal

3. One measure that the nurse will implement as part of a care plan for the client with intestinal infections is:
   1. Sponge baths
   2. Ostomy Care
   3. High fiber diet
   4. Private bathroom

RATIONALE

(4) When possible, the client with intestinal infection should not share bathroom facilities until the infection subsides.

1. These are unnecessary.
2. Many clients will not have an ostomy.
3. These foods increase intestinal irritation.

> Planning
> Medicine/Surgery
> Physiologic and Anatomic Equilibrium
> Acute Care
> Gastrointestinal

4. Nursing care for the client with inflammatory bowel disease is planned to achieve the outcome of:
   1. Weight loss
   2. Minimal anal ulceration
   3. Hard, well formed stools
   4. Maintenance of a well-balanced diet

RATIONALE

(4) A well-balanced diet is essential to minimize symptoms of the disease.

1. Clients usually have altered nutrition and need to gain weight.
2. Intact anal skin is the goal of treatment.

3. Soft, formed stools indicate normal bowel functioning.

> Assessment
> Medicine/Surgery
> Physiologic and Anatomic Equilibrium
> Acute Care
> Gastrointestinal

5. **The client experiencing appendicitis has pain, nausea and rebound tenderness in the lower right quadrant. Objective data will include:**
   1. Rigid abdomen, fever
   2. Increased red blood cells, temperature of 102° F
   3. Increased white blood cells, temperature of 101° F
   4. Decreased white blood cells, hypotension

RATIONALE

(3) Temperature may range from 100° to 101° F, and increases if perforation occurs; blood studies indicate leukocytosis.
   1. This is a sign of peritonitis.
   2. This may occur later.
   4. The white blood cells increase and the blood pressure is usually not affected.

> Analysis
> Medicine/Surgery
> Physiologic and Anatomic Equilibrium
> Acute Care
> Gastrointestinal

6. **In assessing clients with possible inflammatory bowel disease, the nurse recognizes that it is most frequently identified in:**
   1. Jews
   2. Blacks
   3. White female
   4. Native Americans

RATIONALE

(1) Ulcerative colitis and Crohn's disease have an increased incidence in the Jewish population and in higher socioeconomic groups.
   2. There is a lower incidence of this disease in the noncaucasian population.
   3. This group is not the one most often affected.
   4. The incidence is low in this group.

> Assessment
> Medicine/Surgery
> Physiologic and Anatomic Equilibrium
> Acute Care
> Gastrointestinal

7. **In the emergency room, the nurse is caring for a client who has cramping abdominal pain because of an intestinal obstruction, according to the history. On auscultation of the abdomen the nurse will hear:**
   1. Absence of sounds
   2. Splashing sounds
   3. Hypoactive sounds
   4. Hyperactive sounds

RATIONALE

(4) Bowel sounds may increase proximal to the obstruction because of increased peristaltic activity.
   1. This occurs later.
   2. This is not a typical finding.
   3. Hypoactivity occurs as the obstruction progresses.

> Implementation
> Medicine/Surgery
> Physiologic and Anatomic Equilibrium
> Acute Care
> Gastrointestinal

8. **In assisting with the diagnosis of intraperitoneal bleeding in the client with blunt trauma to the abdomen, the nurse would most likely be asked to obtain supplies for:**
   1. Foley catheter
   2. Nasogastric tube insertion
   3. Diagnostic peritoneal lavage
   4. Insertion of a central venous catheter

RATIONALE

(3) This involves instillation of a crystalloid solution into the peritoneal cavity and siphoning it for analysis of white and red blood cells, amylase, bile, bacteria, and foreign matter.
   1. This is done to drain urine.
   2. This is done to decompress the stomach.
   4. This is done to provide venous access for fluids and blood.

CHAPTER 52 Nursing Management of Adults with Disorders of the Liver, Biliary Tract, or Exocrine Pancreas

> Assessment
> Medicine/Surgery
> Physiologic and Anatomic Equilibrium
> Acute Care
> Gastrointestinal

1. **In performing a physical examination of a client who may have cirrhosis of the liver, the nurse will notice jaundice and:**
   1. Paresthesias
   2. Palmar erythema
   3. White facial blotches
   4. Swollen moist skin

RATIONALE

(2) This is redness of the palms that blanches with pressure. This is thought to be caused by an increase in estrogen levels.

1. Pruritus or itching of the skin is common.
3. Spider angiomas or small red dilated pulsating arterioles are common.
4. The skin is usually dry with lesions present.

Implementation
Medicine/Surgery
Physiologic and Anatomic Equilibrium
Acute Care
Gastrointestinal

2. **A client with cirrhosis has developed ascites. In addition to administering a diuretic, the nurse may be asked to administer:**
   1. 0.9% normal saline
   2. 5% dextrose in water
   3. Ringer's lactate
   4. Salt-poor albumin

RATIONALE

(4) This increases the plasma volume and enhances diuresis by draining fluid from the interstitial area into the intravenous area.
   1. This is isotonic fluid and will not have the same effect.
   2. This may complicate the hyperglycemia that may occur because of liver failure.
   3. This is an isotonic solution and will not have the same effect as the albumin.

Evaluation
Medicine/Surgery
Physiologic and Anatomic Equilibrium
Acute Care
Gastrointestinal

3. The nurse is monitoring a client who has had a Leveen shunt placed for ascites. Signs of complications include:
   1. Dyspnea
   2. Hypotension
   3. Hypothermia
   4. Decreased drainage in the collection bag

RATIONALE

(1) Complications such as congestive heart failure and pulmonary edema occur in about 50% of clients who have these shunts.
   2. Hypertension may occur because of the increased intravenous volume.
   3. This does not usually occur.
   4. The fluid drains from the peritoneum into the superior vena cava so no drainage bag is needed.

Evaluation
Medicine/Surgery
Physiologic and Anatomic Equilibrium
Acute Care
Gastrointestinal

4. **The nurse is asked to administer neomycin to a client who has advanced cirrhosis. The drug's**

effectiveness is evaluated by monitoring the serum:
   1. Sodium level
   2. Glucose level
   3. Ammonia level
   4. Potassium

RATIONALE

(3) This antibiotic destroys colonic bacteria and prevents the formation of ammonia, which can cause hepatic encephalopathy.
   1. This is not affected.
   2. This is not evaluated.
   4. This is not affected.

Analysis
Medicine/Surgery
Physiologic and Anatomic Equilibrium
Acute Care
Gastrointestinal

5. **A flight attendant has acquired hepatitis A after a trip abroad. The best way to prevent the spread of this disease is:**
   1. Testing blood supplies
   2. Good personal hygiene
   3. Antibiotic therapy
   4. Respiratory isolation

RATIONALE

(2) The hepatitis A virus is spread through gastrointestinal secretions and urine.
   1. This applies to hepatitis B.
   3. Hepatitis is a viral infection. Antibiotics are not usually given.
   4. This is not necessary.

Planning
Medicine/Surgery
Physiologic and Anatomic E
quilibrium
Acute Care
Gastrointestinal

6. **The major goal after a liver transplant is:**
   1. Prevent all forms of rejection
   2. Encephalopathy
   3. Restore nutritional status
   4. Reduction of jaundice

RATIONALE

(1) This is the primary goal for any transplant client. This is done by massive doses of immunosuppressive agents.
   2. This should not be present before surgery.
   3. This is a secondary goal.
   4. This usually resolves over time.

Implementation
Medicine/Surgery
Physiologic and Anatomic Equilibrium

7. **A client with pancreatitis is complaining of severe pain. The nurse will administer:**
   1. Tigan
   2. Demerol
   3. Morphine
   4. Klonopin

RATIONALE

(2) This does not cause spasm of the sphincter of Oddi.
   1. This is an antiemetic.
   3. This does cause spasms of the sphincter of Oddi and is contraindicated.
   4. This is a antianxiety drug.

UNIT XIII   Reproductive System

CHAPTER 53   Nursing Assessment of the Reproductive System

Implementation
Medicine/Surgery
Physiologic and Anatomic Equilibrium
Acute Care
Reproduction

1. **In educating clients about the causes and the treatments of menstrual irregularities, the nurse begins by telling them that the first day of the menstrual cycle is:**
   1. At the time ovulation occurs
   2. The 28th day after the last cycle
   3. The last day of menstrual bleeding
   4. The first day of menstrual bleeding

RATIONALE

(4) Bleeding is the result of shedding of the superficial layer of the endometrium because of changes in hormone levels. It is clearly identifiable and is called day 1 of the cycle.
   1. This occurs later in the cycle.
   2. This is the last day of the cycle.
   3. The first day of bleeding is identified.

Assessment
Medicine/Surgery
Physiologic and Anatomic Equilibrium
Acute Care
Reproduction

2. **The primary organ of the male reproduction system is:**
   1. Penis
   2. Testes
   3. Vas deferens
   4. Ejaculatory ducts

RATIONALE

(2) The testes are the organs that produce sperm. They are usually 2 degrees below body temperature for optimum sperm viability.
   1. This is a conduit for urine and sperm.
   3. This is a tube that propels the sperm from the epididymis to the ejaculatory duct.
   4. This collects viscous liquid from the seminal vesicles.

Analysis
Medicine/Surgery
Physiologic and Anatomic Equilibrium
Acute Care
Reproduction

3. **The hormone that stimulates the production of milk is:**
   1. Oxytocin
   2. Prolactin
   3. Luteinizing hormone
   4. Follicle-stimulating hormone

RATIONALE

(2) Prolactin is secreted by the anterior lobe of the pituitary gland.
   1. This affects the movement of milk from the mammary gland alveoli to the nipple area.
   3. Luteinizing hormone stimulates the development of the reproductive tract at puberty.
   4. This influences the growth of six primordial follicles.

Implementation
Medicine/Surgery
Physiologic and Anatomic Equilibrium
Acute Care
Reproduction

4. **In preparing a client for a gynecologic examination, the nurse explains that a bimanual examination will be done as a part of it. The purpose of this examination is to:**
   1. Percuss the ovaries
   2. Visualize the uterus
   3. Palpate the uterus and ovaries
   4. Visualize the cervix and vagina

RATIONALE

(3) The examiner places one hand on the abdomen and two fingers inside the vagina and evaluates the size of the uterus, cervix, ovaries, and fallopian tubes.
   1. This is not part of the bimanual examination.
   2. This is not possible with this technique.
   4. This is not possible during this type of examination.

Planning
Medicine/Surgery
Physiologic and Anatomic Equilibrium
Acute Care
Reproduction

5. **In preparing a client for a Papanicolaou (Pap) test, the nurse should give the following instructions:**
   1. Don't douche before the test
   2. The test can be done if menstruating
   3. Take a tub bath before the test
   4. Sexual intercourse is not restricted

RATIONALE

(1) Douching and the use of lubricants are to be stopped 24 hours before the test.
   2. The results may be inaccurate.
   3. Tub baths should also be avoided in the 24 hours before the test.
   4. Sexual activity should be stopped 24 hours before the test.

> Evaluation
> Medicine/Surgery
> Physiologic and Anatomic Equilibrium
> Acute Care
> Reproduction

6. **When the nurse is evaluating the client's compliance with cervical biopsy postprocedure care, a correct statement by the client would be:**
   1. "I left the packing in all day."
   2. "I felt well enough to move my piano."
   3. "Intercourse wasn't painful at all."
   4. "I only needed four tampons to control the bleeding."

RATIONALE

(1) A cervical biopsy involves removing a piece of tissue. Bleeding may occur afterward, so a packing or tampon is left in place for 8 to 24 hours.
   2. Heavy lifting should be avoided for 24 hours.
   3. Intercourse or douching is avoided until the physician indicates otherwise.
   4. Continued use of tampons is to be avoided, because it may provide irritation and provoke bleeding.

> Analysis
> Medicine/Surgery
> Physiologic and Anatomic Equilibrium
> Acute Care
> Reproduction

7. **A client arrives at the clinic to have a specimen drawn for alpha-fetoprotein level and asks why this is necessary. The nurse explain that it assists in detecting:**
   1. Cervical cancer
   2. Testicular cancer
   3. Protein deficiency
   4. Lowered sperm count

RATIONALE

(2) This protein is produced primarily by embryonic and fetal cancer cells. It is elevated with testicular and primary liver cancer, pregnancy, and abortion.
   1. This is not diagnostic for this disease.
   2. This will not be identified by this test.
   4. The sperm count is not determined by this test.

> Implementation
> Medicine/Surgery
> Physiologic and Anatomic Equilibrium
> Acute Care
> Reproduction

8. **As a client goes home after a prostate biopsy, the nurse gives instructions to:**
   1. Report any sign of bleeding
   2. Expect an elevated temperature
   3. Anticipate changes in the voiding pattern
   4. Follow regular perineal hygienic practices

RATIONALE

(3) There may be changes in the frequency and amount of urine voided for 2 to 3 days after the biopsy.
   1. Some bleeding is normal.
   2. Any elevated temperature should be reported to the doctor.
   4. The scrotal area is to be washed with soap and water after bowel movements to reduce the chance of infection.

CHAPTER 54 Sexuality and Reproductive Health

> Analysis
> Medicine/Surgery
> Physiologic and Anatomic Equilibrium
> Acute Care
> Reproduction

1. **The basic physiologic changes that occur during the excitement or arousal phase of the sexual response cycle are:**
   1. Myotonia and vasoconstriction
   2. Myotonia and vasocongestion
   3. Myoclonus and vasoconstriction
   4. Myoclonus and vasocongestion

RATIONALE

(2) Vasocongestion in the genital area is the major physiologic change that occurs in the excitement or arousal phase; myotonia or muscular tension develops through out the body, particularly in the thighs, abdomen, and pelvic area.
   1. Vasocongestion occurs in the genital area.
   3. Vasoconstriction occurs in the plateau phase.
   4. Myoclonus does not occur.

> Assessment
> Medicine/Surgery

Physiologic and Anatomic Equilibrium
Acute Care
Reproduction

2. **The nurse is counseling an older client about the sexual response. One change in females that occurs as a result of aging is:**
   1. Decreased vaginal lubrication
   2. Longer orgasmic experience
   3. Increased expansion of vaginal space
   4. Orgasm does not occur after menopause

RATIONALE

(1) Vaginal lubrication is reduced in amount, and the time it takes to be produced is prolonged. Decreased vaginal lubrication can make penetration uncomfortable or even painful.
2. The orgasmic phase may be shortened.
3. This does not occur.
4. This is false. The orgasmic phase is shortened but not absent.

Implementation
Medicine/Surgery
Physiologic and Anatomic Equilibrium
Acute Care
Reproduction

3. **A client has come to the clinic for evaluation of erectile dysfunction (impotence). After the nurse obtains a sexual history, one of the first aspects of therapy will be suggesting:**
   1. Less sleep
   2. Abstaining from sex
   3. Abstaining from alcohol
   4. Increasing antidepressant dose

RATIONALE

(3) The chemical influences of alcohol and drugs are known to be causative factors to erectile dysfunction.
1. Fatigue can contribute to this disorder. More sleep is recommended.
2. This is not a part of the therapy.
4. Antidepressants can cause this disorder. Decreasing the dose if possible would be more beneficial.

Planning
Medicine/Surgery
Physiologic and Anatomic
   Equilibrium
Acute Care
Reproduction

4. **In a care plan for a client with erectile dysfunction (impotence), one appropriate goal is:**
   1. Minimize discussion of the problem
   2. Avoid involving the partner in sexual problems
   3. Internalize feelings about sexual performance
   4. Maintain a positive attitude toward sexuality

RATIONALE

(4) The expected outcomes of the client are to be able to maintain an erection and resume normal sexual performance. Having a positive attitude about sexuality will contribute to this goal.
1. The client should be comfortable discussing his problem.
2. Communication with the partner about sexual dysfunction is beneficial.
3. Verbalization of feelings and perceptions about sexual performance is healthy.

Assessment
Medicine/Surgery
Physiologic and Anatomic Equilibrium
Acute Care
Reproduction

5. **A client is being assessed for a problem with sexual intercourse. The symptoms involve involuntary spasms of the outer vagina. This is called:**
   1. Vaginitis
   2. Vaginismus
   3. Dyspareunia
   4. Female arousal disorder

RATIONALE

(2) This is a recurrent or persistent involuntary spasm of the genital musculature at the outer third of the vagina that interferes with coitus.
1. This is inflammation of the vagina.
3. This is pain associated with intercourse in either men or women.
4. This is an inability to maintain sexual arousal.

Evaluation
Medicine/Surgery
Physiologic and Anatomic Equilibrium
Acute Care
Reproduction

6. **In evaluating the benefits of a Masters and Johnson seminar, the nurse would expect that the client would be using more:**
   1. Biofeedback
   2. Nongenital pleasuring
   3. Verbal communication
   4. Power play between partners

RATIONALE

(2) The Masters and Johnson method focuses on exploring sensual pleasure and assisting the person or couple to learn what stimuli are pleasurable to each other before any genital contact occurs.
1. This is not a part of the therapy.
3. The nonverbal or physical communication is emphasized.
4. This is definitely not a part of the therapy.

7. **Premature ejaculation is the most common sexual dysfunction in the male. The plan of therapy for the client will include counseling to:**
   1. Abstain from alcohol
   2. Use an anesthetic gel
   3. Refrain from use of vaginal lubricants
   4. Use condom to decrease sensitivity

RATIONALE

(4) Techniques to delay ejaculation were developed by Masters and Johnson and include condom use.
   1. Drinking an alcoholic beverage may be helpful.
   2. This is not recommended.
   3. Ensuring sufficient vaginal lubrication is important.

Analysis
Medicine/Surgery
Physiologic and Anatomic Equilibrium
Acute Care
Reproduction

8. **Problems with ejaculation are often associated with:**
   1. Physical findings
   2. Lack of sex education
   3. Anxiety and fatigue
   4. Lack of meaningful relationships

RATIONALE

(3) Performance anxiety can block the persons ability to prolong sexual performance; stress reduction will help with fatigue.
   1. Many psychologic factors are associated with this disorder.
   2. This is not always a part of the problem.
   4. Sexual dysfunction can occur in casual or meaningful relationships.

CHAPTER 55 Nursing Management of Women with Reproductive System Disorders

Evaluation
Medicine/Surgery
Physiologic and Anatomic Equilibrium
Acute Care
Reproduction

1. **An elderly client with vaginitis has returned for a follow-up evaluation of her disease. If the therapy has been effective, the nurse will observe:**
   1. Grayish white secretions
   2. White curdlike secretions
   3. Clear vaginal secretions
   4. Reddish tinged secretions

RATIONALE

(3) Clear, odorless secretions indicate an absence of infection.
   1. This indicates a purulent discharge.
   2. This indicates an infective process.
   4. This may indicate bleeding.

Evaluation
Medicine/Surgery
Physiologic and Anatomic Equilibrium
Acute Care
Reproduction

2. **A client with pelvic inflammatory disease has achieved a planned goal of compliance with treatment regimen. This is evidenced by:**
   1. Use of tampons without irritation
   2. Continuous urinary catheterization
   3. Continuing bed rest in semi-Fowler's position
   4. Minimal vaginal itching and inflammation

RATIONALE

(3) Clients are placed in this position to provide dependent drainage so that abscesses will not form high in the abdomen.
   1. Tampon use is avoided to prevent the spread of infection.
   2. This is also avoided to prevent the spread of infection.
   4. No lower abdominal pain, vaginal drainage, pruritus, inflammation, or excoriation of the vulva is expected.

Planning
Medicine/Surgery
Physiologic and Anatomic Equilibrium
Acute Care
Reproduction

3. **In planning the care of a client with toxic shock syndrome the nurse will anticipate:**
   1. Hypothermia
   2. Puncture site oozing
   3. Cardiac arrest or dysrhythmias
   4. White patches on the genital area

RATIONALE

(2) Disseminated intravascular coagulopathy (DIC) has been observed in clients with toxic shock syndrome. The nurse should observe for hematomas, petechiae, cyanosis, and oozing from puncture sites.
   1. A sudden high fever may develop.
   3. This is not an immediate finding. It may develop if the septic shock is not treated.

4. A red macular palmar or diffuse rash is common.

> Assessment
> Medicine/Surgery
> Physiologic and Anatomic Equilibrium
> Acute Care
> Reproduction

4. **The nurse is assessing a client for possible cervical cancer. One of the early signs of this disease is:**
   1. Back pain
   2. Leukorrhea
   3. Normal period
   4. Breast tenderness

RATIONALE

(2) Early cancer of the cervix is usually asymptomatic. The two chief symptoms are leukorrhea (vaginal discharge) and irregular vaginal bleeding or spotting.
1. This may occur when the cancer has invaded other organs.
3. Usually vaginal bleeding or spotting occurs.
4. This is associated with breast disease.

> Planning
> Medicine/Surgery
> Physiologic and Anatomic Equilibrium
> Acute Care
> Reproduction

5. **In preparing instructions to be given to clients who experience premenstrual syndrome (PMS), the nurse would appropriately include:**
   1. Eat three, large meals a day
   2. Restrict caffeine, sugar, and nicotine
   3. Use sanitary pads rather than tampons
   4. Limit exercise to non–weight bearing exercises

RATIONALE

(2) Limiting the use of these substances may minimize the symptoms of PMS.
1. Eating small meals is recommended.
3. This restriction is limited to clients with toxic shock syndrome.
4. Daily exercise and relaxation are recommended.

> Analysis
> Medicine/Surgery
> Physiologic and Anatomic Equilibrium
> Acute Care
> Reproduction

6. **The community center is offering a seminar on women's health. The nurse, who is going to speak on endometriosis, will explain that this is:**
   1. Erosion of cervical tissue

2. An enlargement of ovarian tissue
3. Seeding of endometrial cells in the pelvis
4. Overgrowth of endometrial cells in the uterus

RATIONALE

(3) Endometriosis is a condition in which endometrial cells that normally live in the uterus are seeded throughout the pelvis and extend to the umbilicus.
1. This is cervical dysplasia or a change in the cells of the cervix.
2. This may describe an ovarian tumor.
4. This may be a type of uterine polyp.

> Evaluation
> Medicine/Surgery
> Physiologic and Anatomic Equilibrium
> Acute Care
> Reproduction

7. **When the nurse is evaluating a client's progress after a hysterectomy, one favorable sign would be:**
   1. Negative Homan's sign
   2. Positive Homan's sign
   3. Decreased urinary output
   4. Acceptance of end of sex life

RATIONALE

(1) Homan's sign indicates the development of thrombophlebitis in the calf. The absence of pain on dorsiflexion of the foot is a negative finding.
2. A negative sign is expected.
3. The urinary output should be normal in amount, color, and frequency.
4. Sexual activity is not limited by the loss of the uterus.

> Implementation
> Medicine/Surgery
> Physiologic and Anatomic Equilibrium
> Acute Care
> Reproduction

8. **One postoperative instruction that should be given to a client who has undergone a dilation and curettage is:**
   1. Do not douche for 2 weeks
   2. Discontinue birth control pills
   3. Continue birth control pills
   4. Report any vaginal bleeding

RATIONALE

(3) If a client has been taking birth control pills, they should be continued as prescribed. The menstrual cycle will continue as before and the possibility of pregnancy will remain.

1. Douching, sexual intercourse, and tampon use are restricted for 1 week.
2. They should be continued as prescribed.
4. Some vaginal bleeding is expected. All vaginal bleeding should disappear in 7 to 10 days. Excessive amounts of bleeding, recurrence of bleeding, or development of a vaginal discharge should be reported to the health care provider.

CHAPTER 56 Nursing Management of Men with Reproductive System Disorders

Analysis
Medicine/Surgery
Physiologic and Anatomic Equilibrium
Acute Care
Reproduction

1. **An expected effect of the drug finasteride, given to clients with benign prostatic hypertrophy, is:**
   1. Urinary bladder filling
   2. Decreased urinary flow
   3. Enlargement of the prostate gland
   4. Reduction of the prostate gland

RATIONALE

(4) This drug inhibits the enzyme 5-alpha reductase, preventing the conversion of testosterone to dihydrotestosterone in the prostate gland. It reduces the size of the prostate.
   1. The urinary bladder is not affected because the urinary flow is unobstructed.
   2. Urinary flow is slightly increased.
   3. The gland size is reduced.

Assessment
Medicine/Surgery
Physiologic and Anatomic
   Equilibrium
Acute Care
Reproduction

2. **Six hours after a transurethral resection of the prostate, the nurse assesses vital signs and empties the urinary drainage bag. One expected finding is:**
   1. Clear, yellow urine
   2. Bright red, bloody urine
   3. Urinary output of 1000 ml/day
   4. Blood pressure 100/60, pulse 120

RATIONALE

(2) The prostate is a vascular organ and bleeding may continue for some time, resolving completely within 7 to 10 days after resection.
   1. This is not likely for a week to 10 days after the procedure.
   3. The urinary output should be between 1500 to 2000 ml/day.

4. A rapid pulse with a drop in blood pressure is a potential sign of excessive blood loss; the surgeon should be notified.

Implementation
Medicine/Surgery
Physiologic and Anatomic Equilibrium
Acute Care
Reproduction

3. **Potential fluid volume excess related to transurethral resection of the prostate (TURP) syndrome from irrigation fluid can occur after a TURP. The nurse should monitor for:**
   1. Tachypnea and confusion
   2. Tachycardia and diarrhea
   3. Increased urinary output and hematuria
   4. Decreased urinary output and bladder spasms

RATIONALE

(1) When excessive irrigating solution is absorbed through the prostatic vascular bed, it causes tachypnea, agitation, and confusion.
   2. Bradycardia is produced.
   3. These are expected outcomes.
   4. These are not symptoms produced by the TUR syndrome.

Planning
Medicine/Surgery
Physiologic and Anatomic Equilibrium
Acute Care
Reproduction

4. **The client after a prostatectomy has a nursing diagnosis of altered prostatic bed tissue perfusion. One aspect of care related to this problem is to leave the catheter in place. This is because doing so will:**
   1. Ensure patency of urine
   2. Catch clots in the Foley bag
   3. Ensure gentle traction against the urethra
   4. Compare the pre- and postoperative hematocrit

RATIONALE

(3) Gentle traction on the drainage catheter balloon allows hemostasis until the prostatic capsule heals.
   1. The urethral drainage may not be affected.
   2. This is a secondary function.
   4. This is not directly possible with the catheter.

Implementation
Medicine/Surgery
Physiologic and Anatomic Equilibrium
Acute Care
Reproduction

5. **One concern that a client who has had a prostatectomy might have is about sexual functioning. The nurse should explain that:**

1. Sexual activity will increase
2. There will be no change
3. Permanent impotence will occur
4. Fertility potential is decreased

RATIONALE

(4) Altered ejaculatory function is expected after prostatectomy and this will decrease the fertility potential. this occurs because of retrograde ejaculation into the bladder.
1. This may or may not occur.
2. There may be decreased fertility.
3. The surgery is not expected to impair his ability to generate and maintain an erection.

> Implementation
> Medicine/Surgery
> Physiologic and Anatomic Equilibrium
> Acute Care
> Reproduction

6. **A client has continuous bladder irrigation in place after a prostatectomy and is complaining of bladder spasms. The most appropriate nursing action is to:**
1. Administer Demerol
2. Minimize catheter manipulation
3. Discontinue the continuous bladder irrigation
4. Increase the rate of the infusion of the irrigating solution

RATIONALE

(2) Pain caused by irritation from the catheter is alleviated by minimizing manipulation and by promoting adequate rest.
1. Smooth muscle relaxants would be more effective.
3. This is not appropriate.
4. This could be harmful because of the increased risk of transurethral resection (TUR) syndrome.

> Evaluation
> Medicine/Surgery
> Physiologic and Anatomic Equilibrium
> Acute Care
> Reproduction

7. **The primary serum marker for prostate cancer is prostate-specific antigen (PSA). The normal range for PSA is affected by the client's age and the presence of coexisting benign prostatic hypertrophy. Men 40 to 50 years of age should have a serum PSA of less than or equal to:**
1. 2.0 nanograms/ml
2. 4.0 nanograms/ml
3. 6.0 nanogram/ml
4. 10.0 nanograms/ml

RATIONALE

(1) This is the expected range for men in this age group.

2. This is the normal range for men aged 50 to 60 years.
3. This is above normal for men in this age range.
4. This represents an elevated level.

> Planning
> Medicine/Surgery
> Physiologic and Anatomic Equilibrium
> Acute Care
> Reproduction

8. **General goals of care for the client with prostatic cancer who is undergoing radiation therapy include:**
1. Fluid restriction
2. Complete bladder emptying every 6 hours
3. Less than 4 episodes of nocturia per night
4. Consumes 2000 to 2500 ml of fluid per day

RATIONALE

(4) Diarrhea and irritative voiding symptoms are common. The diarrhea is usually transient, and the nurse should ensure an adequate fluid intake.
1. This should be avoided. Hydration is very important.
2. This should occur every 2 to 4 hours during waking hours.
3. This should be 2 or fewer episodes of nocturia per night.

CHAPTER 57 Nursing Management of Adults with Sexually Transmitted Diseases

> Analysis
> Medicine/Surgery
> Physiologic and Anatomic Equilibrium
> Acute Care
> Reproduction

1. **In conducting an educational program on sexually transmitted disease (STD), the nurse advises the attendees that the most prevalent STD is:**
1. Chlamydia
2. Syphilis
3. Gonorrhea
4. Herpes genitalis

RATIONALE

(1) An estimated 4 million Americans develop chlamydia each year.
2. Recent statistics indicate approximately 80,000 cases of syphilis are reported annually.
3. One-half million people a year are infected with gonorrhea.
4. Herpes is a frequently occurring disease, but the incidence is less than that of chlamydia.

2. **A client has been treated for trichomoniasis. On a return visit the nurse would expect the eradication of the characteristic symptom:**
   1. Beefy ulcer
   2. Scanty white discharge
   3. Cauliflower growths
   4. Strawberry patches

RATIONALE

(4) These are petechiae which may be present on the cervix or vagina.
   1. This is characteristic of Donovanosis.
   2. This is characteristic of chlamydia in men.
   3. Venereal warts are raised, rough, cauliflower-like fleshy growth on the genitalia.

Analysis
Medicine/Surgery
Physiologic and Anatomic
    Equilibrium
Acute Care
Reproduction

3. **In conducting a health history, the nurse learns that a client has had a sexually transmitted disease, probably herpesvirus. The client is at increased risk for:**
   1. Cervical cancer
   2. Multiple births
   3. Kaposi's sarcoma
   4. Reduced sexual response

RATIONALE

(1) Recently, cervical cancer has been strongly associated with herpesvirus, human papillomavirus, and HIV infection.
   2. There is not a link between these two things.
   3. This is common in clients with HIV, which can be acquired through sexual transmission.
   4. This does not usually occur.

Implementation
Medicine/Surgery
Physiologic and Anatomic
    Equilibrium
Acute Care
Reproduction

4. **In teaching a client practices to prevent sexually transmitted disease (STD), the nurse would include:**
   1. Douche frequently
   2. Do not urinate after intercourse
   3. Gargle with warm salt water
   4. Seek an STD examination twice per year

(4) Having this examination twice a year or more often as needed will contribute to early diagnosis of STDs.
   1. Excessive douching may reduce the normal bacterial balance in the vagina.
   2. Urinating after intercourse reduces the risk of contracting some forms of STDs.
   3. Using a mouthwash or gargle with hydrogen peroxide or antiseptics may possibly reduce the risk of oropharyngeal STD infection.

5. **In assessing a client for herpes genitalis, the nurse would expect to see:**
   1. Flat, soft ulcers
   2. Purulent penile discharge
   3. A painless indurated ulcer
   4. Clusters of 2 mm blisters

RATIONALE

(4) Primary herpes has an incubation period of 2 to 12 days. Local lesions appear from 2 to 8 mm in size, preceded by a prodrome of tingling, itching, or burning pain.
   1. This is characteristic of a chancroid lesion.
   2. This is characteristic of gonorrhea.
   3. This is characteristic of syphilis.

Assessment
Medicine/Surgery
Physiologic and Anatomic
    Equilibrium
Acute Care
Reproduction

6. **Syphilis is a disease of several stages. A client with syphilis is complaining of headache, weight loss, fever, anorexia, and sore throat. These symptoms are characteristic of:**
   1. Late
   2. Latent
   3. Primary
   4. Secondary

RATIONALE

(4) Flu-like symptoms described are found in the secondary stage of the disease, as is a maculopapular rash.
   1. A variety of nervous system syndromes including dementia, leg pain, and aortic destruction are characteristic of this stage.
   2. The latent stage may last 20 or more years, may be asymptomatic, or have relapsing lesions.

3. This usually appears as a painless, indurated ulcer with serous exudate on the skin or mucous membrane.

> Planning
> Medicine/Surgery
> Physiologic and Anatomic Equilibrium
> Acute Care

7. **In a treatment plan for the client with active syphilis, the goal is to eradicate the disease. This is best accomplished by administering:**
   1. Gentamicin
   2. Cephalosporin
   3. Penicillin
   4. Erythromycin

RATIONALE

(3) Penicillin is the drug of choice for syphilis and is usually given intramuscularly or intravenously because of the consequences of inadequate treatment.
   1. This is not prescribed.
   2. This is not the primary drug of choice.
   4. This is prescribed when the client is allergic to penicillin.

> Evaluation
> Medicine/Surgery
> Physiologic and Anatomic Equilibrium
> Acute Care
> Reproduction

8. **Successful treatment of syphilis is evidenced by:**
   1. Shrinkage of ulcer
   2. Rash localized to the palms
   3. Minimal episodes of confusion
   4. Minimal fatigue or fever

RATIONALE

(1) The size of the primary chancre should be evaluated and documented and should have reduced in size or disappeared.
   2. This is one sign of secondary syphilis and should have been eliminated by the treatment.
   3. Dementia is associated with tertiary syphilis. No possible symptoms of it should be noted.
   4. Fatigue, fever, and lymph node enlargement should be eradicated by the treatment.

Unit XIV   Integumentary System

CHAPTER 58   Nursing Assessment of the Integumentary System

> Analysis
> Medicine/surgery
> Physiologic and Anatomic Equilibrium
> Acute Care
> Integumentary

1. **The pigment of the skin is determined by:**
   1. Dermis
   2. Epidermis
   3. Melanocytes
   4. Stratum corneum

RATIONALE

(3) Melanocytes found in the epidermal layers near the dermis produce melanin granules; the larger the number of granules and the more the melanin is dispersed through the epidermis, the darker the appearance of the skin.
   1. This is the skin layer below the epidermis and has a rich blood supply.
   2. This is the top layer of skin.
   4. This is the outermost layer of the epidermis.

> Assessment
> Medicine/Surgery
> Physiologic and Anatomic Equilibrium
> Acute Care
> Integumentary

2. **Changes in blood composition can alter skin color. Deoxygenated hemoglobin gives the skin a bluish tint called:**
   1. Cyanosis
   2. Vitiligo
   3. Jaundice
   4. Erythema

RATIONALE

(1) The skin appears blue when the partial pressure of oxygen is low and the absolute amount of deoxygenated hemoglobin exceeds 5 g/100 ml.
   2. This is patches of whiteness in otherwise darkly pigmented skin.
   3. This is a yellowish discoloration of the skin.
   4. This is redness of the skin.

> Analysis
> Medicine/Surgery
> Physiologic and Anatomic Equilibrium
> Acute Care
> Integumentary

3. **The skin helps to regulate body temperature by:**
   1. Heat loss and production
   2. Stimulation of the hypothalamus
   3. Decrease of sweat gland secretion
   4. Control of voluntary mechanisms

RATIONALE

(1) Heat is lost through the skin by conduction, convection, radiation, and evaporation. Heat production is proportional to the metabolic rate.
   2. This occurs because of changes in the core temperature.

3. Increasing sweat gland secretion decreases the skin temperature.
4. This is not a function of the skin.

> Implementation
> Medicine/Surgery
> Physiologic and Anatomic Equilibrium
> Acute Care
> Integumentary

4. **In performing a physical assessment in the dark-skinned client, the nurse identifies the best location for assessing pallor as:**
   1. Lips
   2. Nose
   3. Eyelids
   4. Forehead

RATIONALE

(1) Skin color changes are best observed in the sclera, conjunctiva, oral mucosa, tongue, lips, nail bed, palms, and soles. Normal variations in pigmentation also occurs in the mouth.
2. This is not a reliable area to assess.
3. Subtle color changes may not be visible here.
4. This is not a reliable assessment site.

> Assessment
> Medicine/Surgery
> Physiologic and Anatomic Equilibrium
> Acute Care
> Integumentary

5. **In assessing a client for a skin disorder, the nurse observes an elevated, circumscribed, superficial sac filed with serous fluid that is less than 1 cm in diameter. This is called a:**
   1. Macule
   2. Vesicle
   3. Pustule
   4. Lichenification

RATIONALE

(2) A vesicle greater than 1 cm is called a bulla.
1. This is a discolored spot that is not elevated.
3. This is an elevated, superficial sac filled with purulent fluid.
4. This is roughening or thickening of the epidermis.

> Planning
> Medicine/Surgery
> Physiologic and Anatomic Equilibrium
> Acute Care
> Reproduction

6. **In planning for an examination of the skin with a Wood's light, the nurse instructs the client to:**
   1. Bathe with an antiseptic soap and brush
   2. Apply mineral oil to the surface
   3. Avoid bathing for 48 hours before the test
   4. Avoid shampooing for 24 hours before the test

RATIONALE

(4) Bathing and applying makeup to the area should be avoided for 24 hours before the test.
1. This may remove cells from the skin surface.
2. This will mask the condition of the skin.
3. Baths should be avoided for 24 hours only.

> Analysis
> Medicine/Surgery
> Physiologic and Anatomic Equilibrium
> Acute Care
> Integumentary

7. **The Wood's light is useful in visualizing skin disorders including:**
   1. Sunburn
   2. Clubbing
   3. Fungal infections
   4. Cancerous lesions

RATIONALE

(3) The light is useful in detecting bacterial and fungal infections, porphyria, and pigmentary alterations.
1. This is not the primary disorder identified with this device.
2. This is not evaluated with the Wood's light.
4. These are examined under a microscope.

> Implementation
> Medicine/Surgery
> Physiologic and Anatomic Equilibrium
> Acute Care
> Integumentary

8. **In administering an intradermal skin test the nurse should inject the allergen:**
   1. At a 90-degree angle
   2. 3 mm below the skin
   3. Into a hairy area
   4. After rubbing the skin vigorously

RATIONALE

(2) The nurse should use the nondominant hand to stretch the client's skin and insert the needle no more than 3 mm below the skin surface.
1. The angle should be almost parallel to the skin.
3. Hairy, blemished areas should be avoided.
4. The skin should not be rubbed to the point where it produces redness.

CHAPTER 59 Nursing Management of Adults with Skin Disorders

> Planning
> Medicine/Surgery
> Physiologic and Anatomic Equilibrium
> Older Adult Care
> Integumentary

1. **A nurse in a long-term care facility has noticed several clients with very dry skin. An intervention that might help to alleviate this problem is:**
   1. Keep the skin warm
   2. Keep the skin covered
   3. Cool mist vaporizer
   4. Warm mist vaporizer

   RATIONALE

   (3) Dryness causes itching, which can be aggravated during winter months by hot, dry air. Lubricating the skin and increasing the room humidity is recommended.
   1. This is not a suggested intervention.
   2. This is unnecessary.
   4. Cool mist is recommended.

   > Evaluation
   > Medicine/Surgery
   > Physiologic and Anatomic Equilibrium
   > Acute Care
   > Integumentary

2. **When the nurse is evaluating the care of a client who has undergone surgical resection of a malignant melanoma, a desired outcome would be the client's statement that:**
   1. "I am so glad that this was something minor."
   2. "My incision looks like it did the day after surgery."
   3. "My granddaughter has a spot on her arm but I don't think it is important."
   4. "I went camping this week but I wore sunscreen at all times and hiked only in the early morning."

   RATIONALE

   (4) Malignant melanoma is an aggressive cancer that is thought to be related to sun exposure. Clients should limit sun exposure and use sun screen at all times when outdoors.
   1. Malignant melanoma is a deadly, metastatic disease that must be treated aggressively.
   2. The incision should show evidence of increased healing without infection.
   3. Family members with suspicious lesions should see a physician.

   > Assessment
   > Medicine/Surgery
   > Physiologic and Anatomic Equilibrium
   > Acute Care
   > Integumentary

3. **The Skin Cancer Foundation has published the ABCDs of malignant melanoma to assist with early detection of the disease. One identifying feature is:**
   1. A - asymmetry
   2. B - bright
   3. C - crusty
   4. D - dimpled

   RATIONALE

   (1) Malignant melanoma appears in many forms, but the lesions are usually circular with irregular borders.
   2. B is for border irregularity.
   3. C is for color variations, which include brown, black, blue, red, or white. The lesions are not always crusty.
   4. D is for diameter, which is usually greater than 5 mm. The lesions are not always dimpled.

   > Assessment
   > Medicine/Surgery
   > Physiologic and Anatomic Equilibrium
   > Long-term Care
   > Integumentary

4. **A client who is a golfer comes to the clinic because of a lesion on the nose. The dermatologist tells the client that it is a basal cell carcinoma. This common form of skin cancer usually appears as a:**
   1. Finely mottled, white and brown pigmented area
   2. Thick, rough, horny, shallow lesion
   3. Waxy-looking nodule with a translucent border
   4. Mole that changes in size, color, or shape

   RATIONALE

   (3) This is a basal cell carcinoma. It is a slow growing cancer usually found on the exposed areas of the face and neck.
   1. This describes lesions typical of dermatomyositis
   2. These lesions are typical of squamous cell carcinoma.
   4. This describes malignant melanoma lesions.

   > Planning
   > Medicine/Surgery
   > Physiologic and Anatomic Equilibrium
   > Long-term Care
   > Integumentary

5. **In planning the care for a client with scleroderma, the nurse knows that one intervention will be:**
   1. Surgical resection
   2. Penicillamine
   3. Steroids, immunosuppressive drugs
   4. Regional lymph node dissection

   RATIONALE

   (2) This has been proven effective in reducing skin thickness and slowing progression of visceral disease.
   1. This is used to treat malignant melanoma and basal and squamous cell carcinomas.
   3. This is part of the treatment protocol for pemphigus vulgaris, an autoimmune disease that causes blistering of the epidermis.
   4. This is one treatment attempted for malignant melanoma.

Evaluation
Medicine/Surgery
Physiologic and Anatomic Equilibrium
Long-term Care
Integumentary

1. **A home health nurse is performing follow-up care on a client who was burned in an airplane crash. If the client has been carrying out the instructions correctly, the nurse should see:**
   1. Client eating diet of choice
   2. Client wearing shorts and a tank top
   3. Gradual weight gain and minimal activity
   4. Application of moisturizer to healed areas

RATIONALE

(4) Once the burn has healed, this may be ordered by the doctor to soften the scar tissue.
   1. A well-balanced diet is important to ensure adequate healing.
   2. Long-sleeved shirt, pants, and a hat should be worn to protect the skin from sunlight.
   3. A drastic weight loss or gain should be avoided so that the pressure garments will fit properly.

Implementation
Medicine/Surgery
Physiologic and Anatomic Equilibrium
Long-term Care
Integumentary

2. **The priorities for a nurse in the burn intensive care unit, for the day that the burn occurred, is:**
   1. Oral fluid replacement
   2. Assist client to chair
   3. Teach burn wound care
   4. Intravenous fluid replacement

RATIONALE

(4) Replacing the massive fluid that is lost from damage to skin and blood vessels is a priority at this time.
   1. This usually occurs on day 3.
   2. This usually occurs on day 2.
   3. This usually occurs on day 3.

Implementation
Medicine/Surgery
Physiologic and Anatomic Equilibrium
Long-term Care
Integumentary

3. **A client who sustained a burn in a house fire required "meshed" skin grafts to the most badly burned areas. Nursing care of these sites will include:**
   1. Gentle massage of the area
   2. Allowing them to dry completely
   3. Leaving dressing intact for 3 days
   4. Beginning range of motion exercise quickly

RATIONALE

(3) Meshed grafts are split-thickness skin grafts that have been perforated with small slits to allow for expansion of the graft to fully cover the open wound and to drain. Leaving the dressing in place for 3 to 5 days allows for optimal adherence.
   1. These grafts are loosely adhered, so minimal manipulation of the graft is important.
   2. Keeping the graft moist is essential so that the graft does not adhere to the dressing and come off when it is changed.
   4. Beginning range of motion exercises before 5 to 7 days may cause the graft not to adhere properly.

Implementation
Medicine/Surgery
Physiologic and Anatomic Equilibrium
Long-term Care
Integumentary

4. **A client has received a partial thickness burn in an industrial accident. The pain is excruciating. The nurse will provide:**
   1. Sedative
   2. Morphine
   3. Nitrous oxide
   4. Hydrotherapy

RATIONALE

(2) This is the initial drug of choice. Others include methadone, codeine, and hydromorphone.
   1. This is used to relieve anxiety but not pain. Psychotropic drugs may be used in combination with narcotics.
   3. This is an inhalation anesthetic that is frequently used during dressing changes but not for routine pain management.
   4. This is one aspect of treatment of burned tissue. It is quite painful and clients must be given adequate analgesia during these times.

Analysis
Medicine/Surgery
Physiologic and Anatomic Equilibrium
Long-term Care
Integumentary

5. **According to the American Burn Association burn classification scale, a minor burn is one in which:**
   1. A small area around the face is burned
   2. Partial-thickness burns of less than 15% of total body surface area
   3. Full thickness burns of less than 10% of total body surface area
   4. An electrical burn to the hands, feet, ears, eyes, and genitalia

RATIONALE

(2) This burn category does not include full-thickness burns or those involving the eyes or ears. Clients are treated in the emergency room and as outpatients.

1. Facial burns are considered major because the airway may be involved.
3. These are moderate burns that may be treated at general hospitals.
4. This is also considered a major burn, requiring treatment in a burn unit.

CHAPTER 61 Nursing Management of Adults Undergoing Cosmetic or Reconstructive Surgery

Implementation
Medicine/Surgery
Physiologic and Anatomic Equilibrium
Acute Care
Plastic Surgery

1. **In the postoperative area of an outpatient surgery unit, the nurse is caring for a client who has undergone a blepharoplasty. The nurse's actions will include:**
1. Warm compresses to eye
2. Iced compresses to eye
3. Bed rest in the flat, supine position
4. Bed rest in a side-lying position

RATIONALE

(2) This will reduce edema and bruising.
1. Ice is recommended.
3. The head of the bed should be elevated to reduce edema.
4. This increases edema in the dependent eye. Clients should sleep supine with two pillows under the head.

Planning
Medicine/Surgery
Physiologic and Anatomic Equilibrium
Acute Care
Plastic Surgery

2. **A client with a previous nasal fracture has arrived in the outpatient surgery area for a rhinoplasty. Expected outcomes after the surgery include:**
1. No ecchymosis or edema
2. Absence of nasal packing
3. Minimal nasal bone displacement
4. Absence of respiratory distress

RATIONALE

(4) Clients should be able to breathe without difficulty through their mouths.
1. Some ecchymosis and edema around the eye are inevitable.

2. The nasal packing remains in place overnight, nasal splints for 1 week.
3. There should be no displacement of nasal bones.

Analysis
Medicine/Surgery
Physiologic and Anatomic Equilibrium
Acute Care
Plastic Surgery

3. **A former tennis professional has arrived for a face lift. The medical name for this procedure is:**
1. Dermabrasion
2. Mentoplasty
3. Rhytidectomy
4. Abdominoplasty

RATIONALE

(3) This is the removal of loose skin associated with aging from around the face.
1. This is the abrasion of the skin to remove fine wrinkles around the mouth, forehead, or corners of the eyes.
2. This is surgical reshaping of the chin.
4. This is the removal of loose abdominal tissue and skin.

Implementation
Medicine/Surgery
Physiologic and Anatomic Equilibrium
Acute Care
Plastic Surgery

4. **Preoperative instructions to a client who is about to undergo a rhytidectomy should include:**
1. Avoid aspirin
2. No sex for 24 hours before surgery
3. Avoid the sun for 1 month before surgery
4. Wear light make-up only for the day of surgery

RATIONALE

(1) This can increase the risk for bleeding.
2. This is irrelevant.
3. The client should avoid getting a sun burn for at least 2 weeks before surgery.
4. No cosmetics or toiletries are to be worn the morning of surgery.

Analysis
Medicine/Surgery
Physiologic and Anatomic Equilibrium
Acute Care
Plastic Surgery

5. **A client undergoing a phenol chemical peel to remove fine facial wrinkles will have this done in the operating room and not in the surgeon's office because of the risk of:**
1. Dysrhythmias
2. Hypothermia

3. Malignant hyperthermia
4. Respiratory distress

RATIONALE

(1) Phenol is absorbed into the blood stream and can cause systemic toxicity, including cardiac dysrhythmias.
2. This is not a complication of this procedure.
3. This occurs as a result of the usage of general anesthetics, not phenol.
4. This does not usually occur.

> Assessment
> Medicine/Surgery
> Physiologic and Anatomic Equilibrium
> Acute Care
> Plastic Surgery

6. **In assessing a client who had an abdominoplasty 6 hours ago, the nurse would expect to find:**
1. Edema and pallor at the incision site
2. Voiding 200 ml yellow urine
3. Diminished breath sounds bilaterally
4. 200 ml of fluid in the drainage bag within 1 hour

RATIONALE

(2) The client should void within 6 to 8 hours after surgery.
1. These are signs of possible incisional ischemia.
3. The client should have clear, audible, bilateral breath sounds. Diminished sounds may indicate early atelectasis.

4. This is an increased amount of output. Depending on the continued amount of drainage, and the color and consistency of it, this may indicate hemorrhage.

> Implementation
> Medicine/Surgery
> Physiologic and Anatomic Equilibrium
> Acute Care
> Plastic Surgery

7. **The nurse iscaring for a client who has had reconstructive surgery of the leg for a deformity resulting from a skiing accident. The surgery involved the placement of a flap and skin graft. Nursing actions will include:**
1. Offer tea or coffee
2. Keep leg flat
3. Assess circulation
4. Place sheet loosely over graft

RATIONALE

(3) Checking color, temperature, sensation, and capillary refill frequently and reporting adverse changes will ensure continued circulation to the reconstructed area.
1. Caffeine and nicotine cause venous constriction and may decrease blood flow to the surgical site.
2. The extremity should be elevated at all times.
4. Bed covers should be kept off the surgical site with the use of a cradle.

Appendixes

Appendix A: Nursing and Health Science Internet Sites

Site name and address	Contents
NURSING	
American Nurses Association Nursing World http://www/nursingworld.org	Information about ANA publications, "Captiol Watch" featuring government and political information, "Reading Room" section containing ANA fact sheets and numerous references
Nurseweek http://www.nurseweek.com	*Nurseweek* publication news, articles (columns, editorials, features, and interviews), and continuing education information and links.
Nursing Net http://www.nursingnet.org	Chat room, employment information, links to nursing unions, journals, references, nursing specialties, and more.
Health Web Nursing Page http://www.lib.umich.edu/hw/nursing.html	Links to continuing education, research, career information, and clinical nursing information.
NCLEX and CAT http://www.kaplan.com:80/nclex/nclex_and_cat.html	Information about taking NCLEX: Computer Adaptive Test, as well as sample NCLEX questions with answers.
The "Virtual" Nursing Center http://www-sci.lib.uci.edu/HSG/Nursing/html	Interactive case studies, protocols, and procedures, and much more.
Galexy Index of Nursing-Related Services on the Internet http://galexy.einet.net/galaxy/Medicine/Nursing.html	Links to nursing academic organizations and periodicals.
MedWeb: Nursing http://www.gen.emory.edu/medweb/medweb.nursing.html	Links to nursing conferences, associations, and publications.
HEALTH SCIENCE & HEALTH PROMOTION	
National Institutes of Health http://www.nih.gov/	Directory of NIH health information resources, scientific resources, directory of news and events, NIH press releases, and information about the Visible Human project.
NOAH (New York Online Access to Health) http://www.noah.cuny.edu/	"Health topics and research" section contains comprehensive information about various disorders (AIDS and HIV, cancer, the eye, and mental health), covering treatment, prevention, glossaries, and news updates. "Most Read Documents" section contains commonly requested information, such as "How your baby grows" and "Chronic fatigue syndrome."
World Health Organization http://www.who.org	Information about WHO programs, publications and policy documents, reports, link to the WHO library and database, and links to other health care sites.

Site name and address	Contents
Mayo Health O@sis Resource Center http://healthnet.ivi.com/mayo/common/html	Health care news updates, a library containing reference articles categorized by condition or disorder, quizzes, an "ask the Mayo physician or dietician" feature, and links to special Cancer Center, Heart Center, Women's Health, Diet and Nutrition, Medicine Center, and Pregnancy and Children pages.
U.S. Centers for Disease Control (CDC) http://www.cdc.gov	Infection control guidelines and CDC's journals, *Morbidity and Mortality Weekly Report* and *Emerging Infectious Diseases.*
MedAccess On-Line http://medaccess.com/	A variety of health care resources, including products and services, a directory of health care facilities, a bulletin board, health information, quizzes, and a databank.
Helix Healthcare Education Learning & Information Exchange http://www.helix.com	Glaxo Wellcome continuing education programs, on-line exams and grading, access to MEDLINE, health care news from *The Medical Tribune,* discussion forums, and professional development tools.
Hospital+Net http://hospital.net/home.html	News, numerous links to other health care sites, sites categorized by disorder and specialty, and links to hospitals on the web.
Agency for Health Policy and Research http://www.ahcpr.gov/	Links to AHCPR clinical practice guidelines and outcomes, as well as news and resources.
Department of Health and Human Services http://www.os.dhhs.gov	Links to many DHHS agencies and publications, a News and Public Affairs page with press releases and fact sheets, and a link to Healthfinder, a government-sponsored consumer information resource.
Med Help http://medhlp.netusa.net/index.html	Health care news and a library of articles including hundreds of patient handout documents on various disorders and conditions.
Global Health Network http://www.pitt.edu/HOME/GHNet/GHNet.html	A variety of health care resources, including information on women and minorities considerations, tips for travelers, as slide show on the Internet and health care, and links to disorder-specific online/electronic resources.
Food and Nutrition Information Center http://www.nal.usda.gov/fnic/	Nutrition guidelines, searchable database, and links to other related government sites.
PharmInfoNet http://pharminfo.com/	Frequently updated drug information news, research, and discussion groups.
FDA-Approved Drugs http://www.fda.gov/cder/da96.htm	Recent FDA-approved drugs by month, including drug name, indication, sponsor, treatment potential, and chemical type.

DON'T FORGET! The Mosby Nursing web page (http://www.mosby.com/Mosby/Nursing/) features updated information about nursing publications, special offers, contests, and much more!

Appendix B:
Images in Mosby's Medical-Surgical Nursing VIEWSTUDY

VS figure no.*	Abbreviated legend	Beare/ Myers chapter no.
1	Nursing process	—
2	Cognitive appraisal process	—
3	Neurochemical links among the nervous, endocrine, and immune systems	6
4	The cerebral cortex processes stressful stimuli	—
5	Alarm reaction responses	—
6	Current concepts of the stress syndrome	—
7	Five components of pain	3
8	Peripheral terminals are sensitive to direct heat, mechanical pressure, and chemicals released in response to tissue damage	3
9	Dorsal root nociceptive afferents	3
10	Schematic representation of two pathways that lead to the production of chemicals that cause the peripheral afferent nociceptors to be more easily excited.	3
11	Typical areas of referred pain	3
12	Nociceptive pathways and synaptic connections of selected pain pathways	3
13	Descending pain-modulation system at receptors in the dorsal horn of the spinal cord	3
14	Descending pathway and endorphin response	3
15	Sites of commonly used pharmacologic and nonpharmacologic analgesic therapies	3
16	Mechanism of acute pain	3
17	Sites of neurosurgical procedures for pain relief	3
18	Adaptive alterations in simple cuboidal epithelial cells	24
19	Vascular response in inflammation	24
20	Cellular response in inflammation	24
21	Margination, diapedesis, chemotaxis of white blood cells	24
22	Sequential activation and biologic effects of the complement system	24
23	Pathway of arachidonic acid oxygenation and generation of prostaglandins and leukotrienes	24
24	When monocytes and macrophages are activated, they secrete interleukin-1	24

Continued

Continued

Continued

A-5

Continued

Continued

Continued

Continued

Continued

Continued

Continued

Continued

A-13

Continued

Continued

VS figure no.*	Abbreviated legend	Beare/ Myers chapter no
345	Development of osteomyelitis infection	42
346	Location and description of amputation sites of upper and lower extremities	42
347	Stump bandaging for above-the-knee stump	42
348	Compression of spinal cord caused by herniation of nucleus pulposus into spinal cord	43
349	Joints most frequently involved in osteoarthritis	43
350	Typical deformities of rheumatoid arthritis	43
351	Common extraarticular manifestations of rheumatoid arthritis	43
352	Tophaceous gout	43
353	Multisystem involvement in systemic lupus erythematosus	25
354	Scleroderma skin changes	59
355	Components of a pressure monitoring system	30
356	Venous infusion port pulmonary artery catheter	30
357	Position of the pulmonary artery flow directed catheter	30
358	During systole the balloon is deflated	18
359	Intracranial volume-pressure curve	30
360	Effects of independent changes in arterial blood pressure, oxygen, or carbon dioxide on cerebral blood flow	30
361	Intracranial pressure waveform noted on fast time scale recording	30
362	Causes of systemic inflammatory response syndrome and multiple organ dysfunction syndrome	6
363	Pathophysiology of systemic inflammatory response syndrome and multiple organ dysfunction system	6
364	Jaw-thrust maneuver	30
365	Tension pneumothorax	11
366	Pulmonary effects of water aspiration	—

*Please note: this log lists each main figure, but not the separate pieces and legends contained within each figure; overall, Mosby's Medical-Surgical Nursing VIEWSTUDY contains 533 illustrations and photos. To conserve space, the abbreviated legends here have been significantly reduced; the actual VIEWSTUDY legends are much longer and more descriptive.